Handbuch der experimentellen Pharmakologie

Vol. 40 Heffter-Heubner New Series

Handbook of Experimental Pharmacology

Add : NEED —, Philip editor

Organic Nitrates

Contributors

W. S. Aronow · M. G. Bogaert · C. J. Carr
G. R. Heyndrickx · E. M. Johnson, Jr. · J. C. Krantz, Jr.
P. Needleman · B. Pitt · S. F. Vatner

Editor

Philip Needleman

With 51 Figures

Springer-Verlag Berlin Heidelberg New York 1975

PHILIP NEEDLEMAN, Ph. D., Associate Professor of Pharmacology, Pharmacology Department, Washington University, 4566 Scott Avenue, St. Louis, MO 63110/USA

ISBN 3-540-07048-6 Springer-Verlag Berlin · Heidelberg · New York
ISBN 0-387-07048-6 Springer-Verlag New York · Heidelberg · Berlin

Library of Congress Cataloging in Publication Data Main entry under title: Organic nitrates. (Handbook of experimental pharmacology. New series; 40) 1. Nitrates—Physiological effect. 2. Nitrates. I. Aronow, W.S. II. Needleman, Philip, 1939— ed. III. Series: Handbuch der experimentellen Pharmakologie. New series; 40. [DNLM: 1. Glyceryl trinitrate. 2. Nitrates. 3. Nitrites. QV34 H236 new ser. v. 40] QP905.H3 Bd. 40 [QP913.N1] 615'.1'08s [574.1'924] 74-30332.

Typesetting, printing, and binding: Brühlsche Universitätsdruckerei, Gießen.

Preface

Nitroglycerin and other organic nitrates have been used for over a century in the treatment of angina pectoris. Millions of patients, throughout the world, have placed nitroglycerin tablets under the tongue and have experienced rapid and dramatic relief from the chest pain that frequently occurs as a manifestation of disease of the coronary arteries. The empirical observation of the safe use of nitrates for the alleviation of the symptoms of angina have led to their widespread medical acceptance. The use of organic nitrates preceded any knowledge of their mechanism of action or their ultimate metabolic fate. Thus, more simply stated, although sublingual nitrates helped the patients, little was known concerning what these drugs do to the body or what the body does to the drugs.

A substantial number of investigators have focused on these questions especially during the last two decades. We now have considerably more insight into the pathways of degradation of organic nitrates and the relationship of the metabolic processes to the biological action of these agents. Similarly, considerable effort has been expended in understanding the mechanism of action of these agents directly on vascular smooth muscle and on cardiac work and performance. Finally, there is a more substantive understanding of the physiology of the coronary circulation as well as the pathophysiologic manifestations of myocardial disease. The above advances will be reviewed in this text; however, a number of questions concerning (a) the mechanism of action, (b) the effectiveness of these agents by various routes of administration, and (c) their utility as prophylactic agents, remain to be resolved completely.

The present volume was written by a number of highly competent scientists and clinicians who are intimately involved in investigations of the basic mechanisms of action and the therapeutic utility of organic nitrates. The monograph is designed to give an over-view, as well as considerable detail concerning and exhaustive referencing of the investigational status of research in the area of organic nitrates. The chapter contributions primarily reflect the viewpoints of the authors and editing was limited, with a view to achieving continuity and avoiding unnecessary overlap. Differences in opinion have not been omitted and in certain areas different approaches to the same subject seemed worthwhile and were left intact. The pathophysiology of angina pectoris and the clinical pharmacology and therapeutic application of organic nitrates can be found in several portions of the text. Indeed, the current surge of clinical interest in the intravenous administration of nitroglycerin in the treatment of myocardial infarction is detailed and supported by the work of several of the chapter contributors.

The editor wishes to acknowledge the assistance of JAMES R. DOUGLAS, JR., BARBARA A. JAKSCHIK, PRASAD KULKARNI, and SHARON L. KEY for their assistance in proof-reading and the preparation of the index.

St. Louis, Winter 1974/75

PHILIP NEEDLEMAN

Table of Contents

CHAPTER 5

Biotransformation of Organic Nitrates. PHILIP NEEDLEMAN. With 19 Figures

CHAPTER 6

The Pharmacological and Biochemical Interaction of Organic Nitrates with Sulfhydryls: Possible Correlations with the Mechanism for Tolerance Development, Vasodilation, and Mitochondrial and Enzyme Reactions. PHILIP NEEDLEMAN and EUGENE M. JOHNSON, JR. With 5 Figures

CHAPTER 7

Physiology and Pathophysiology of the Coronary Circulation and the Role of Nitroglycerin. BERTRAM PITT. With 11 Figures

CHAPTER 8

Mechanism of Action of Nitroglycerin: Coronary, Cardiac, and Systemic Effects. STEPHEN F. VATNER and GUY R. HEYNDRICKX. With 14 Figures

CHAPTER 9

Use of Nitrates as Antianginal Agents. WILBERT S. ARONOW

List of Contributors

Dr. WILBERT S. ARONOW, Cardiology Section, Veterans Administration Hospital, 5901 East Seventh Street, Long Beach, CA 90801/USA

Dr. MARK G. BOGAERT, J. F. & C. Heymans Instituut voor Farmakodynamie en Terapie der Rijksuniversiteit, De Pintelaan 135, B–9000 Gent, Belgium

Dr. C. JELLEFF CARR, Life Science Research Office, Federation of American Societies for Experimental Biology, 9650 Rockville Pike, Bethesda, MD 20014/USA

Dr. GUY R. HEYNDRICKX, Dept. of Cardiology, State University of Ghent, Ghent/Belgium

Dr. EUGENE M. JOHNSON, JR., Department of Pharmacology, Medical College of Pennsylvania, 3300 Henry Avenue, Philadelphia, PA 19129/USA

Dr. JOHN C. KRANTZ, JR., Box 84, Gibson Island, MD 21056/USA

Dr. PHILIP NEEDLEMAN, Associate Professor of Pharmacology, Pharmacology Department, Washington University, 4566 Scott Avenue, St. Louis, MO 63110/USA

Dr. BERTRAM PITT, Associate Professor of Medicine, Division of Cardiology, Department of Medicine, Johns Hopkins University, Medical School, Baltimore, MD 21205/USA

Dr. STEPHEN F. VATNER, Department of Medicine, Harvard Medical School, 25 Shattuck Street, Boston, MA 02115/USA

CHAPTER 1

Historical Background

JOHN C. KRANTZ, JR.

I. Nitrogen and Its Compounds

The existence of nitrogen was observed by CARL W. SCHEELE in 1772. He called it foul air, as it remained as an atmospheric residue after the removal of oxygen. Lavoisier independently discovered the element and named it *azote* owing to its inability to support life. Chemical historians attribute the actual discovery of nitrogen to Dr. DANIEL RUTHERFORD, a Scottish physician, botanist and chemist. Dr. RUTHERFORD's distinguished nephew, Sir WALTER SCOTT, wrote about his uncle and physician, "Prosecuting medical studies at the University of Edinburgh he early discovered the existence of a gaseous fluid now known as nitrogen gas." Although many distinguished chemists almost simultaneously recognized the presence of this substance in the air, Sir WILLIAM RAMSAY stated, "Rutherford may well be credited with the discovery of nitrogen." The name nitrogen was suggested by the distinguished chemist J. A. C. CHAPTAL, after CAVENDISH had prepared niter (potassium nitrate or salt petre) by sparking the new gas with oxygen in the presence of caustic potash. (WEEKS, 1960).

The fact that air contains about 78% by volume in an uncombined state indicates the lack of chemical activity of the element. However combinations of nitrogen with other elements are abundant in nature in all living matter. Protein contains about 16% of the element.

The atom of nitrogen has an atomic number of 7. It unites readily with hydrogen appropriating 3 electrons from 3 hydrogen atoms to form the well known gas ammonia NH_3. The gas is freely soluble in water and combines with it to form the base ammonium hydroxide. Under specific conditions nitrogen and oxygen combine to form 6 different oxides of nitrogen with widely varying properties. The two oxides of nitrogen pertinent to this discussion are N_2O_3 and N_2O_5. Nitrogen trioxide is the anhydride of nitrous acid that is the source of the medicinal nitrites. The second oxide nitrogen pentoxide is the anhydride of nitric acid from which the medicinal nitrates are formed.

II. Biological Occurrence of Nitrites and Nitrates

The ions of nitrous and nitric acids are not foreign constituents of the blood of many species of animals, for example the nitrate ion is present in the blood of man in a concentration of 1 in 10^6 (WHALEN, 1935). The nitrite ion is also present, but to a lesser extent, in man and other species (STIEGLITZ and PALMER, 1934). RATH and KRANTZ (1942) showed that the blood of *rhesus* monkeys, dogs, cattle, and man contain levels of the nitrite of 1 in 10^7. These investigators found a correlation between the blood-level of the nitrite ion and age. The blood of persons in the eighth decade of life contained nitrite levels of approximately one-half of those of individuals of younger age groups. This finding could not be correlated with the blood pressure levels of the various age groups. It was interesting to note that the level of nitrite in the blood remained unaltered by adding various nitrogen-containing agents to the diet such as sodium nitrate, ammonium chloride and amino acids.

III. The Synthesis of Nitrite and Nitrate Esters

Since the experiment of WÖHLER, who in the laboratory of BERZELIUS in 1828, destroyed the "vital force concept" of science by synthesizing urea from ammonium cyanate, the field of organic chemistry pushed forward with breath-taking strides. Under the leadership of JUSTUS VON LIEBIG, WÖHLER, PASTEUR and others organic chemistry became a flourishing science. Germane to this topic, M. BERTHELOT and L. PÉAU DE ST. GILES (1862) pointed out that the union of an acid with an alcohol enters into an equilibrium and no more ester is formed until removal of one of the products of reaction.

IV. Discovery of Amyl Nitrite

The first ester synthesized of interest to this treatise is amyl nitrite made by treating amyl alcohol with nitrous acid. It was prepared by A. J. BALARD in 1844 with Montpellier who was distinguished for his discovery of bromine in 1826.

Fifteen years later GUTHRIE (1859) made amyl nitrite and observed that the inhalation of its vapors caused flushing of the face, throbbing of the carotids and acceleration of the pulse rate. He recommended its use in resuscitation in threatened drowning, suffocation and protracted fainting.

BRUNTON (1867) mentions in his work with amyl nitrite that some years after GUTHRIE's observations a Dr. B. W. RICHARDSON observed that the ester caused paralysis of the nerves from the periphery inward. It also evoked diminished contractility of the muscles and dilation of the capillaries as observed in the web of the frog's foot.

V. T. LAUDER BRUNTON, England's Leading Therapist

THOMAS LAUDER BRUNTON, the son of JAMES BRUNTON, was born at Bowdon, Roxburghshire on March 14, 1844. He was destined to become one of England's most distinguished physicians of the nineteenth century. He qualified in 1866 as a physician by taking the M. B. and C. M. at Edinburgh with honors. He was awarded the M.D. degree for his work on the urinary effects of digitalis. This was the beginning of his intense interest in the action of drugs. His interest deepened into investigating the mechanism of action of various drugs.

Later BRUNTON was to write a classical textbook on "Therapeutics and Materia Medica". This book of over 1000 pages appeared in 1885. It marked him as England's greatest therapist of the nineteenth century. He received the honor of knighthood at the turn of the century and in 1908 he was made a baronet. He traveled extensively in Europe and was responsible for conveying much of England's knowledge of drugs to the profession on the continent and in turn bringing the medical knowledge of the great clinics in Vienna and Berlin back to England.

He led an active life in practice, teaching and investigation. It does appear that the salient drive in his active life was a deep seated desire to alleviate human pain and suffering. His health was shaken by the World War I. He was emotionally disturbed owing to the fact that he had numerous friends among the German scientists and their attitude toward England caused him great remorse. When his son Lieutenant HENRY POLLACK BRUNTON was killed in France October 8, 1915, it was like a body blow to Sir LAUDER. His health precipitously failed and he died quietly in his residence in London on September 15, 1916.

Of all the interesting and thought-provoking studies conducted by this distinguished physician in his multiplicity of efforts the one event that has survived the pruning knife of science was his observation that amyl nitrite was useful in the treatment of angina pectoris.

VI. Sir LAUDER BRUNTON and Amyl Nitrite

The disease angina pectoris has been described by WILLIAM HEBERTON in the Medical Transactions of the College of Physicians in 1768. His classical description of the anginal attack, which summarized his observations after treating more than 100 patients, would fit into any modern textbook on that subject. One statement made by HEBERTON was changed a century later by T. LAUDER BRUNTON. HEBERTON stated, "With respect to this complaint, I have little or nothing to advance." Several paragraphs from Dr. BRUNTON's paper are quoted indicating his experiences in the first use of amyl nitrite in angina pectoris.

"Perhaps there is no class of cases in which such occurrences as this take place so frequently as in some kinds of cardiac disease, in which angina pectoris forms at once the most prominent and the most painful and distressing symptom. This painful affection is defined by Dr. WALSHE as a paroxysmal neurosis, in which the heart is essentially concerned, and the cases included in this definition may be divided into two classes."

"In the first and most typical there is severe pain in the precordial region, often shooting up the neck and down the arms, accompanied by dyspnoea and a most distressing sense of impending dissolution. The occurrence and departure of the attack are both equally sudden, and its duration is only a few minutes."

"In the second class, which from its greater frequency is probably the more important, though the pain and dyspnoea may both be very great, the occurrence of the attack is sometimes gradual, and its departure generally so; its duration is from a few minutes to an hour and a half or more, and the sense of impending dissolution is less marked or altogether absent."

"Brandy, ether, chloroform, ammonia, and other stimulants have hitherto been chiefly relied upon for the relief of angina pectoris; but the alleviation which they produce is but slight, and the duration of the attack is but little affected by them."

"During the past winter there has been in the clinical wards one case in which the anginal pain was very severe, lasted from an hour to an hour and a half, and recurred every night, generally between two and four a.m.; besides several others in whom the affection, though present, was less frequent and less severe. Digitalis, aconite, and lobelia inflata were given in the intervals, without producing any benefit; and brandy and other diffusible stimulants during the fit produced little or no relief. When chloroform was given so as to produce partial stupefaction, it relieved the pain for the time; but whenever the senses again became clear, the pain was as bad as before. Small bleedings of three or four ounces, whether by cupping or venesection, were, however, always beneficial; the pain being completely absent for one night after the operation, but generally returning on the second. As I believed the relief produced by the bleeding to be due to the diminution it occasioned in the arterial tension, it occurred to me that a substance which possesses the power of lessening it in such an eminent degree as nitrite of amyl would probably produce the same effect, and might be repeated as often as necessary without detriment to the patient's health. On application to my friend Dr. Gamgee, he kindly furnished me with a supply of pure nitrite which he himself had made; and on proceeding to try it in the wards, with the sanction of the visiting physician, Dr. J. Hughes Bennett, my hopes were completely fulfilled. On pouring from five to ten drops of the nitrite on a cloth and giving it to the patient to inhale, the physiological action took place in from thirty to sixty seconds; and simultaneously with the flushing of the face the pain completely disappeared, and generally did not return till its wonted time next night. Occasionally it began to return about five minutes after its first disappearance; but on giving a few drops more it again disappeared, and did not return. On a few occasions I have found that while the pain disappeared from every other part of the chest, it remained persistent at a spot about two inches to the side of the right nipple, and the action of the remedy had to be kept up for several minutes before this completely subsided. In almost all other cases in which I have given it, as well as in those in which it has been tried by my friends, the pain has at once completely disappeared. In cases of aneurism, where the pain was constant, inhalation of the nitrite gave no relief, but where it was spasmodic or subject to occasional exacerbations it either completely removed or greatly relieved it. It may be as well to note that in those cases in which it failed, small bleedings were likewise useless."

"From observations during the attack, and from an examination of numerous sphygmographic tracings taken while the patients were free from pain, while it was coming on, at its height, passing off under the influence of amyl, and again completely gone, I find that when the attack comes on gradually the pulse becomes smaller, and the arterial tension greater as the pain increases in severity. During the attack the breathing is quick, the pulse small and rapid, and the arterial tension high, owing, I believe, to contraction of the systemic capillaries. As the nitrite is inhaled the pulse becomes slower and fuller, the tension diminished, and the breathing less hurried. On those occasions when the pain returned after an interval of a few minutes, the pulse, though showing small tension, remained small in volume, and not till the volume as well as tension of the pulse became normal, did I feel sure that the pain would not return."

"It is of interest that an epidemic of cholera occurred in Edinburgh about at this period. Dr. ARTHUR GAMGEE recommended amyl nitrite to be used in the stage of collapse of the disease. It did not prove of value. After the ester was used in the collapse phase of cholera, no "well marked" cases occurred and the trial of amyl nitrite in the real epidemic was impossible. BRUNTON commented, "Should another epidemic occur it might prove our most valuable remedy."

If one peruses the older treatises on materia medica, there are few maladies in which amyl nitrite has not been tried. On all of these cases the remedy was chosen on an empirical basis and likely owing to its prompt and dramatic effect upon the heart and circulation. In coronary artery insufficiency amyl nitrite and its congeners nitroglycerin, isosorbide dinitrate and octyl nitrite have been the drugs of choice in most cases for more than a century. Sir LAUDER led a vigorous life and developed angina pectoris. He used amyl nitrite repeatedly in terminating the attack of the disease.

One of the specific uses for amyl nitrite in modern toxicology is in cyanide poisoning. The nitrite ion converts hemoglobin to methemoglobin, and the latter combines readily with the cyanide ion to form cyanomethemoglobin. Thus protecting the cytochrome oxidase from being inactivated by the cyanide ion.

VII. The Discovery of Nitroglycerin

It does appear that Sir LAUDER was either unacquainted with the discovery of nitroglycerin or he did not consider it to be useful in the treatment of anginal syndrome. His work in this malady was confined to amyl nitrite.

Nitroglycerin was synthesized first by A. SOBRERO in 1846. By mixing cold concentrated sulfuric and nitric acids and allowing them to act on glycerin he obtained an oily liquid that was not miscible with water. He observed that the oily liquid was soluble in ether and alcohol and evoked an aromatic taste. A small quantity placed on the tip of the tongue elicited severe throbbing of the temples and a severe headache which persisted for a considerable period of time. These findings were confirmed by several of his associates. MUNCH and PETTER (1965) recorded that SOBRERO reported his observations in a chemical journal in Turin but they were unable to find it as a reference.

In 1847 a French group of chemists reported to THEOPHILE PELOUZE in the (Comptes rendus) Academy of Sciences, the synthesis of a group of nitrated explosives including nitroglycerin. This prompted SOBRERO to claim priority for the synthesis of the ester and his letter and claim was published in the Comp. rendus which established him as the discoverer of the compound.

The comparatively safe use of nitroglycerin as a blasting agent attracted the attention of ALFRED B. NOBEL, a Swedish engineer. He mixed such materials as charcoal or diatomaceous earth with nitroglycerin and produced *dynamite*. He also made many modifications of dynamite to serve for various types of blasting. One of these was *blasting gelatin* which NOBEL patented in 1876. From these patents and the exploitation of the Baku oil fields NOBEL amassed an enormous fortune. He suffered with ill-health most of his life and remained a bachelor. In the seventh decade of his life he became extremely pessimistic about the future of mankind. This, coupled with his failing health, prompted him to leave the greater mass of his fortune for the creation of the Nobel prize, its purpose was for the betterment of the human race. He died December 10, 1896, at St. Remo, Italy. The five prizes in chemistry, physics, medicine, literature and peace have been the incentives for many great advances in the sciences and arts and have redowned to the betterment of mankind. At this point in time one might conjecture, had SOBRERO not made nitroglycerin, would there have been a Nobel Prize?

VIII. Early Studies on Nitroglycerin in America

CONSTANTIN HERING, the professor of materia medica at the Hahnemann Medical School in Philadelphia read and was intrigued by the paper of SOBRERO on the preparation of nitroglycerin. He decided to repeat the synthesis. His endeavors were unsuccessful, likely owing to the fact that he could not obtain pure glycerin and did not chill the reaction mixture sufficiently. HERING's attempt was made during the summer.

The following winter MORRIS DAVIS, a chemist acquainted with Professor HERING, repeated the experiment taking special caution to keep the reaction mixture cold. He obtained 20 drops of the desired product, presumably nitroglycerin. Application to the tip of the tongue evoked intense throbbing in the temples and severe headache. Professor HERING had the same experience with the DAVIS product.

Professor HERING showed the new product to an associate, Dr. JEANES, who disregarded the potency of the agent and applied a comparatively large dose to his tongue. He became visibly agitated and suffered with an intense headache. The experimenters observed that strong coffee was useful in mitigating the headache.

After this experience Professor HERING was convinced that a more satisfactory method of administering nitroglycerin had to be devised. They had observed marked variation in the susceptibility of various individuals to the drug. This was an appropriate place for such a study, since the Hahnemann Medical School was a homepathic school skilled in administering small quantities of medicaments.

This was achieved by dissolving the nitroglycerin in alcohol and allowing the solution to be absorbed on sugar pellets. Each pellet contained from 1/300th to 1/5000th of a drop. The pellets were administered sublingually. Possessed now with a more dependable dosage form, these investigators observed that nitroglycerin evokes a more decisive effect on the pulse and heart than any other substance known. It is interesting to note how well these early investigators approached and solved the problem of administering nitroglycerin. The alcoholic solution (Spirit of Nitroglycerin 1%) was a standard product for years. The sugar pellet under the tongue is the present day sublingual milk sugar or other excipient tablet.

In the winter of 1847 HERING and DAVIS made an additional supply of nitroglycerin and supplied it in dosage forms to 100 physicians. They were requested to record the effects of the drug. Most of the physicians reported their findings to Professor HERING. The outstanding symptoms were headache, throbbing of the temples, increased pulse rate and diffuse pains in the chest and other areas of the body. "It was suggested that this new product should be helpful in the treatment of coronary involvements, angina pectoris, cardiac edema, headache, epilepsy and cerebral involvements, among other disease conditions" (thru MUNCH and PETTER 1965). A review of the therapeutic uses of nitroglycerin in the older treatises on materia medica will indicate that nitroglycerin has been recommended in a host of common maladies, in which later studies showed that it was of no value.

IX. Nitroglycerin or Glonoin

It appears that Professor HERING did not know the composition of nitroglycerin and did not wait for the determination of its composition before assigning a name to the product. This name tenaciously remained with the product for a century and is still used by some physicians of the older school today.

In 1853 Professor CONSTANTIN HERING wrote the following:

"Before all things the child had to receive a name. SOBRERO didn't think it necessary since the explosive had not even a chemical name yet. So I proceeded to prepare a name existing from the components. Glycyloxydhydrat or glycerin gives the product with nitro-sulfuric acid. Sulfuric acid and the water remained, therefore, for our matter *Gl*ycyl *O*xyd and *N*itrogen *O*xygen, the latter may be as nitrous acid, the elements of the first may be pushed over to the alkaline side; all that we actually did not understand even to analyze and we had to wait until the experts did investigate it; but we could not wait with a name, and so we added them to the Gl. O. N. O. the inum which illustrates what it came from, and we had a well-sounding and effective descriptive name *Glonoin*, with the i long and stressed."

X. Nitroglycerin in England

Nitroglycerin was being investigated by Professor HERING in Philadelphia as previously discussed in 1847. This was two decades prior to Sir LAUDER BRUNTON'S use of amyl nitrite in the treatment of angina pectoris. It appears that Sir LAUDER was unfamiliar with the existence of nitroglycerin. There was work on the compound going on in England that might have prompted him to use nitrolgycerin for the treatment of angina pectoris as he had used amyl nitrite.

For example FIELDS (1858a) published on the medicinal and toxic properties of the "Nitrate of Oxyde of Glycyl" which was undoubtedly nitroglycerin likely with other products of the reaction. A year later he again published a paper in 1859b entitled "Nitroglycerine or Glonoin". He had likely become acquainted with investigations of Professor HERING. No definite progress was made in the use of the agent in angina pectoris until the concept reached the fertile mind of WILLIAM MURRELL.

XI. WILLIAM MURRELL

WILLIAM MURRELL was born November 26, 1853, the son of KERRICK MURRELL, M.A. barrister-at-law. He received his early education at Murray's School, Wimbleton and later the University College, London. He then went in training in the University

College Hospital. He qualified as a L.S.A. in 1874 and received the diplomas of M.R.C.S. Eng. and L.R.C.P. Lon. in 1875. Two years later the enterprising young MURRELL became a member of the Royal College of Physicians and was elected a Fellow in 1883. He obtained the degree of M.D. from the University of Brussels in 1879.

MURRELL was a scientifically minded physician. He became a demonstrator in physiology in the Medical School of the University College Hospital. He had been awarded the Sharpey Physiological Scholarship. MURRELL worked under Dr. SIDNEY RINGER and assisted him in his researches. This association undoubtedly influenced MURRELL to take a keen interest in pharmacology.

He later associated himself with the Westminster Hospital Medical School. He taught histology and was elected physician to the hospital in 1896. Dr. MURRELL was a physician who exhibited intense concern for his patients. His life was in work. Unfortunately early in his career he suffered with cardiac insufficiency and after a short rest, against medical advice, returned to his work at the hospital. There was a second occurrence of his illness with extreme edema. He was forced to stop work and returned to his home and died on June 28, 1912.

MURRELL was a prolific writer and acquired a felicity of diction that made his writings popular. His best known books are "A Manual of Pharmacology and Therapeutics" and "What To Do in Cases of Poisoning". The latter went through ten editions. The world is most indebted to him for his classical paper on the use of nitroglycerin in angina pectoris written when he was 26 years old. It was his first independent publication.

Young MURRELL became interested in the subject of nitroglycerin from a controversy that was published in "Medical Times and Gazette" two decades before. Mr. A. G. FIELD of Brighton described his sensation in detail after taking two drops of a one percent alcoholic solution of nitroglycerin. Among the effects reported were fullness about the neck, throbbing of the temples, headache and nausea. Dr. MURRELL ingested a comparable dose of nitroglycerin and confirmed the typical nitroglycerin effect. The controversy in which Mr. FIELD was engaged stemmed from the fact that certain subjects experienced a typical amyl nitrite syndrome and others did not.

MURRELL was convinced that the action of nitroglycerin emulated that of amyl nitrite used by Sir LAUDER BRUNTON a decade before in the treatment of angina pectoris: cogent paragraphs from Dr. MURRELL'S paper in Lancet in 1879, follow:

"From a consideration of the physiological action of the drug and more especially from the similarity existing between its general action and that of nitrite of amyl, I concluded that it would probably prove of service in the treatment of angina pectoris, and I am happy to say that this anticipation has been realied.

"As a preliminary step I was anxious to obtain a comparative series of sphygmographic tracings ... Judged by the sphygmographic tracings, the effects of nitrite of amyl and of nitro-glycerine on the pulse are similar. Both drugs produce a marked state of dicrotism and both accelerate the rapidity of the heart's action. They differ, however, in the time they respectively take to produce these effects. The full action of the nitro-glycerine is not observed in the sphygmographic tracings until six or seven minutes after the dose has been taken. In the case of nitrite of amyl, the effect is obtained in from fifteen to twenty seconds after an inhalation or a dose has been taken on sugar. The influence of the nitrite of amyl is extremely transitory, a tracing taken a minute and a half after the exhibition of the drug being perfectly normal. In fact, the full effect of the nitrite of amyl on the pulse is not maintained for more than fifteen seconds. The nitro-glycerine produces its effects much more slowly; they last longer and disappear gradually, the tracing not resuming its normal condition for nearly half an hour. The effect may be maintained for a much longer time by repeating the dose. Nitro-glycerine is more lasting in its power of producing a dicrotic form of pulse beat, and consequently in cases where the conditions of relaxation and dicrotism are desired to be maintained for a space of time, its exhibition is to be preferred to that of nitrite of amyl."

"During the last nine months I have treated three cases of undoubted angina pectoris with nitro-glycerine with what success the cases themselves will show."

"There could be no possibility of doubt respecting the diagnosis. It was a typical uncomplicated case of angina pectoris.

Patient was placed for a week on infusion of quassia in order that he might be observed and also to eliminate the effects of expectation. It need hardly be said that he derived no benefit from this treatment. He was then ordered drop doses of the one per cent nitro-glycerine solution in half an ounce of water three times a day. At the expiration of a week he reported that there had been a very great improvement. The attacks had been considerably reduced in frequency and for two or three days he had only one attack in the morning after breakfest. The attacks, when they did occur, were much less severe. He found, too, that a dose of medicine taken during an attack would cut it short. He had tried it several times, and it had always succeeded. It would not act instantly, but still very quickly; so that the attacks were considerably shortened. He was thoroughly convinced that the medicine had done him good and said he was better than he had been since first he had the attacks ..."

"... Patient had adopted the plan of carrying his medicine with him in a phial and taking a dose if an attack seized him in the street. It never failed to afford relief."

XII. Amyl Nitrite and Nitroglycerin in Angina Pectoris

Although the precise etiology of angina pectoris is not definitively understood it is generally agreed that the attack is due to the failure of the coronary arteries to dilate and supply a greater quantity of blood to the heart under a condition of stress. The cause of the poignant pain is controversial. Cardiac hypoxia and an increase of lactic acid formation each has been incriminated.

Regardless of the exact origin of the pain, Sir LAUDER BRUNTON'S amyl nitrite inhalation or WILLIAM MURRELL'S nitroglycerin sublingually will, as a rule, terminate the attack. And we now have a century of clinical history confirming this statement. Each drug dilates the coronary vessels, reduces the workload on the heart and improves the distribution of coronary flow in the ischemic areas of the heart. These drug induced changes appear to be the factors responsible for the termination of the anginal attack. It is interesting that these two compounds of different chemical constitution should evoke identical pharmacologic syndromes in diseases of coronary insufficiency. This unusual activity of these two drugs intrigued the author a third of a century ago and led to his investigation of the problem.

XIII. Organic and Inorganic Nitrites and Nitrates

Although the nitrate ion does not evoke any definitive effect on the circulation or other functions of the body, the ester nitroglycerin and many other nitrate esters elicit profound circulatory activity. In contrast to the nitrate ion the nitrite ion does produce a circulatory response similar to amyl nitrite and nitroglycerin, however it is much less potent. The structural formulae of the various organic nitrates are shown in the Chemistry Chapter.

Since the discovery of the use of nitroglycerin a century ago until about three decades ago most texts on pharmacology attributed the vasodilating action of nitroglycerin to its reduction to nitrite. The author taught this concept to many classes of medical students. The concept stemmed from the fact that $NaNO_2$ evoked a vasodilating action and $NaNO_3$ produced no circulatory response. Besides upon hydrolysis with alkali one molecule of nitroglycerin yields 2 molecules of alkali nitrate and one of alkali nitrite. This is due to the reduction of nitrate to nitrite by the liberated glycerin.

In the decade 1940 to 1950, the author and his associates at the University of Maryland Medical School were concerned with the metabolism of the sugar alcohols such as sorbitol and mannitol. In addition we prepared their anhydrides and studied their fate in the body. These two sugar alcohols each form mono and di anhydrides named mannide and isomannide and sorbide and isosorbide respectively. Since mannitol hexanitrate was being used in the treatment of hypertension, we thought it would be of interest to prepare the nitrates of the anhydrides of mannitol and sorbitol. The di anhydrides were used since these were more easily prepared and nitrated.

KRANTZ et al. (1940) studied the effect of alkali hydrolysis upon isosorbide dinitrate and compared it with nitroglycerin. It was observed that isosorbide dinitrate yielded no nitrite when treated with diluted alkali at 100° as does nitroglycerin. The work was extended by injecting intravenously into an anesthetized dog a solution of nitroglycerin 1:10000. A characteristic depressor response was produced. A portion of the solution was boiled with dilute sodium hydroxide, cooled, neutralized with hydrochloric acid and injected into the same animal. No depressor response was observed. Isosorbide dinitrate was subjected to the same treatment and its depressor response was not affected. We concluded that the depressor response was an action of the intact molecule of nitroglycerin.

A consideration of the well established clinical experience with these drugs indicates the validity of the conclusion drawn from the foregoing experiment. When sodium nitrite is used in hypertension and/or angina pectoris the average effective dose is 60 mg. When nitroglycerin is employed 1/100 of the dose or 0.6 mg. is considered effective. If all the nitroglycerin were instantly converted to nitrite the quantity would be insufficient for an effective dose if either organic or inorganic nitrite is formed.

HEPPEL and HILMOE (1950) isolated an enzyme from hog's liver which catalyzes the reduction of nitroglycerin to glyceryl trinitrite by glutathione. Glutathione appeared to react with nitroglycerin to form the trinitrite before hydrolysis occurred. The reaction of nitroglycerin with glutathione is an orderly time process, whereas the vasopressor response of nitroglycerin is immediate and evanescent. As glyceryl trinitrite is very unstable and decomposed immediately by water and air, it appears that the response of nitroglycerin is due to the intact molecule and not to its reduction product or the product of hydrolytic cleavage.

XIV. The Influence of Oil Solubility on Nitrate Ester Response

Nitroglycerin is freely soluble in many organic solvents and oil. It is nearly insoluble in water. For example at 20°. 1 liter of water will dissolve only 1.8 g of nitroglycerin, hence its oil/water coefficient is very high. In our studies we found that high oil/water coefficients were essential for a typical nitroglycerin pharmacological response. For example we prepared the nitrate of hydroxy acetic acid, glycolic acid. The sodium salt was water soluble, evoked a negligible depressor response. Its oil/water coefficient was 0.9. The butyl ester of the nitrate of glycolic acid had on oil/water coefficient of 108 and evoked a marked depressor response when injected intravenously into a dog. It appears that the receptor sites in the vessels that accept the nitrites and nitrates are lipophilic in character.

XV. Nitrites and Nitrates in Hypertension

For a century it has been known that a reduction of blood pressure occurs when esters of nitrous or nitric acid are administered. The author has been unable to find an account of the first use of sodium nitrite in hypertension. It was extensively used during the first four decades of this century for the want of any superior agent. Mannitol hexanitrate made by SOBRERO in 1847 was found to give a more prolonged effect with less severe side effects and it largely replaced sodium nitrite until the advent of reserpine in 1949. The great disadvantages of the drugs of the nitrite series are headache, throbbing in the temples, methemoglobin formation and the rapidity of tolerance development. ELLIS and WEISS (1932) carried out a thorough clinical investigation of the action of sodium nitrite and revealed certain untoward effects of the drug that had not been recorded previously. To my knowledge sodium nitrite is no longer used in hypertension and mannitol hexanitrate, although available for this purpose, is seldom used.

In addition to the use of mannitol hexanitrate, erythrityl tetranitrate and more extensively pentaerythritol tetranitrate were used in the treatment of hypertension and angina pectoris. This last mentioned nitrate was patented in 1895 by the Rheinisch-Westfälische Sprengstoff-Aktiengesellschaft for the purpose of making a smokeless powder. BJERLÖV (1943) used the drug in the treatment of angina pectoris under the name of "Nitropent". This compound is used today in the treatment of coronary insufficiency disease under the name "Peritrate".

XVI. Extending the Duration of Action of Nitroglycerin

In spite of the fact that much controversy has surrounded the value of the use of the drugs of nitrite-nitrate series in coronary insufficieny disease, the drugs after a century remain pre-eminent in this field. Even the most critical authorities (A.M.A., 1971) recognize the value of nitroglycerin and isosorbide dinitrate.

The ideal method of administering either of these two drugs is sublingually. This method avoids the rigorous effects of peptic digestion and the hydrolytic cleavage produced in the liver. When given orally the drug must survive each of these hazards before reaching the heart. Despite these means of destroying the therapeutic usefulness of the drug enough may survive to achieve its effect. The author and his associates (1962) perfused the coronary vessels of an isolated beating rabbit's heart. To the perfusion fluid was added a definite quantity of nitroglycerin. The coronary vessels dilated to about 50%, but only 14% of the nitroglycerin was fixed by the tissues of the coronary vessels. The remainder was recovered in the perfusate. It is probable that this condition might also prevail in the intact human body. It suggests that only a small fraction of the orally ingested dose is required to provide maximal coronary response. This lends justification to the use of oral controlled release nitroglycerin dosage forms that have been so widely used in recent years.

XVII. Summary

One who has watched this field of medicine change from empiricism to scientific exactness is still awed by the fact that nitroglycerin, the active principle in dynamite, dilates the coronary vessels of man. At present this remains an enigma enveloped in an inscrutable puzzle. Perhaps some day the puzzle will be solved by the repetitious researches of man (KRANTZ, 1972). The story of a century of nitrites and nitrates reminds one again of those immortal words of PASTEUR, "In the field of observation chance favors only the mind that is prepared."

References

A.M.A. Drug Evaluations. Chicago: Amer. Med. Ass. Publ. 1971.

BALARD, J. M.: Sur la décomposition du bioxalatée d'ammonique par la chaleur, et les produits qui en résultent. Ann. Chimie et de Physique. **4**, 93—104 (1842).

BALARD, J. M.: Premier memoire sur l'alcool amylique. Ann. Chim. Phys. **12**, 294—330 (1844).

BERTHELOT, M. ST., GILLES, P.: Annuaire Chim. **65**, 385 (1862).

BJERLÖV, H.: A new drug against angina pectoris: Svenska Läk.-Tidn. **40**, 649—697 (1943).

BRUNTON, T. L.: Use of nitrite of amyl in angina pectoris. Lancet **1857II**, 97—98, 561—564.

FIELD, A. G.: On toxical and medicinal properties of oxyde glycyl. Med. Times Gaz. **16**, 291 (1858a).

FIELD, A. G.: Nitroglycerin or glonoin. Med. Times Gaz. **18**, 339 (1859b).

GUTHRIE, FREDERICK: Nitrite of amyl and its derivatives. chem. Soc. **11**, 245—252 (1859).

HEBERTON, W.: Angina pectoris: Medical transactions of the College of Physicians 1768 through commentaries on the history and cure of Diseases, p. 292. Boston: Wells and Lilly 1818.

HEPPEL, L. A., HILMOE, R. J.: Metabolic reduction of inorganic nitrate esters: J. biol. Chem. **183**, 129—138 (1950).

HERING, C.: Glonoin: Kirby's N. Am. J. Homeopathy, May (1849).

HERING, C.: Glonoin or nitroglycerin. Amerikanische Arzneiprüfungen und Vorarbeiten zur Arzneilehre als Naturwissenschaft, Erstes Heft. Leipzig: Schäfer 1853.

KRANTZ, J. C., JR., Action and nomenclature of nitroglycerin and nitrate esters. Amer. J. Card. **29**, 436—438 (1972).

KRANTZ, J. C., JR., CARR, C. J., FORMAN, S. E., CONE, N.: Mechanism and action of organic nitrates. J. Pharmacol. exp. Ther. **70**, 323—327 (1940).

KRANTZ, J. C., JR., LU, G. G., BELL, F. K., CASCORBI, H. F.: Nitrites XIX studies of the mechanism of action of glyceryl trinitrate: Biochem. Pharmacol. **11**, 1095—1099 (1962).

MUNCH, J. C., PETTER, H. H.: The story of glyceryl trinitrate (development of glonoin). J. Amer. pharm. Assoc. N.S. **5**, 494—495 (1965).
MURRELL, W.: Nitroglycerine as a remedy for angina pectoris. Lancet *1879I*, 80, 113, **225**, 642—646.
RATH, M., KRANTZ, J. C., JR.: The blood-nitrite content of man and other species. J. Pharmacol. exp. Ther. **76**, 27—31 (1942).
RICHARDSON, Sir BENJAMIN WARD. Report on the Physiological Action of Nitrite of Amyl. British Association for the Advancement of Science. Ann. Reports. **34**, 120—129 (1864).
SOBRERO, A.: Sur pluriers composes detonants produc avec l'acide nitrique et le sucre, la dextrine, la lactine, la mannite et la glycerine. R. Acad. Sci. (Paris) **24**, 247—248 (1847).
STIEGLITZ, E. J., PALMER, A. E.: The blood-nitrite content. Arch. intern. Med. **69**, 620—630 (1937).
WEEKS, M. E.: Discovery of the elements. J. Chem. Ed. 6th Ed. Easton, Pa.: Mack Printing Comp. 1960.
WEISS, S., ELLIS, L. B.: Influence of sodium nitrite on the cardiovascular system and renal activity. Arch. intern. Med. **52**, 105—119 (1933).
WHALEN, M.: Determination of nitrates in animal tissues. J. Lab. clin. Med. **20**, 755—757 (1935).

CHAPTER 2

Chemistry of Organic Nitrates

EUGENE M. JOHNSON, JR.

With 1 Figure

It is the purpose of this chapter to discuss the physical and chemical properties of organic polynitrates of pharmacological interest (Fig. 1). This chapter is not designed as a thorough review of the chemistry of all organic nitrates, most of which have been prepared for studies of explosive properties. For more complete reviews and more theoretical considerations the reader is referred to the reviews by BOSHAN et al. (1955); CANNON (1970), and the books by URBANSKI (1965) and SMITH (1966).

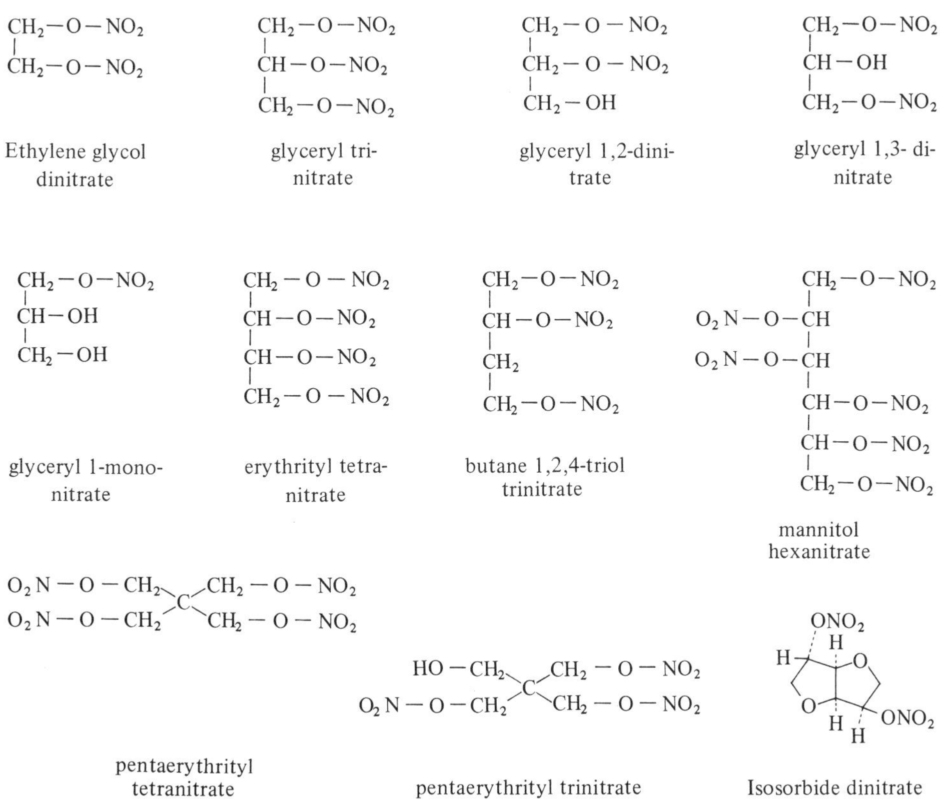

Fig. 1. Structures of some organic nitrates of pharmacological interest

I. General Properties

A. Structure

Organic nitrates are esters of nitric acid:

$$-C-O-NO_2 .$$

They thus contain a nitroxy group. This grouping is distinguished from nitrites (–C–O–NO) which are esters of nitrous acid and from nitro compounds ($C-NO_2$) in which the carbon and nitrogen are directly bonded.

B. Physical State

Organic nitrates formed by esterification of lower alcohols or polyols are liquids (colorless oils, e.g., ethylene glycol dinitrate, glyceryl trinitrate) whereas those formed from higher molecular weight polyols form crystalline solids (e.g. mannitol hexanitrate, isosorbide dinitrate). The nitrate esters which are liquids have boiling points slightly higher than their corresponding alcohols. Because the alcohols are more associated through hydrogen bonding, the alcohols are more viscous than their nitric acid esters. Because of the semi-polar bond in the nitro group, organic nitrates have a higher vapor pressure than their corresponding alcohols, and are therefore more volatile.

The organic nitrates have a higher specific gravity than their corresponding alcohols. Within a series of non-nitrated, partially nitrated, and completely nitrated polyol, the more completely nitrated compound will have the highest specific gravity. For example the specific gravity of glyceryl trinitrate (1.60) > glyceryl dinitrates (1.47) > glycerol (1.25).

C. Water Solubility

The nitric acid esters of polyols have low water solubility. As the molecular weight of completely nitrated polyols increase, water solubility decreases. For example, the water solubility of ethylene glycol dinitrate is 6.8 g/liter, glyceryl trinitrate is 1.2 to 1.8 g/liter, whereas pentaerythrityl tetranitrate is almost completely insoluble (0.1 g/liter at 50°) in water (URBANSKI, 1965). They are much more soluble in alcohol and other organic solvents.

Incompletely nitrated polyols are more water soluble than the completely nitrated polyols: the more free OH groups, the more water soluble the compound. For example, in the series of glyceryl nitrates, glyceryl mononitrates are very soluble in water, glyceryl dinitrates are of intermediate solubility (glyceryl 1,2-dinitrate, 65.7 g/liter, glyceryl 1,3-dinitrate 78.4 g/liter, DUNSTAN et al. 1965) and glyceryl trinitrate has a low solubility (1.2 to 1.8 g/liter).

D. Spectral Characteristics

The absorption spectrum of the nitroxy group of organic nitrate yields an absorbance maximum at 270 nm. The absorption, however, is very low ($E = 10$ to 20). The infrared absorption spectrum shows maxima at 1675 to 1610 (assymetric-NO_2 stretch), 1300 to 1250 (symmetric-NO_2 stretch) and 870 to 840 cm^{-1} (broad CO–N stretch) (BROWN, 1955; CANNON, 1970). The assymetric NO_2 vibrations are subject to change depending upon the positive or negative inductive effect of *R* in the molecule $R–O–NO_2$. This makes it possible to distinguish between primary, secondary, and tertiary nitrates (URBANSKI, 1965). A compilation of infrared absorbtion spectra of many of the compounds shown in Fig. 1 is provided in the paper by SAMMUL et al. (1964).

Table 1. Some physical properties of organic nitrates

Compound	Physical state at room temp.	m.p. °C	Specific gravity	Water solubility g/liter	Ethanol solubility g/liter 30°C	References
Ethylene glycol dinitrate	Oil	−22°	1.489	6.8		a
Erythrityl tetranitrate	Solid	61°		0.12	60.53	a, c
Glyceryl 1,2-dinitrate	Oil	−40°	1.47	65.7		a, b
Glyceryl 1,3-dinitrate	Oil	−40°	1.47	78.4		a, b
Glyceryl trinitrate	Oil	2.2° (labile) 13.2° (stable)	1.60	1.2—1.8	350 (approx.)	a, c
Isosorbide dinitrate	Solid	68—71°		0.68	41.87	c
Mannitol hexanitrate	Solid	112—113°	1.60			a
		108—110°	1.77	0.05	19.62	c
Pentaerythrityl tetranitrate	Solid	140—142°	1.77	0.01	0.69	c
					0.275	a
Pentaerythrithyl trinitrate	Solid	27—28°				a

References: [a] URBANSKI (1965). — [b] DUNSTAN et al. (1965). — [c] Information supplied by T. Z. Ball, Atlas Powder Company, Wilmington, Del.

II. Methods of Laboratory Synthesis

A. Mixed Acid Synthesis

The most common method of converting alcohols (including polyols) to nitric acid esters involves the use of a mixture of acids, usually nitric and sulfuric acids (BOSCHAN et al., 1955; LAWRIE, 1928). The nitrating mixture consists of equal parts of sulfuric and nitric acids such that a slight excess of nitric acid with respect to alcohol is provided. The alcohol is added slowly to the mixed acids in an ice bath. The nitrate ester forms rapidly providing good yields of primary and secondary esters [Eq. (1) and (2)].

$$2H_2SO_4 + HNO_3 \longrightarrow NO_2^+ + H_3^+O\,2HSO^-, \quad (1)$$

$$NO_2^+ + R\text{–}OH \longrightarrow R\text{–}O\text{–}NO_2 + H^+. \quad (2)$$

After the nitration reaction is complete the polynitrate can be readily isolated by pouring the reaction mixture into cold water and stirring. After decanting the upper aqueous phase, the polynitrate is washed with dilute Na_2CO_3 solution (to neutralize remaining acid) and water. The water is decanted and the polynitrate is dried over an appropriate dessiccant. The solid polynitrates will recrystallize from ethanol.

The completeness of the nitration can be easily determined by thin layer chromatography of the product on silica gel using solvents such as benzene: ethylacetate (4:1) or similar systems. In these nonpolar solvent systems the more completely nitrated polyols (e.g. glyceryl-trinitrate) can be separated from the less completely nitrated products (e.g. glyceryl 1,3- or 1,2-dinitrate) which remain closer to the origin.

Nitric acid generally contains nitrous acid. In addition, nitrous acid may also be formed by the reduction of nitric acid by the alcohol. In the presence of nitrous acid the alcohol is violently oxidized, so that the yield of nitrate ester is diminished and explosion may occur. Hence, there is a possibility that such reactions can get out of control if not properly monitored. These reactions should be carried out behind appropriate explosion shields and the worker should abandon the area if the reaction gets out of control. In order to reduce the chances of explosion and to increase the yield of desired product, urea or urea nitrate is often added as a nitrous acid scavenger [Eq. (3)].

$$CO(NH_2)_2 + 2\,HNO_2 \longrightarrow CO_2 + 2N_2 + 3H_20\,. \qquad (3)$$

Esterification may also be carried out using mixtures of nitric acid and acetic anhydride (BOSCHAN, 1955; MALNS et al., 1964). Techniques similar to those described for the nitric acid: sulfuric acid mixed acid procedure may be used.

B. Preparation of Incompletely Nitrated Polyols

1. Partial Nitration or Denitration

Preparation of completely nitrated polyols (e.g. glyceryl trinitrate) are readily accomplished on a laboratory scale by the mixed acid methods. Several methods of preparation of partially nitrated polyols (e.g. glyceryl 1,3-dinitrate) are available. The partially nitrated polyols are of great pharmacological interest because they represent the metabolites of the parent (completely nitrated) organic nitrates. The partially nitrated metabolites are pharmacologically active, although they are much less potent than the completely nitrated parent compound.

The partially nitrated polyols can be prepared by (1) incomplete nitration of the polyol; or (2) partial denitration of the completely nitrated polyol. Partial denitration can be carried out using acid or base hydrolysis or by reaction with sodium nitrite. Conditions for these procedures in the preparation of the glyceryl dinitrates from glyceryl trinitrate and expected yields have been described (DUNSTAN et al., 1965). These partial nitration or partial denitration procedures produce mixtures of the possible isomers. For example, partial nitration of glycerol or denitration of glyceryl trinitrate yields a mixture of glyceryl 1,3-dinitrate, glyceryl, 1,2-dinitrate, glyceryl 1-mononitrate and possibly glyceryl 2-mononitrate. The desired product may not be readily separated from the parent nitrate and the other nitrate esters by simple differential solvent separation. Chromatographic separation may be necessary. These mixtures can be separated by column or thin layer chromatography using silica gel and development with non-polar solvents (see Chapter on Analytical Techniques).

2. Reaction of Alkyl Halides and Silver Nitrate

A more direct method of producing the partially nitrated polyol is the reaction between silver nitrate and an alkyl halide [Eq. (4)] to produce the corresponding nitrate ester.

$$R\text{–}Cl + AgNO_3 \longrightarrow R\text{–}O\text{–}NO_2 + AgCl\,. \qquad (4)$$

The high solubility of silver nitrate in acetonitrile affords a method of nitrate ester synthesis from silver nitrate and alkyl halides in which the reaction mixture is homogeneous (FERRIS et al., 1953). Most primary and secondary iodides, many bromides, and active chlorides react rapidly enough at room temperature or slightly above to be useful in preparative work. DUNSTAN et al. (1965) have described a procedure for the preparation of glyceryl 1,3-dinitrate [Eq. (5)] and glyceryl 1,2-dinitrate from 1,3-dibromohydrin and 1,2-dibromhydrin respectively.

$$\begin{array}{l} CH_2\text{—}Cl \\ \;| \\ CH\text{—}OH \\ \;| \\ CH_2Cl \end{array} + 2AgClAgNO_3 \longrightarrow \begin{array}{l} CH_2\text{—}O\text{—}NO_2 \\ \;| \\ CH\text{—}OH \\ \;| \\ CH_2\text{—}O\text{—}NO_2 \end{array} \qquad (5)$$

The desired dinitrate can be isolated free of side products of the reaction by solvent extraction. This procedure has been successfully used by others (CREW and DICARLO, 1968; NEEDLEMAN and JOHNSON, 1973) in the preparation of these compounds for pharmacological study.

A thorough discussion of methods of separating and identifying the various organic nitrates and their denitrated metabolites is provided elsewhere in this book.

III. Chemical Properties

A. Acid and Base Hydrolysis of Nitric Acid Esters

Organic nitrates, like any other ester, undergo hydrolysis. This reaction occurs more rapidly in alkaline than acid solution, and only very slowly in a neutral medium. Nitrate esters can undergo hydrolysis by several possible pathways (BOSCHAN et al., 1955; CANNON, 1970) to yield products of elimination as well as the expected alcohol. Primary mononitrate esters undergo alkaline hydrolysis to produce only negligible quantities of the elimination products and the alcohol is essentially the only product formed (BOSCHAN et al., 1955; CANNON, 1970). Alkaline hydrolysis of secondary and tertiary nitrate esters yields more complicated reaction products. In some cases, the hydrolysis process does not yield any initial alcohol. As early as 1885 hydrolysis of glyceryl trinitrate in aqueous or alcoholic solution of sodium or potassium hydroxide was shown to yield a complex mixture of organic acids without the formation of glycerol (URBANSKI, 1965).

The rate of alkaline hydrolysis is much greater than acid hydrolysis. A comparison of the rates of hydrolysis of glyceryl trinitrate (CREW and DICARLO, 1968) showed that incubation the trinitrate in 4N NaOH for 15 min at 37° produced almost complete denitration whereas treatment in 4N HCl for six hours produced only a 28% decrease in glyceryl trinitrate. Most of the decrease in glyceryl trinitrate under the acid condition was accounted for as dinitrates and only 0.5% was completely denitrated. Incubation at 37° for six hours in water produced no detectable denitration.

It is important to note that alkaline hydrolysis of organic nitrates does not yield stoichiometric amount of inorganic nitrite. This must be considered when concentrations of organic nitrates are determined by measuring the amount inorganic nitrite (BELL et al., 1963) formed upon alkaline hydrolysis of the ester. The standard curve of the assay must be generated from simultaneously hydrolyzed organic nitrate and not inorganic nitrite.

B. Reductive Hydrolysis

In contrast to the complex products produced by hydrolysis of polynitrates obtained in simple basic solution, the alcohol can be obtained by alkaline hydrolysis of the ester if the reaction is carried out in the presence of a readily oxidizable substance. This was originally shown by the production of glycerol and diphenylsulfide when glyceryl trinitrate was hydrolyzed in the presence of phenylmercaptan (KLASON and CARLSON, 1906). This reaction may be analogous to the metabolic reactions *in vivo* whereby reductive hydrolysis of glyceryl trinitrate and other organic nitrates proceed with the formation of inorganic nitrite and oxidized glutathione (see Biotransformation Chapter). The reductive hydrolysis of organic nitrates is facilitated by an increase in the pH of the medium (NEEDLEMAN and JOHNSON, 1973). Reductive hydrolysis of nitrate esters can occur in the presence of other reducing agents such as sodium hydrosulfide and ammonium hydrosulfide. These reactions also yield inorganic nitrite and take place more readily at elevated pH (MERROW et al., 1953).

C. Acid Decomposition

Organic nitrates contaminated with acid due to incomplete washing during mixed acid synthesis or due to acid released due to thermal decomposition undergo acid catalyzed decomposition. Decomposition in unconfined samples is not dangerous. In a sealed container, however, the reaction produces increasing quantities of gaseous products and thereby produces increasing pressure. The increased pressure further stimulates decomposition, and this can be dangerous. Eventually the heat caused by decomposition is not removed quickly enough and an explosion can occur. For example, placing 0.3 g of glyceryl trinitrate with an admixture of 5% HNO_3 in a sealed ampoule at 41° resulted in an explosion in 320 min (URBANSKI, 1965). The presence of water greatly shortens the time necessary for autocatalytic decomposition and will hence accelerate explosion.

Well purified glyceryl trinitrate does not undergo decomposition under storage. Some organic nitrates decompose even more rapidly than glyceryl trinitrate. Impure preparations of mannitol hexanitrate are such an example. Repeated recrystallization is required to obtain high enough purity for the compound to have a high chemical stability.

D. Explosiveness

Explosives are compounds or mixtures which undergo a very rapid exothermic decomposition and generate a large volume of heated gas when they are subjected to some initiating disturbance (detonation) such as by heating, mechanical impact, or explosion of some other compound. In almost all cases of classical explosives the decomposition is an oxidation, the combined oxygen in the compound being roughly sufficient for the whole explosive to be transformed into gaseous products (MILLAR and SPRINGALL, 1966). The performance of a nitrate ester as an explosive is related to its oxygen balance, which is defined as the percentage of oxygen needed for complete combustion that is not available from the nitrate group (LOTHROP and HANDRICK, 1949; CANNON, 1970). The power of an explosion will theoretically be close to maximum when the oxygen balance is close to zero. Such is the case when the oxygen of the nitrate groups are the sole sources of oxygen in the combustion products. Hence esters of nitric acid, including the clinically used organic nitrates, have more explosive strength than other nitrocompounds such as TNT. Organic nitrates are very sensitive to shock and friction and to thermal decomposition at high temperatures. The more powerful the explosive the more sensitive it will be to initiators of explosion (LOTHROP and HANDRICK, 1949).

Although incompletely nitrated polyols do not possess the explosive strength of the completely nitrated polyols, the incompletely nitrated compounds may still be powerful explosives. For example, the sensitivity to shock of the glyceryl dinitrates are only slightly less than glyceryl trinitrate and they have about 80% of the explosive strength of the trinitrate (NAOUM, 1924). Glyceryl mononitrates are stable substances when heated to a moderate temperature; however, they will decompose explosively if heated to 170° in a sealed tube. Glyceryl mononitrates are weak explosives and sensitiveness to shock is very low. In contrast, ethylene glycol mononitrate, because of its favorable oxygen balance still detonates with enough force to be classed as a high explosive.

In addition to the sensitivity to shock, organic nitrates are very sensitive to friction. Glyceryl trinitrate can explode simply as the result of rubbing it in a porcelain mortar with a rough surface (URBANSKI, 1965).

IV. Cautions in Handling

A. Storage

Organic nitrates for use in experimentation can be obtained either as the clinically used tablets or from a manufacturer in larger quantities. When working with quantities of compound large enough such that the tablets are not practical, the compounds can be obtained adsorbed onto a suitable diluent, usually one part organic nitrate to approximately ten parts lactose. The compounds will not explode when so prepared. Other diluents such as mannitol or starch may be added to these mixtures, but other ingredients, especially alkaline or abrasive materials should not be added without consulting the manufacturer. These mixtures, like any light powder, should not be used near a source of static electricity. Deterioration and instability of these preparations is indicated by the development of an acidic condition or by the evolution of gas or odor. The organic nitrate mixtures are supplied in polyethylene bags which are impermeable to the agent. In the instances where the organic nitrate is a liquid, it is important to avoid leakage since concentration of the organic nitrate outside of the polyethylene bagging is hazardous (Atlas Bulletin, 1959).

B. Isolation

The organic nitrate may be removed from the adsorbant by repeated extraction with organic solvents (usually acetone, ether, or petroleum ether). The organic nitrate may then be isolated by evaporation of the organic solvent using a stream of dry air in a tared container. *In this form, the organic nitrates are powerful explosives and must be handled with extreme caution.* After weighing, solutions of known concentration may be prepared by dissolving the compound in methanol, ethanol or other suitable solvent. Upon dissolution in a large volume of ethanol, the compounds no longer represent an explosion hazard.

Solid organic nitrates can be readily isolated by addition of a large volume of water to a concentrated solution of the nitrate in acetone or other solvent. The organic nitrate will precipitate out of solution and can be isolated by filtration. *Again, this leaves the nitrate in a state which is highly explosive and caution must be used in handling the compound.*

C. Disposal

Free organic nitrates should be destroyed prior to disposal. This may be accomplished by dissolving the nitrate is fresh 2% sodium sulfide and heating at 70° for four hours (approximately one gram or organic nitrate per 100 ml of sodium sulfide solution, Atlas Bulletin, 1959). All glassware used to handle organic nitrates should be rinsed in acetone to insure removal of all organic nitrate. An oily residue of nitroglycerin can easily be overlooked if the glassware is simply washed in water.

D. Handling of Solutions

When handling pure organic nitrates or solutions of organic nitrates, it must be remembered that these agents can be absorbed through the skin in large enough amounts to exert a systemic pharmacological response, especially headache. Hence, it may be advisable to wear rubber gloves when handling solutions. Spills of these solutions should be cleaned up quickly and in such a way that a residue is not left on work surfaces.

References

Atlas Pharmaceutical Bulletin, Atlas Powder Company, Wilmington, Delaware, 1959.

BELL, F. K., O'NEILL, J. J., BURGISON, R. M.: Determination of the oil/water distribution coefficients of glyceryl trinitrate and two similar nitrate esters. J. Pharm. Sci. **52**, 637—641 (1963).

BOSHAN, R., MERROW, R. T., DOLAH, R. W., VAN: The chemistry of nitrate esters. Chem. Rev. **55**, 485—510 (1955).

BROWN, J. F.: The infrared spectra of nitro and other oxidized nitrogen compounds. J. Amer. chem. Soc. **77**, 6341—6349 (1955).

CANNON, N. W.: Nitrate esters. Eastman Organic Chemical Bull. **42**, (1970).
CREW, M. C., DICARLO, F. J.: Identification and assay of isomeric ^{14}C-glyceryl nitrates. J. Chromatog. **35**, 506—512 (1968).
DUNSTAN, I., GRIFFITHS, J. V., HARVEY, S. A.: Nitric esters. Part I. Characterization of the isomeric glycerol dinitrates. J. chem. Soc. (Lond.) 1319—1324 (1965).
FERRIS, A. F., MCLEAN, K. W., MARKS, I. G., EMMON, W. D.: Metathetical reactions of silver salts in solution III. The synthesis of nitrate esters. J. Amer. chem. Soc. **75**, 4078—4079 (1953).
KLASON, P., CARLSON, T.: Kenntniss der organischen Nitrate. Chem. Ber. **39**, 2752—2755 (1906).
LAWRIE, J. W.: Glycerol and the glycols, p. 377. New York: Chemical Catelog Co. 1928.
LOTHROP, W. C., HANDRICK, G. R.: The relationship between performance and constitution of pure organic explosive compounds. Chem. Rev. **44**, 419—445 (1949).
MALNS, D. C., WEKELL, J. C., HOULES, C. R.: Reaction of acetyl nitrate with alcohol derivatives of fatty acids: a synthesis of nitrate esters. J. Amer. Oil chem. Soc. **41**, 44—46 (1964).
MERROW, R. T., CRISTOL, S. J., DOHAH, R. W., VAN: The reaction of n-butyl nitrate with alkaline hydrosulfides. J. Amer. chem. Soc. **75**, 4259—4263 (1953).
MILLAR, I. T., SPRINGALL, H. D., EDS.: Sidgwick's organic chemistry of nitrogen. Third edition, p. 87—94. Oxford: Clarenden Press 1966.
NEEDLEMAN, P., JOHNSON, E. M., JR.: Mechanism of tolerance development to organic nitrates. J. Pharm. exp. Ther. **184**, 709—715 (1973).
SAMMUL, OSCAR R., BRANNON, W. L., HAYDEN, A. L.: Infrared spectra of some compounds of pharmaceutical interest. J. Ass. Offic. Agr. Chem. **47**, 918—991 (1964).
SMITH, P. A. S.: Open-chain nitrogen compounds, Vol. 2, pp. 483—490. New York: W. A. Benjamin 1966.
URBANSKI, T.: Chemistry and technology of explosives. New York: MacMillan Co. 1965.

CHAPTER 3

Organic Nitrates: Analytical Techniques

MARC G. BOGAERT

With 1 Figure

Most analytical techniques in the field of organic nitrates have been developed for the study of explosives or for pharmaceutical purposes; therefore, these techniques are often only qualitative or, if quantitative, their limit of detection is far above the concentrations one can expect to occur in biological fluids.

It was only in the 1960's that the search for the fate of organic nitrates in animals or humans fully started, with the use of analytical methods that are sensitive enough, and, on the other hand, allow distinction between a given organic nitrate and its breakdown products.

In this survey, attention will be mainly focused on those methods of analysis that are of interest for the study of organic nitrates in the living organism, i.e., for detection and quantitation in different biological fluids and tissues. This survey will practically be limited to the nitrates of glycerol, of isosorbide and of pentaerythritol, as only for these products is relevant information found in the literature.

I. Extraction Procedures

Most extraction procedures separate organic nitrates from inorganic nitrate or nitrite ions; these inorganic molecules are endogenous (CARR, 1958) or are due to breakdown of the organic nitrate administered. Furthermore, sometimes an extraction procedure can be found that allows separation of an organic nitrate from its more polar breakdown products.

A. Glyceryl Nitrates

For glyceryl trinitrate, CRANDALL et al. (1929) and CRANDALL (1933) reported quantitative extraction from blood with diethyl ether. In NEEDLEMAN'S work (NEEDLEMAN and HUNTER, 1965; NEEDLEMAN and KRANTZ, 1965) diethyl ether is used for extraction of glyceryl trinitrate and of the lower glyceryl nitrates, whereas some of the fully denitrated breakdown products are not extracted (NEEDLEMAN et al., 1971). CREW and DICARLO (1968) however warn that the efficiency of the extraction with diethyl ether is only 69% for the glyceryl mononitrates. Ethyl acetate can be used for extraction of glyceryl tri-, di- and mononitrates, without at least some of the denitrated products (NEEDLEMAN et al., 1972; ROSSEEL and BOGAERT, 1973b). Petroleum ether quantitatively separates glyceryl trinitrate from its metabolites (NEEDLEMAN et al., 1972). Using labeled material, DICARLO et al. (1968) could show that dioxane removes glyceryl nitrates and glycerol from homogenized tissues, without the metabolic products formed from glycerol.

B. Isosorbide Nitrates

Ethyl acetate extracts the dinitrate as well as the 2 mononitrates of isosorbide from biological material (NEEDLEMAN et al., 1972; ROSSEEL and BOGAERT, 1973a). Ethyl acetate was also used for removal of isosorbide dinitrate from human plasma by SHERBER et al. (1970) and GÖBBELER (1971). SISENWINE and RUELIUS (1971) used methanol for extraction of isosorbide dinitrate and mononitrates from lyophilized plasma or urine. Petroleum ether can be used selectively to extract the parent molecule, isosorbide dinitrate, without its lower esters, just as for the glyceryl nitrates (NEEDLEMAN et al., 1972).

The isosorbide mononitrates are excreted in the urine partly as glucuronides (REED et al., 1971): extraction solvents such as ethyl acetate can be used after previous incubation of the urine with glucuronidase or glusulase (REED et al., 1971; ROSSEEL and BOGAERT, 1973a); it is not surprising that, after administration of isosorbide dinitrate in man, no metabolites were detected in some subjects after ethyl acetate extraction of non-incubated urine (DIETZ, 1967).

For the dinitrate and the mononitrate of each of the 2 isomers of isosorbide, namely isomannide and isoidide, ethyl acetate can be used for extraction, as is the case for the isosorbide nitrates (ROSSEEL and BOGAERT, 1973a, 1973b).

C. Pentaerythritol Nitrates

Extraction procedures used in studies of the metabolic pathways in animals or man after administration of pentaerythritol tetranitrate or pentaerythritol trinitrate are described by the group of DICARLO (DICARLO et al., 1966, 1969; DAVIDSON et al., 1970, 1971b; CREW et al., 1971).

For the study of urinary excretion, urine samples were evaporated to dryness, and the residues were taken up in methanol-ethyl acetate (1/1); for faeces, an extract with dioxane was obtained, and then treated like the urine. Glucuronides of the different pentaerythritol nitrates were extracted with ethanol-ether (1/1), after ammonium sulfate saturation of material from bile or urine. For study of the different pentaerythritol nitrates in blood a "far more difficult and tedious" procedure had to be used, due to the very low levels in blood and the presence of blood components preventing resolution of the metabolites by subsequent thin layer chromatography. This procedure described in detail, e.g., by DICARLO et al. (1966) involves several extractions [with dioxane, with methanol, with methanol-ethyl acetate (1/1)], with filtrations and evaporations, in order to get rid of lipid material.

II. Spectrometric Methods

Whereas visible spectrometry has been used again and again in attempts (that were often fruitless) to measure the concentration of "nitrate", e.g. in plasma, other forms of spectrometry have mainly been employed for identification of large concentrations, often of pure material, without direct application to the study of nitrates in the living organism.

A. Visible Spectrophotometry

Innumerable reports have been written about colorimetric methods for quantitation of the nitrate and nitrite ions that are found after hydrolysis of the organic compounds. These methods were originally developed for use under conditions that are quite different from those encountered in biological studies.

Some of these methods are based upon the formation of nitrocompounds. In the so-called xylenol procedure, the organic nitrates are hydrolyzed with sulfuric acid; the nitrate ions formed react with 2,4-xylenol and the nitroxylenol formed is quantitated in the visible spectrum range (YAGODA, 1943); use of 2,6-xylenol instead of 2,4-xylenol is said to enhance the sensitivity of the procedure (ANDREWS, 1964). The phenoldisulfonic acid method, with colorimetric determination of nitrophenoldisulfonic acid (OSOL and FARRAR, 1950) has also been used in biological work.

In most biological work on nitrates, colorimetric methods based upon the classical Griess-reaction (GRIESS, 1879) are applied. The original Griess-reaction involved the diazotation, in acid conditions, of sulfanilic acid by the nitrite ion, followed by coupling with α-naphthylamine; the colored compound formed is measured. Various modifications of the Griess-reaction have been proposed; SHINN (1941) e.g. uses sulfanilamide as reacting agent and N-(l-naphthyl)-ethylenediamine as coupling agent; LAMBERT and ZITOMER (1960) propose (4-aminophenyl)trimethylammonium as reacting agent and N, N-dimethyl-1-naphthylamine as coupler. These are only two of the multiple variations on the Griess-reaction. In these Griess-procedures, the nitrite ions are measured; the nitrate ions can be quantitated after reduction to nitrite, e.g. with zinc. Organic nitrates are first hydrolyzed, usually by alkalinization. If both nitrite and nitrate ions are present, nitrate ions can be measured after removing the nitrites. Applications of these methods for biological work can be found in CASS et al. (1962); BELL et al. (1963); BELL (1964); LORENZETTI et al. (1966). An automated procedure was described by LITCHFIELD (1967). This author mentions the problem of transformation of nitrite to nitrate in blood at 37°.

The whole procedure for determination of nitrates, e.g., in plasma, can be performed as follows (see LORENZETTI et al., 1966): Add to 1 ml of plasma and 1 ml of bidistilled water, at 0° C, 10 ml 0.2% sulphanilamide, 2 ml of 50% concentrated HCl and 2 ml 5% $HgCl_2$ (to precipitate proteins). Centrifuge; add to the clear supernatant 0.5 g Amberlite IR 120 AA, an acidic, sulfonic cation exchange resin: precipitate the complex Amberlite-diazonium by centrifugation. To the nitrite-free supernatant add 5 ml 12% NH_4OH and 1 ml 1% $MnCl_2$. Leave in ice for 10 min; add 0.1 g zinc dust and stir for 10 min. Filter; acidify with 0.5 ml 50% concentrated HCl and add 1 ml of 0.1% N-(l-naphtyl)-ethylenediamine dihydrochloride; read the color at 538 mμ after 10 min.

These colorimetric methods have been used extensively in work on animals and humans, mainly for plasma or blood, but these methods lack sensitivity and specificity. The lack of specificity is an obvious handicap. In many instances there is a certain background of nitrate and nitrite ions, e.g., in blood (CARR, 1958; LORENZETTI et al., 1966), and this background changes during the day, e.g., with intake of food. Previous extraction of the material with one of the usual solvents eliminates this problem (LITCHFIELD, 1967), as well as the problem of distinguishing between the organic material and the inorganic ions formed by hydrolysis of the esters. But even then the concentration measured is made up by the parent drug that was given, and its break-down products, the lower nitrate esters. Quantitating this bulk of organic nitrates, e.g. in plasma, is not very meaningfull, as the levels of break-down products can be much higher than those of the parent product, as shown e.g. for glyceryl trinitrate by NEEDLEMAN et al. (1972), for isosorbide dinitrate by SISENWINE and RUELIUS (1971) and ROSSEEL and BOGAERT (1973b), and for pentaerythritol tetranitrate by DAVIDSON et al. (1970). Use of an extraction procedure that separates the parent molecule from the metabolites, e.g. with petroleum ether, can help (NEEDLEMAN et al., 1972).

Lack of sensitivity is another problem with the colorimetric method. Although very low limits of detection are often claimed, mainly for pure solutions, but also in blood, see e.g. the micromethod for determination of nitrite of SHECHTER et al. (1972), based on the Griess-reaction (with detection of 0.01 μg/ml in 0.1 ml of blood), there is not much hope that with these colorimetric methods the very low concentrations that are obtained in plasma after administration of reasonable doses, can be measured accurately. The fallacies of the colorimetric methods for work with biological material are illustrated by publications such as those of BERRY and ROACH (1958), RITSCHEL and CLOTTEN (1970) and RITSCHEL (1971) on plasma concentrations of "nitrate" after oral administration of organic nitrates: these authors find in plasma much more nitrate than the amount administered, even if one assumes that all nitrate given is present in the plasma, without any distribution to other tissues.

The colorimetric methods have only proven to be of value in a few selected circumstances, where high amounts of nitrate are present, and where colorimetry is used in conjunction with other techniques: determinations on urine, coupled with thin layer chromatography (ROSSEEL et al., 1970); assay of perfusion fluid after specific extraction (NEEDLEMAN and HARKEY, 1971; JOHNSON et al., 1972); study of nitrite formation *in vitro* (DICARLO and MELGAR, 1970).

B. Spectrometric Techniques Outside the Visible Range

These techniques are not used for quantitative work on the fate of the organic nitrates in the living organism, and therefore only a few selected references are given:

Infrared spectrometry: JACKSON and HAYWARD (1960); PRISTERA et al. (1960); SHERBER et al. (1970); WOO et al. (1973).

U.V. spectrometry: WEISS and BOLTZ (1971); TINGSTAD et al. (1972).

Mass spectrometry: FRASER and PAUL (1968a, 1968b).

Nuclear magnetic resonance spectrometry: ANTEUNIS et al. (1971); GARRIGOU-LAGRANGE et al. (1971); SCHIRMER et al. (1972).

III. Chromatographic Procedures

A. Column Chromatography

DICARLO et al. (1968) used ion exchange chromatography for separation of acidic material from neutral material, in order to study the fate of the ^{14}C after administration of labeled glyceryl trinitrate to rats. REED et al. (1971) separated neutral compounds from charged molecules (mainly glucuronides) in the urine of animals treated with labeled isosorbide dinitrate, with a combination of ion exchange and molecular sieve chromatography. Column chromatography of organic nitrates has also been described for the study of explosives (see e.g., OVENSTON, 1949) or for pharmaceutical purposes (see e.g., HOHMANN and LEVINE, 1964).

B. Paper Chromatography

Paper chromatography has been applied for separation of explosives (KRIEN, 1963). JACKSON and HAYWARD (1961) separated the dinitrates of isosorbide, isomannide and isoidide by paper chromatography, but did not mention the problem of the respective mononitrates.

C. Thin Layer Chromatography

This technique has been extensively used for study of mixtures of explosives; the following papers can be consulted for details how to separate glyceryl trinitrate or pentaerythritol tetranitrate from other explosives: HANSSON (1963); BÖHM (1966); BARNES (1967); PARIHAR et al. (1967); YASUDA (1970).

In the last ten years, thin layer chromatography has also been applied for separation of the different nitrates of a given series (parent compound and break-down products) in biological material. The material is spotted as such on the plates if the concentration is high enough and a sensitive quantitation method is present (e.g. study of urinary excretion after administration of labelled products); usually, however, preliminary extraction and concentration procedures are necessary.

Thin layer chromatography is usually done by the ascending technique, mostly on silica gel plates of 250 μ thickness.

1. Glyceryl Nitrates

For the glyceryl nitrates, a commonly used solvent is the mixture benzene-ethyl acetate (4/1, v/v), sometimes used in conjunction with acetic acid, e.g. benzene-ethyl acetate-acetic acid (16/4/1 or 16/4/4) (NEEDLEMAN and HUNTER, 1965; NEEDLEMAN et al., 1972), with satisfactory resolution of the different nitrates, except for the mononitrates that are not separated from each other and move very slowly. In such solvent systems, the greater the esterification, the faster the migration on the plate, as there is an increase in water solubility with de-esterification. CREW and DICARLO (1968), working with labeled glyceryl nitrates, tested 7 different solvent systems; here too, migration increases with degree of esterification. In a subsequent paper of DICARLO's group (DICARLO et al., 1968) on the urinary excretion after glyceryl trinitrate administration in the rat, three of these solvents were used: the above mentioned benzene-ethyl acetate-acetic acid (16/4/1) with chamber saturation is satisfactory, except for the mononitrates; ethyl acetate-n-heptane (9/1) without chamber saturation, gives a faster migration and a good resolution of the mononitrates; finally, 1-butanol-acetic acid-water (5/1/4) allows separation of 3 radioactive unidentified areas, probably neutral or amphoteric compounds.

2. Isosorbide Nitrates

For the isosorbide nitrates benzene-ethyl acetate-acetic acid (16/4/1) was found by NEEDLEMAN and HUNTER (1965) to separate two nitrated breakdown products from the parent isosorbide dinitrate. DIETZ (1967) used benzene-ethyl acetate (1/1) for separation of isosorbide dinitrate, 5-mononitrate and 2-mononitrate after extraction and concentration from urine; with isopropanol-concentrated ammonium hydroxide (4/1) the 3 products moved more closely together. SISENWINE and RUELIUS (1971), using labeled material, found that benzene-ethyl acetate (1/1) could resolve isosorbide as well as the nitrated derivatives of isosorbide; the same authors saw with isopropanol-concentrated ammonium hydroxide (4/1) 2 radioactive spots, supposed to be glucuronides. Good separation of parent nitrate and nitrated break-down products with benzene-ethyl acetate (1/1) was found by ROSSEEL and BOGAERT (1973a) for the nitrates of isosorbide, isoidide and isomannide.

In all these solvents the dinitrated products move faster than their respective mononitrates; isosorbide-2-mononitrate, with its nitrate group in the exo-position, usually moves faster than the 5-mononitrate; for the isopropanol-ammonium hydroxide solvent, DIETZ (1967) reports that 5-mononitrate moves faster than 2-mononitrate, while SISENWINE and RUELIUS (1971) saw, for with the same solvent mixture, the opposite result.

REED et al. (1971) used thin layer chromatography in conjuntion with column for separation of urine: they used as thin layer solvent trichloroethylene-acetone (4/1) on unactivated silica gel plates, or ethyl acetate-glacial acetic acid-formic acid-0.02 M boric acid (pH 8.2)(14/4/2/5), with heating of the plates; details about the actual chromatograms were not given.

3. Pentaerythritol Nitrates

For the pentaerythritol nitrates, apart from fragmentary data of NEEDLEMAN and HUNTER (1965) and YASUDA (1970), all information comes from the work done with labeled material by DICARLO's group.

In a study of hydrolysis of pentaerythritol tetranitrate (DICARLO et al., 1964), it can be seen that among 5 solvent systems used, combination of two of them gives good results: with toluene-ethyl acetate (1/1) the pentaerythritol nitrates are separated from each other, but pentaerythritol is not separated from the mononitrate; ethyl acetate saturated with water is better in that regard but here the tetranitrate and the trinitrate move very closely together. Later on DICARLO's group showed that good resolution of the whole series, pentaerythritol included, could be obtained with toluene-ethyl acetate-butanol-water (10/5/2/2, upper phase) (DICARLO et al., 1966) or (5/5/1/1, upper phase) (DAVIDSON et al., 1970). These two solvents were used for urine after the usual extraction-concentration procedures. For blood, after the extraction-concentration procedures, the material was spotted on a thin layer plate, and developed in one of these two solvents, but then redeveloped successively three times, with intermediate drying, with n-butanol-ammonium hydroxide-water (4/1/3, upper phase); after transfer of the radioactive material to a fresh thin layer plate, development was done with the solvent used the first time. This procedure resulted in elimination of interfering material (DICARLO et al., 1966, 1969; DAVIDSON et al.,

1970). Finally, CREW et al. (1971) used a number of solvents in order to deal with the problems of separation and identification of different pentaerythritol compounds and their glucuronides in bile and urine.

4. Visualization

Localization of nitrated compounds on thin layer plates is often done in biological work by coloring them with a spray of diphenylamine, usually 1% in ethanol or methanol, followed by U.V. irradiation for a few minutes (COLDWELL and MCLEAN, 1958, 1959; COLDWELL, 1959), although numerous other coloring methods can be found in the literature (e.g. those based on the Griess-reaction, LLOYD, 1967; YASUDA, 1970). The limit of detection with these methods lies below 1 µg.

5. Quantitation

For quantitation on the plate, radioscan and autoradiography have been used in the case of labeled material (e.g. for glyceryl nitrates, NEEDLEMAN et al., 1971, and DICARLO et al., 1968; for isosorbide dinitrate, SISENWINE and RUELIUS, 1971; for pentaerythritol nitrates, DICARLO et al., 1964). After coloration of the nitrates, quantitation on the plate of non-labeled nitrates can be done with visible reflectance scanning (YASUDA, 1970) or spectrophotometric scanning (ROSSEEL et al., 1970); in this last paper the problems of sensitivity, of plate-to-plate variation, and of variation on a given plate are discussed; a good quantitation in the µg range can be obtained. Other methods have been suggested, such as quantitation by area-measuring (KOHLBECK, 1965).

Finally, quantitation is often done by scraping off selected areas of the plate, and measuring the nitrate content by a classical colorimetric determination. In the case of labeled products, the radioactivity that is scraped off can be counted.

D. Gas Liquid Chromatography (GLC)

A number of papers have appeared on this method of separation and detection of organic nitrates outside the biological field, and a few of these references are cited here.

EVERED and POLLARD (1960) gave retention data for flame ionization detection of different alkyl nitrates. Catharometer detection of glyceryl trinitrate and other explosives was discussed by WILLIAMS and MURRAY (1963), CAMERA and PRAVISANI (1964) and FOSSEL (1965). WILLIAMS and MURRAY (1963) used also flame ionization detection, and in 1966, WILLIAMS et al. mentioned that electron capture GLC allows detection of less than 1 ng of glyceryl trinitrate.

TROWELL and PHILPOT (1969) and ALLEY and DYKES (1972) discussed technical aspects of GLC with flame ionization detection for glyceryl trinitrate and other explosives with emphasis on the problem of thermal decomposition of glyceryl trinitrate on the column.

GLC separation of an organic nitrate from its degradation products, again without direct application to biological problems, was studied by a few authors. TROWELL (1970), in a paper on aged propellant samples, saw, with flame ionization detection, separation of glyceryl trinitrate from the trimethylsilyl derivatives of the glyceryl dinitrates and of glyceryl-1-mononitrate; he noted a "lack of response" of the flame detector for glyceryl trinitrate. In a paper on the technique of selective purging from a GLC column, WARNER et al. (1973) showed, as illustration, chromatograms with separation of the trimethylsilyl derivatives of the 2 mononitrates of isosorbide, with flame ionization detection. DAVIDSON et al. (1971 a) studied GLC separation and quantitation of mixtures of the 4 nitrates of pentaerythritol and of pentaerythritol itself; trifluoroacetyl derivatives were formed, except, of course, for the tetranitrate. With flame ionization detection, both SE-30 and Dexsil columns gave good separation of the 5 products; lower limits of detection ranged between 5 ng (for pentaerythritol) and 50 ng (for the tetranitrate), with the other products in between. With electron capture detection, picogram amounts of the products can be seen; with both SE-30 and Dexsil columns, working at 2 selected temperatures is necessary for satisfactory chromatography of the 5 compounds. In the same paper DAVIDSON et al. (1971a) reported separation of a mixture of pentaerythritol tetranitrate, erythritol tetranitrate, isosorbide dinitrate and mannitol hexanitrate.

Reports on application of GLC for biological work are limited. SHERBER et al. (1970) showed fragmentary data, obtained with GLC with flame ionization detection, on the assay of isosorbide dinitrate in rabbit blood, and said that with electron capture detection, a very high sensitivity should be obtained; no mention was made of the metabolites of isosorbide dinitrate. GÖBBELER (1971) showed chromatograms of isosorbide dinitrate in dog blood, obtained with electron capture detection with ^{63}Ni source. This author claims a very high sensitivity of his method (40 pg), but this is not substantiated by the fragmentary, mostly qualitative data given.

In our laboratory we developed a procedure for GLC of the glyceryl and isosorbide nitrates, and showed that, with electron capture detection, the method is suitable for quantitation of the substances in plasma after administration of therapeutic doses in man (ROSSEEL and BOGAERT, 1972, 1973b; BOGAERT and ROSSEEL, 1972). In the preparation of the sample to be injected, care should be taken to eliminate endogenous interfering substances and to avoid introduction of impurities during the procedure. All glassware is silanized; the ethyl acetate used for the extraction is shaken with ferrous sulfate and with distilled water, and distilled immediately before use; the organic extraction phase is filtered through charcoal. The column used is 3.5% of QF-1 on 60 to 80 mesh Gaschrom Q; column temperature is around 120°. With this system, a good separation is obtained between glyceryl trinitrate, its 2 dinitrates (that are only partially separated from each other), glyceryl-1-mononitrate and glycerol, and on the other hand, the 3 nitrates of isosorbide and isosorbide itself are well separated from each other. Although the base line is far from perfect, no endogenous substances were found to interfere with the peaks of the nitrates studied when extracts of human plasma are injected.

For quantitation, an internal standard was added to the plasma samples before the extraction procedure: isosorbide dinitrate was the standard for glyceryl nitrate studies, isomannide or isoidide dinitrate the standard for studies with isosorbide nitrates. Peak areas were measured; the relationship between the ratio of peak areas and the ratio of the quantities was linear.

When 5 ml of plasma is available, quantitation is possible for amounts as low as 1 ng/ml plasma, this for the parent products. As illustration of the method, in Fig. 1

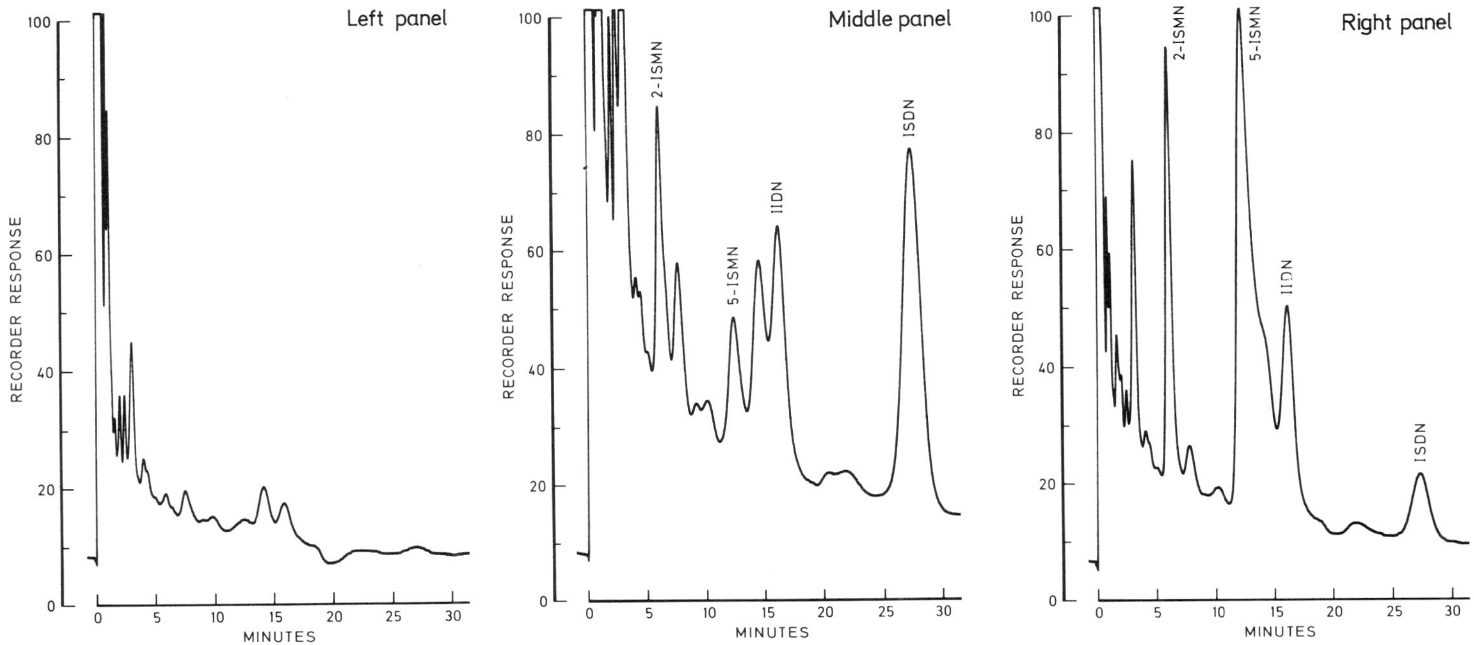

Fig. 1. Gas chromatograms of extracts of 5 ml plasma samples of a healthy volunteer. *Left panel:* blank plasma. *Middle panel*, 15 min and *right panel*, 60 min after oral administration of 5 mg of isosorbide dinitrate; to these 2 plasma samples isoidide dinitrate, 5 ng, was added as internal standard before the extraction. 2-ISMN: 2-isosorbide mononitrate; 5-ISMN: 5-isosorbide mononitrate; IIDN: isoidide dinitrate; ISDN: isosorbide dinitrate. Note the decrease of concentration of the parent molecule and the increase of the concentration of the mononitrates between 15th and 60th min. Instrument: Packard Series 7400 gas chromatograph with tritium electron capture detector. Column: 1.83 m × 2 mm I.D.; 3.5% of QF-1 on 60 to 80 mesh Gaschrom Q; column temperature: 117° C. Pulse voltage 25 V; electrometer range 1×10^{-9}

chromatograms of plasma extracts from a human volunteer are shown, before and after oral administration of 5 mg isosorbide dinitrate.

In another study, the possibility of separating with GLC a mixture of the di- and mononitrates of isosorbide, isomannide and isoidide, was demonstrated (ROSSEEL and BOGAERT, 1973a).

IV. Use of Labeled Products

For the different series of nitrates, labeled compounds have been used. They can be prepared by nitration (LAWRIE, 1928) of ^{14}C-glycerol (CREW and DICARLO, 1968), ^{14}C-pentaerythritol (DICARLO et al., 1964) or ^{14}C-isosorbide (REED et al., 1971). Work with labeled glyceryl trinitrate has been reported, e.g., by CREW and DICARLO (1968); DICARLO et al. (1968); DICARLO and MELGAR (1969, 1970); NEEDLEMAN et al. (1971, 1972); LANG et al. (1972). Labeled isosorbide dinitrate was used by REED et al. (1971); SISENWINE and RUELIUS (1971) and NEEDLEMAN et al. (1972). DICARLO's group worked extensively with labeled pentaerythritol nitrates (for references see the section on thin layer chromatography of these substances).

References

ALLEY, B. J., DYKES, H. W. H.: Gas-liquid chromatographic determination of nitrate esters, stabilizers and plasticizers in nitrocellulose-base propellants. J. Chromatog. **71**, 23—37 (1972).

ANDREWS, D. W. W.: A sensitive method for determining nitrate in water with 2,6-xylenol. Analyst **89**, 730—734 (1964).

ANTEUNIS, M., VERHEGGHE, G., ROSSEEL, M. T.: Configurational and conformational insights on exo- and endo-1, 4:3, 6-dianhydroglucitol mononitrate. Org. magn. Resonance **3**, 693—701 (1971).

BARNES, R. W.: Identification of the nitrate esters of five alkyl alcohols by thin-layer chromatography. J. Chromatog. **31**, 606—608 (1967).

BELL, F. K.: Spectrophotometric method for the assay of individual nitroglycerin tablets. J. pharm. Sci. **53**, 752—755 (1964).

BELL, F. K., O'NEILL, J. J., BURGISON, R. M.: Determination of the oil/water distribution coefficients of glyceryl trinitrate and two similar nitrate esters. J. pharm. Sci. **52**, 637—639 (1963).

BERRY, J. W., ROACH, T. C.: An evaluation of blood nitrate levels. Circulation **17**, 1041—1046 (1958).

BÖHM, O.: Dünnschichtchromatographie einiger Nitroverbindungen und Salpetersäureester an Kieselgel G. Explosivstoffe **15**, 97—106 (1966).

BOGAERT, M. G., ROSSEEL, M. T.: Plasma levels in man of nitroglycerin after buccal administration. J. Pharm. Pharmacol. **24**, 737—738 (1972).

CAMERA, E., PRAVISANI, D.: Separation and analysis of alkylpolynitrates by gas chromatography. Anal. Chem. **36**, 2108—2109 (1964).

CARR, C. J.: The pharmacology of the vasodilator nitrate-nitrite drugs. Int. Rec. Med. **171**, 121—129 (1958).

CASS, L. J., FREDERIK, W. S., DELUCIA, H.: The metabolic fate of nitrate esters. Angiology **13**, 469—473 (1962).

COLDWELL, B. B.: The application of ultra-violet light and diphenylamine to spot tests for explosives. Analyst **84**, 665—667 (1959).

COLDWELL, B. B., MCLEAN, S. R.: A new spot test for nitrate ion. Canad. J. Chem. **36**, 652—655 (1958).

COLDWELL, B. B., MCLEAN, S. R.: The reaction between diphenylamine and nitrates in ultraviolet light. Canad. J. Chem. **37**, 1637—1643 (1959).
CRANDALL, L. A.: The fate of glyceryl trinitrate in the tolerant and non-tolerant animal. J. Pharmacol. exp. Ther. **48**, 127—140 (1933).
CRANDALL, L. A., LEAKE, C. D., LOEVENHART, A. S., MUEHLBERGER, C. W.: The rate of elimination of glyceryl trinitrate from the blood stream after intravenous administration in dogs. J. Pharmacol. exp. Ther. **37**, 283—296 (1929).
CREW, M. C., DICARLO, F. J.: Identification and assay of isomeric ^{14}C-glyceryl nitrates. J. Chromatog. **35**, 506—512 (1968).
CREW, M. C., GALA, R. L., HAYNES, L. J., DICARLO, F. J.: Biliary excretion and biotransformation of pentaerythritol trinitrate in rats. Biochem. Pharmacol. **20**, 3077—3089 (1971).
DAVIDSON, I. W. F., DICARLO, F. J., SZABO, E. I.: Gas chromatographic separation and detection of pentaerythritol nitrates and other organic nitrate esters. J. Chromatog. **57**, 345—352 (1971a).
DAVIDSON, I. W. F., MILLER, H. S., DICARLO, F. J.: Absorption, excretion and metabolism of pentaerythritol tetranitrate by humans. J. Pharmacol. exp. Ther. **175**, 42—50 (1970).
DAVIDSON, I. W. F., MILLER, H. S., DICARLO, F. J.: Pharmacodynamics and biotransformation of pentaerythritol tetranitrate in man. J. pharm. Sci. **60**, 274—277 (1971b).
DICARLO, F. J., CREW, M. C., HAYNES, L. J., MELGAR, M. D., GALA, R. L.: The absorption and biotransformation of glyceryl trinitrate-1,3-^{14}C by rats. Biochem. Pharmacol. **17**, 2179—2183 (1968).
DICARLO, F. J., CREW, M. C., SKLOW, N. J., COUTINHO, C. B., NONKIN, P., SIMON, F., BERNSTEIN, A.: Metabolism of pentaerythritol tetranitrate by patients with coronary artery disease. J. Pharmacol. exp. Ther. **153**, 254—258 (1966).
DICARLO, F. J., HARTIGAN, J. M., PHILLIPS, G. E.: Analysis of pentaerythritol tetranitrate and its hydrolysis products by thin layer chromatography and radio scanning. Anal. Chem. **36**, 2301—2303 (1964).
DICARLO, F. J., MELGAR, M. D.: Binding and metabolism of nitroglycerin by rat blood plasma. Proc. Soc. exp. Biol. (N.Y.) **131**, 406—408 (1969).
DICARLO, F. J., MELGAR, M. D.: Nitroglycerin biotransformation by rat blood serum. Biochem. Pharmacol. **19**, 1371—1379 (1970).
DICARLO, F. J., MELGAR, M. D., HAYNES, L. J., GALA, R. L., CREW, M. C.: Metabolism of pentaerythritol trinitrate and pentaerythritol by dogs. J. Pharmacol. exp. Ther. **168**, 235—239 (1969).
DIETZ, A. J.: The biotransformation of isosorbide dinitrate in dogs and humans. Biochem. Pharmacol. **16**, 2447—2448 (1967).
EVERED, S., POLLARD, F. H.: The application of gas chromatography to the determination of retention data and activity coefficients of some alkanes, alkyl nitrates, nitroalkanes and alcohols on selected stationary phases. J. Chromatog. **4**, 451—457 (1960).
FOSSEL, E. T.: A rapid, accurate determination of glyceryl trinitrate and chloroglyceryl dinitrate in pharmaceutical preparation. J. Gas Chromatog. **3**, 179 (1965).
FRASER, R. T. M., PAUL, N. C.: The mass spectrometry of nitrate esters and related compounds. Part I. J. Chem. Soc. 659—663 (1968a).
FRASER, R. T. M., PAUL, N. C.: The mass spectrometry of nitrate esters and related compounds. Part II. J. Chem. Soc. 1407—1410 (1968b).
GARRIGOU-LAGRANGE, C., ULHRICH, M., SALIER, B., BOILOT, J. C.: Étude conformationnelle de la nitroglycérine et de quelques esters nitriques des propanols. C. R. Acad. Sci. (Paris) **273**, 925—928 (1971).
GÖBBELER, K. H.: Gaschromatographische Bestimmung von Isosorbiddinitrat im Blut mit Hilfe des electron-capture-Detectors. Pharm. Z. **116**, 961—962 (1971).
GRIESS, P.: Cited by LAMBERT and ZITOMER (1960).
HANSSON, J.: Dünnschichtchromatographische Analysenmethode für die Trennung der gewöhnlichsten Sprengstoffe. Explosivstoffe **11**, 73—77 (1963).
HOHMANN, J. R., LEVINE, J.: Partition column for determination of glyceryl trinitrate in tablets. J. Ass. off. agr. Chem. **47**, 471—473 (1964).
JACKSON, M., HAYWARD, L. D.: The action of pyridine on the dinitrate esters of 1,4;3,6-dianhydrohexitols. Canad. J. Chem. **38**, 496—502 (1960).
JACKSON, M., HAYWARD, L. D.: Paper chromatography of nitrate and tosylate esters. J. Chromatog. **5**, 166—169 (1961).

JOHNSON, E. M., HARKEY, A. B., BLEHM, D. J., NEEDLEMAN, P.: Clearance and metabolism of organic nitrates. J. Pharmacol. exp. Ther. **182**, 56—62 (1972).
KOHLBECK, J. A.: Determination of nitroglycerin and resorcinol in double-base propellant following separation by thin layer chromatography. Anal. Chem. **37**, 1282—1283 (1965).
KRIEN, G.: Über die papierchromatographische Analyse von Sprengstoffen. Explosivstoffe **11**, 207—209 (1963).
LAMBERT, J. L., ZITOMER, F.: Differential colorimetric determination of nitrite and nitrate ions. Anal. Chem. **32**, 1684—1686 (1960).
LANG, S., JOHNSON, E. M., NEEDLEMAN, P.: Metabolism of and vascular responses to glyceryl trinitrate in the eviscerated rat. Biochem. Pharmacol. **21**, 422—424 (1972).
LAWRIE, J. W.: Nitroglycerol, its manufacture, properties and analysis. In: Glycerol and the glycols, p. 337—360. New York: Chemical Catalog Co. 1928.
LITCHFIELD, M. H.: The automated analysis of nitrite and nitrate in blood. Analyst **92**, 132—136 (1967).
LLOYD, J. B. F.: Detection of microgram amounts of nitroglycerin and related compounds. Forens. Sci. Soc. **7**, 198 (1967).
LORENZETTI, O. J., TYE, A., NELSON, J. W.: Blood nitrite and nitrate concentration after oral and intravenous administration of glyceryl trinitrate in rabbits. J. pharm. Sci. **55**, 105—106 (1966).
NEEDLEMAN, P., BLEHM, D. J., HARKEY, A. B., JOHNSON, E. M., LANG, S.: The metabolic pathway in the degradation of glyceryl trinitrate. J. Pharmacol. exp. Ther. **179**, 347—353 (1971).
NEEDLEMAN, P., HARKEY, A. B.: Role of endogenous glutathione in the metabolism of glyceryl trinitrate by isolated perfused rat liver. Biochem. Pharmacol. **20**, 1867—1876 (1971).
NEEDLEMAN, P., HUNTER, F. E.: The transformation of glyceryl trinitrate and other nitrates by glutathione-organic nitrate reductase. Molec. Pharmacol. **1**, 77—86 (1965).
NEEDLEMAN, P., KRANTZ, J. C.: The biotransformation of nitroglycerin. Biochem. Pharmacol. **14**, 1225—1230 (1965).
NEEDLEMAN, P., LANG, S., JOHNSON, E. M.: Organic nitrates: relationship between biotransformation and rational angina pectoris therapy. J. Pharmacol. exp. Ther. **181**, 489—497 (1972).
OSOL, A., FARRAR, G. E.: The dispensatory of the United States, p. 432. Philadelphia: Lippincott Company 1950.
OVENSTON, T. C. J.: A scheme for the chromatographic examination of propellant explosives. Analyst **74**, 344—351 (1949).
PARIHAR, D. B., SHARMA, S. P., VERMA, K. K.: Rapid estimation of explosive nitrates. J. Chromatog. **31**, 551—556 (1967).
PRISTERA, F., HALIK, M., CASTELLI, A., FREDERICKS, W.: Analysis of explosives using infrared spectroscopy. Anal. Chem. **32**, 495—508 (1960).
REED, D. E., MAY, J. F., HART, L. G., MCCURDY, D. H.: Identification of the urinary metabolites of isosorbide dinitrate in dogs. Arch. int. Pharmacodyn. **191**, 318—336 (1971).
RITSCHEL, W. A.: Influence of formulating factors on drug safety of timed-release nitroglycerin tablets. J. pharm. Sci. **60**, 1683—1685 (1971).
RITSCHEL, W. A., CLOTTEN, R.: Entwicklung einer peroralen Nitroglycerin-Proxyphyllin-Retard-Form. Arzneimittel-Forsch. **20**, 1180—1187 (1970).
ROSSEEL, M. T., BOGAERT, M. G.: Gas chromatography of the nitrate esters of glycerol, isosorbide and isomannide. J. Chromatog. **64**, 364—367 (1972).
ROSSEEL, M. T., BOGAERT, M. G.: Isosorbide, isomannide and isoidide dinitrate: urinary excretion in the rat. Biochem. Pharmacol. **22**, 67—72 (1973a).
ROSSEEL, M. T., BOGAERT, M. G.: GLC determination of nitroglycerin and isosorbide dinitrate in human plasma. J. pharm. Sci. **62**, 754—758 (1973b).
ROSSEEL, M. T., BOGAERT, M. G., MOERMAN, E. J.: Quantitative analysis of glyceryl nitrates on thin-layer chromatograms. Comparison of colorimetry and densitometry. J. Chromatog. **53**, 263—268 (1970).
SCHIRMER, R. E., ZEMER, R. E., COOKE, G. G.: NMR stability assay for amyl nitrite ampuls. J. pharm. Sci. **61**, 428—429 (1972).
SHECHTER, H., GRUENER, N., SHUVAL, H. I.: A micromethod for the determination of nitrite in blood. Anal. chim. Acta **60**, 93—99 (1972).
SHERBER, D. A., MARCUS, M., KLEINBERG, S.: Rapid clearance of isosorbide dinitrate from rabbit blood. Determination by gas chromatography. Biochem. Pharmacol. **19**, 607—612 (1970).

SHINN, M. B.: Colorimetric method for determination of nitrite. Ind. eng. Chem. **13**, 33—35 (1941).

SISENWINE, S. F., RUELIUS, H. W.: Plasma concentrations and urinary excretion of isosorbide dinitrate and its metabolites in the dog. J. Pharmacol. exp. Ther. **176**, 296—301 (1971).

TINGSTAD, J., GROPPER, E., LACHMAN, L., SHAMI, E.: Dissolution rate studies II: modified column apparatus and its use in evaluating isosorbide dinitrate tablets. J. pharm. Sci. **61**, 1985—1990 (1972).

TROWELL, J. M.: Gas chromatographic determination of nitrated derivatives of glycerine in aged double-base propellants. Anal. Chem. **42**, 1440—1442 (1970).

TROWELL, J. M., PHILPOT, M. C.: Gas chromatographic determination of plasticizers and stabilizers in composite modified double-base propellants. Anal. Chem. **41**, 166—168 (1969).

WARNER, C. R., JOHNSON, M. C., PRUE, D. G., KHO, B. T.: A dcvicc which permits selective purging of the solvent and other components from a gas-liquid chromatographic column. J. Chromatog. **82**, 263—268 (1973).

WEISS, K. G., BOLTZ, D. F.: The ultraviolet spectrophotometric determination of nitrite by the antipyrine method. Anal. chim. Acta **55**, 77—82 (1971).

WILLIAMS, A. F., MURRAY, W. J.: The accuracy of gas chromatography. Talanta **10**, 937—959 (1963).

WILLIAMS, A. F., MURRAY, W. J., GIBB, B. H.: Determination of traces of ethyleneglycol dinitrate (and nitroglycerine) in blood and urine. Nature (Lond.) **210**, 816—817 (1966).

WOO, D., YEN, J. K. C., SOFRONAS, P.: Quantitative analysis of 1,3;4,6-dianhydro-d-glucitol 2,5-dinitrate (isosorbide dinitrate) by infrared spectrometry. Anal. Chem. **45**, 2144—2145 (1973).

YAGODA, H.: Determination of aliphatic nitrate esters. A colorimetric method. Ind. eng. Chem. **15**, 27—29 (1943).

YASUDA, S. K.: Identification and determination of impurities in pentaerythritol tetranitrate. J. Chromatog. **51**, 253—260 (1970).

CHAPTER 4

Pharmacological Properties

C. JELLEFF CARR

The most prominent pharmacologic effects of the nitrate-nitrite drugs are manifested on the vasculature: the small blood vessels, arterioles, capillaries, and venules. The details of these actions and the response of the cardiovascular system will be considered in this chapter. Other pharmacologic properties include actions on bronchial smooth muscle and cardiovascular enzyme systems.

Workers have not yet applied the analytical methods used by RATH et al. (1942a, b) to measure blood nitrate and nitrite levels to correlate these with the pharmacologic effects observed after drug administration. The availability of the various organic nitrate or nitrite drugs, or their active components, at the target cell sites is a fundamental requirement of modern pharmacologic evaluation measures. Only rare reports indicate that the dosage form of the drug was analyzed for the content of the organic nitrate in the tablet or solution administered. In view of the now recognized instability of these compounds analytical data of this character should be included in future investigations. Within the past few years analytical methods have been developed that permit correlations to be made between drug plasma levels and pharmacologic effects (See chapter 3).

I. Action on Vasculature

(*In Vitro* Test Systems)

The vascular effects of an organic nitrate or nitrite can be demonstrated using the preparation of VOEGTLIN and MACHT (1913) of rings of the circumflex coronary artery joined in tandem fashion and exposed to a high dilution of the drug in physiological saline at body temperature. Drugs such as glyceryl trinitrate or octyl nitrite will induce a striking relaxation of this smooth muscle preparation. Different species exhibit varying degrees of sensitivity when drugs are tested on the isolated carotid artery strips of the rabbit, dog, or cat BOGAERT (1972). While it is highly unlikely that such *in vitro* test systems bear more than a crude relationship to the action of these drugs *in vivo*, simple tests of this character served for many years as a means of evaluating compounds thought to possess vasoactive properties. Somewhat more satisfactory vascular test systems are the perfused leg vessels of the frog (TAWAB et al., 1949), the vascular bed of the rabbit's ear KRANTZ et al. (1962); BOGAERT (1972), the perfused isolated rabbit heart (BARBOUR and PRINCE, 1915), the circulation of the intact anesthetized dog heart (heart-lung preparation) (MORAWITZ and ZAHN, 1914), and the more elaborate methods that use electrical or physical devices to measure coronary blood flow in the open chest of anesthetized animals (ESSEX et al., 1936 and ECKENHOFF and HAFKENSCHIEL, 1947).

LANGENDORFF'S (1895) method as refined in modern laboratories continues to be a favorite isolated heart test system for screening coronary drugs in a rough quantitative manner (ANDERSON and CRAVER, 1948 and TRUITT, 1955). In this method the dog, guinea pig, or rabbit coronary vessels are "back perfused" by introducing the special LOCKE-RINGER'S solution containing the drug through the aorta into the heart. The entire process may be carried out in simulated natural conditions of temperature and humidity, but the test situation is neither physiologic nor anatomic when contrasted to the circulation of the living animal. The LANGENDORFF method can provide only a preliminary evaluation of a coronary vasoactive drug.

LEIGHNINGER et al. (1959) used a technique to produce localized ischemia in the myocardium and then tested the effects of various drugs, including the organic nitrates, to increase the blood supply to the ischemic area. Ligation of the circumflex or a descending branch of the left coronary artery of the anesthetized dog produced the localized ischemia with its concomitant oxygen differential. Cutting the artery distal to the ligature permitted measurement of the blood that escaped as an index of the blood flow through the ischemic area. The method measured coronary arterial back flow via the circumflex artery by way of the intercoronary arterial communications. If the systemic arterial pressure is maintained at a normal value of 100 mm Hg the coronary back flow will be related to the coronary arteriolar resistance and may be considered to be a measure of "vascular integrity." This arteriolar segment of the coronary vascular tree has been considered to be the chief locus of action of some coronary dilating drugs. Using this technique in experimental animals these investigators reported that glyceryl trinitrate produced a significant increase in coronary back flow. The authors recommended the method as a basis for evaluating other coronary dilating drugs.

A critique of numerous *in vitro* coronary blood flow methods has been published by CHARLIER (1971).

In Vivo Test System

CHARLIER (1971) reviewed 21 methods that have been used to measure the coronary circulation in man or in animals with the heart *in situ*. Only the techniques that have been employed most successfully are discussed, as these relate to studies conducted with the organic nitrates and nitrites.

Coronary flow can only be measured indirectly in human subjects and most of our knowledge of this circulation of the heart has been derived from experimental animals, usually large dogs (HADDY, 1969). Most methods used have limited accuracy and give mean values rather than direct measures in specific regions that may be critical in estimating the vascular effects of drugs. Most coronary flow measurements recorded in the literature are the results of sampling flow through a major epicardial coronary artery or vein. Anatomically, the rich vasculature of the myocardium is reflected in the close association of capillaries and muscle fibers, so that in the adult heart there is about one capillary per muscle fiber VAN CITTERS (1966). It is these small arteriolar twigs and arteriosinusoidal vessels that undoubtedly play a vital role in oxygenating the ever-functioning muscle segments. Investigators have only recently devised techniques to estimate the flow through these important circulatory pathways. Recently also, implanted flow sensing devices have been perfected that permit the estimation of coronary blood flow in animals under ambulatory conditions. The laboratory techniques developed by workers in this field have been reviewed by GREGG (1950) and KHOURI and GREGG (1963). The accurate estimation of the effects of the organic nitrates and nitrites on the circulation, and especially the coronary circulation, will depend in the final analysis upon solving the elaborate physical and physiological problems that arise when attempts are made to determine blood flow in the unrestrained normal animal. The complexities of the subject are illustrated by KOLIN (1960) in his review of the perfection of the electromagnetic flow meter.

Total flow of blood in the coronary circulation as stressed by many workers may not be the most significant factor that can be changed by drugs. Thus WINBURY (1964, 1967, 1971) emphasizes the importance of the "nutritional microcirculation" as a guide in the quest for anti-anginal drugs. Nutritional circulation is that portion of the regional blood flow that supplies the heart tissue with oxygen and its nutritional requirements. Because a considerable portion of blood flow follows via nonfunctional arterio-venous bypasses, the total flow may not reflect the necessary nutritive blood supply to the vital heart muscle tissues. For these reasons WINBURY suggests that many drugs, including the organic nitrates, can influence the nutritive circulation without necessarily changing the arteriolar or total circulation (WINBURY et al., 1967, 1971). This concept assumes that under normal conditions about 75% of the functional myocardial capillaries are open. The remaining may be nonfunctional but capable of providing nutritional circulation if the pre-capillary sphincters relax. Drugs can exert their pharmacologic effects without a marked arteriolar dilation but by diverting the blood supply to the nutritive circulation by relaxing these pre-capillary sphincters. These actions are discussed in the consideration of the effects of the organic nitrates on the coronary circulation and the myocardium.

The discussion of the physiology of the coronary circulation as related to angina pectoris makes clear that changes in the rate of coronary blood flow alone do not constitute a valid criterion of changes in coronary efficiency. This fact must be kept in mind in assessing laboratory methods used to evaluate the pharmacologic actions of the organic nitrates and nitrites.

The proper pharmacologic evaluation then of any drug on the coronary circulation embraces consideration of not only the correct measurement of blood flow but also A/V oxygen differences across the coronary bed, blood pressure, cardiac output, myocardial contractibility, and heart rate. It must be emphasized that oxygen consumption of the heart is determined by the heart rate, the contractile state of the heart, and the *tension* in the myocardial wall (MASON et al., 1971; PARKER et al., 1971). A decrease in oxygen consumption can be more significant than an increase in oxygen delivery. The overall myocardial oxygen availability and consumption, and its relationship to cardiac work and efficiency, ultimately become the pharmacologic criteria in the evaluation of any coronary "vasodilator." For example, while glyceryl trinitrate had no apparent direct effect on the energy released with each contraction of the heart it did reduce the hemodynamic work load by a decrease in left atrial filling pressure according to DARBY and ALDINGER (1960). In the dog these workers showed that glyceryl trinitrate had no effect on the increased force of contraction elicited by sympathetic stimulation with levarterenol. They concluded that the chief pharmacologic effect in relief of anginal pain is related to the drug's ability to decrease the work load imposed on the myocardium by sympathetic stimulation. A similar decrease in left ventricular end-diastolic pressure after glyceryl trinitrate administration has been reported by many authors (ARBORELIUS et al., 1968; PARKER et al., 1969; TAYLOR, 1970).

It is apparent that many physiological factors will change the rate of coronary flow, including myocardial oxygen consumption and cardiac work, and the final pharmacologic effects of any drug acting on the heart and its circulation are unpredictably related to these events. Studies in normal subjects have shown an increased coronary flow with an increased myocardial oxygen uptake, decreased cardiac work and hence decreased cardiac efficiency followed the administration of glyceryl trinitrate BRACHFELD et al. (1959). Unfortunately, in all these studies, the data obtained from normal animals or normal subjects may not be comparable to the effects of drugs in disease states ROBINSON (1968); BOGAERT (1972). This subject is reviewed elsewhere in this volume.

However, in patients with coronary disease, at rest, the coronary flow may be "normal" and glyceryl trinitrate may not change coronary flow and oxygen usage but the systemic blood pressure, cardiac work, and cardiac output will be reduced GORLIN et al. (1959). The end result is decreased efficiency of the heart without a change in coronary resistance. This type of pharmacologic intervention may be appropriate for a short time in disease states, provided the overall effects on the heart are not too drastic.

Attempts have been made to relate the action of some organic nitrates on the myocardium to the oxygen consumption of cardiac muscle. Thus, LEVY (1970) studied the direct effects of various organic nitrates on basal myocardial oxygen uptake in the isolated rabbit left atria. A significant decrease was observed when a 442 μM concentration of glyceryl trinitrate was perfused. However, isosorbide dinitrate, or erythrityl tetranitrate had no significant effect on oxygen uptake, while mannitol hexanitrate, iditol hexanitrate, and sorbitan tetranitrate produced marked increases. Because all these compounds are pharmacologically active, and approximately equipotent, it does not appear that the test system developed by LEVY of measuring oxygen uptake is indicative of the clinical usefulness of these agents.

The nutritive circulation as it relates to the partial pressure of oxygen in the myocardial tissues is a more satisfactory approach to the study of the actions of the organic nitrates. Thus, WINBURY (1971) measured the pO_2 of the deep and superficial regions (endocardial and epicardial) of the heart with small electrodes by polarography. This technique was used to demonstrate that glyceryl trinitrate selectively increased the endocardial pO_2 without a change in coronary flow.

Coronary flow can be studied in unanesthetized animals using the nitrous oxide method as described by ECKENHOFF et al. (1948). The gas is inhaled under standard conditions and the rate of coronary flow is calculated from the rate of absorption of nitrous oxide by the ventricular muscle. Myocardial absorption of the gas is estimated from arteriovenous differences in the femoral artery and the coronary sinus venus blood obtained by catheterization. In the dog, reasonable agreement has been shown between the nitrous oxide method and the bubble flowmeter method that employs direct cannulation of a coronary artery (ECKENHOFF et al., 1948) and the rotameter (GREGG et al., 1951) method. Clinical studies in man have confirmed that the nitrous oxide method is reproducible and does not alter the subject's normal physiological hemodynamics (ROWE et al., 1864).

As reviewed by ROWE (1966), because the nitrous oxide method can be used in experimental animals and man, drugs can be tested first in animals (usually the dog) and subsequently in man if the results of the animal screening process are encouraging. According to ROWE, the pharmacologic effects of drugs that have resulted in changes in coronary flow in experimental animals have produced similar changes in man. For this reason confidence in the nitrous oxide method as a technique to evaluate coronary drugs in man has increased.

ROWE (1959); BING (1965), and CHARLIER (1971) have reviewed the studies that employed the nitrous oxide method to assess the effects of drugs on coronary flow. Although widely used for measuring cerebral blood flow in man, the nitrous oxide method is time consuming and does not permit a continuous recording of coronary flow changes. While the results may be difficult to interpret for these reasons, the procedure is valuable in the overall comparison of changes in coronary efficiency during drug action. It is possible to study simultaneously changes in blood pressure, myocardial oxygen uptake and other facets of heart function and these parameters may be the more important pharmacologic effects of drugs.

Glyceryl trinitrate has been shown to produce an increase in coronary blood flow in 10 normal men as measured by the nitrous oxide method. BRACHFELD et al. (1959) following sublingual administration. However, this effect may be secondary to the increased myocardial oxygen consumption and increased metabolism according to these authors.

ROWE et al. (1961) reported that erythritol tetranitrate administered sublingually to normal subjects and patients with coronary artery disease manifested by angina pectoris, caused a decreased cardiac output, cardiac work, coronary blood flow, coronary sinus oxygen content, and coronary vascular resistance. There was no significant difference between the normal subjects and the patients when these individuals were studied using the nitrous oxide method to determine coronary blood flow.

Visualization of the coronary circulation is possible in the "closed chest" preparation by direct injection of a radiopaque material. The two main coronary arteries are catheterized through the carotid artery fluoroscopically and the contrast medium (e.g., sodium diatrizoate) and drug are injected directly. This technique has been used to study the effect of drugs, including glyceryl trinitrate, in the anesthetized dog (WEST and GUZMAN, 1959). These workers found that direct injection of sodium nitrite or glyceryl trinitrate into the left coronary artery produced dilation and increased flow even in the presence of decreased central coronary pressure, cardiac output and work. This method is essentially a morphologic technique and physiologic deductions must be made cautiously. Changes in the vascular size may be observed visually but the results are difficult to quantify.

Radioisotopes can be used to measure coronary flow in animals and man by external counting. In general, the methods involve the injection of one of the isotopes ^{24}Na, ^{42}K, ^{86}Rb, ^{84}Rb, ^{85}Kr, or ^{131}I-tagged albumin, and measuring the amount of radioactive substance taken up by the myocardium, as contrasted with the amount in the blood. SEVELIUS and JOHNSON (1959) used ^{131}I tagged human serum albumin injected into the antecubital vein of normal human subjects. The passage of the radioactive substance through the heart was measured by a gamma detector placed over the chest wall to signal chronologic changes as a measure of outflow. Three peaks of radioactivity are observed and the third peak is related to coronary blood flow because this peak does not appear in dogs having the main coronary arteries occluded. The values obtained by this method for normal subjects agree well with the nitrous oxide method.

Glyceryl trinitrate caused an increase in coronary flow when measured by the radioactive isotope technique using ^{84}Rb according to BING et al. (1964) and COHEN et al. (1965). However, BERNSTEIN et al. (1966) and ROSS et al. (1964) failed to obtain any increase in coronary flow with glyceryl trinitrate when the radioactive gas ^{133}Xe was dissolved and injected directly into the coronaries. There are many technical difficulties in the use of these methods and results have not been readily reproduced by other workers. Radioisotopes are not employed at the present time to measure coronary flow except in those laboratories possessing the elaborate equipment. However, the methods are the most satisfactory for routine clinical evaluation of the organic nitrates or nitrites based on present methodology. The use of ^{84}Rb as developed by BING et al. (1968) does not require cardiac catheterization and provides a coronary flow estimation in 30 seconds. This method may prove to be the most useful in evaluation of all types of antianginal drugs including the organic nitrates and nitrites.

Coronary arteriography via direct catheterization has been conducted on animals and man ROSS et al. (1964). Catheterization makes possible the injection of a radioactive gas solution and the direct injection of the drug. Employing this technique, ROSS et al. (1964) failed to find an increase in coronary blood flow in patients with coronary artery disease after the injection of glyceryl trinitrate. BERNSTEIN et al. (1966) obtained similar results. As pointed out by ROWE (1966) these findings may not reflect the pharmacologic situation that follows the usual clinical systemic administration of the drug. The liver enzymic changes that are now recognized and dosage form bioavailability factors may determine the ultimate value of these drugs as employed by patients.

Radioactive microspheres have been used in experimental animals to estimate regional myocardial blood flow DOMENECH et al. (1969); FORTUIN et al. (1971); BECKER et al. (1971). The method is based on the principle that a nondiffusible indicator injected into the circulation distributes according to blood flow in an organ during its first transit. Carbonized microspheres of $15 \pm 5\ \mu$ diameter labeled with gamma-emitting nuclides ^{141}Cr, ^{51}Cr or ^{85}Sr were used by BECKER et al. (1971) to study changes in regional myocardial blood flow during acute ischemia induced in the heart of the open-chest dog preparation. Glyceryl trinitrate injection (0.4 mg) intravenously caused a significant increase in the ratio of endocardial to epicardial radioactivity in both ischemic and nonischemic areas. These workers interpret their findings as suggesting that during acute coronary artery occlusion there is a change in the distribution of flow in the ischemic area with a relatively greater endocardial blood flow than epicardial. This observation is supported by similar reports of other workers employing different techniques. Glyceryl trinitrate is capable of preventing this epicardial ischemia. Previous studies FORTUIN et al. (1971) with this technique in nonischemic hearts of dogs have shown that no significant change in the ratio of endocardial to epicardial radioactivity was produced during the peak hypotensive stage after glyceryl trinitrate administration. In this experimental method the degree of radioactivity as measured in a sample of heart tissue removed after sacrifice of the animal, is the indicator of blood flow. Animals can serve as their own control because each isotope is measured individually by differential spectrometry KAIHARA et al. (1968).

Electromagnetic flowmeter methods that permit the study *in vivo* of vascular changes produced by drugs including the organic nitrates, have been developed in several laboratories KOLIN (1960). The electromagnetic flowmeter has been miniaturized to permit implantation to measure blood flow velocity and volume in various intact blood vessels, including the coronary artery of the dog KHOURI and GREGG (1963). It is possible to obtain continuous phasic flow recordings in the unanesthetized state in animals with an implanted unit while the animal is presumably normal in all respects. A variation of this technique permits the use of 0.5 mm flow probes for measuring intralumenal velocity via a catheter and can be employed in the unanesthetized human subject KOLIN (1970).

Glyceryl trinitrate may redistribute the available blood flow to the myocardium in such a way that ischemic zones receive a nutritional circulation at the expense of other areas WINBURY and GOBEL (1967); WINBURY (1971). Thus the drug increases nutritional coronary circulation and lowers vascular resistance without a significant change in total flow. This mechanism is suggested by these workers as an explanation for the antianginal value of the drug. Glyceryl trinitrate intravenously or injected directly into the coronary artery in the dog in low doses (0.005 to 0.02 mg/kg and 0.002 to 0.004 mg respectively), increases the oxygen tension of the subendocardium but not the subepicardium without an increase in coronary blood flow or a decrease in aortic pressure WINBURY et al. (1971). These workers suggest that glyceryl trinitrate causes a redistribution of myocardial blood flow from the epicardium to the ischemic subendocardium. These actions are presumed to be the result of the dilation of the intramural arteries in the left ventricle, a mechanism that determines the distribution of blood between the superficial and the deeper regions of the left ventricle.

Additional evidence that glyceryl trinitrate can increase coronary collateral blood flow has been presented by GOLDSTEIN et al. (1973). The drug was injected as a single 100 μg bolus or at a rate of 100 to 150 μg per minute into the ascending aorta of 27 patients with occlusive disease undergoing saphenous vein bypass surgery. After drug administration the aortic pressure decreased but the retrograde flow was not consistently changed while the collateral resistance fell significantly. The peripheral coronary pressure decreased consistently after glyceryl trinitrate but less than would be anticipated from the fall in aortic pressure. When the results were expressed as a fraction of the aortic pressure, the net peripheral coronary pressure increased and this was consistent with the enhanced flow through the collateral channels. Pharmacologic evidence of the effects of the organic nitrates on diseased hearts is rare and data of this character supports the clinical experience with these drugs.

A novel approach to the study of the effects of glyceryl trinitrate in man was developed by DE MARIA et al. (1974) using ultrasonic techniques. They evaluated the pharmacologic effects on endocardial left ventricular dimensions by ultrasonic echograms in normal subjects and patients with coronary disease after sublingual glyceryl trinitrate dosage. The drug reduced the left ventricular end-diastolic dimension and end-systolic dimension that accounted for a decline in the left ventricular end-diastolic volume and end-systolic volume, with a fall in stroke volume. Since stroke volume fell in patients with minimal heart rate change while the peripheral vascular resistance was unaltered, the extracardiac dilator effects of glyceryl trinitrate are on the systemic venous beds. They conclude that glyceryl trinitrate in man reduces end-diastolic dimensions and end-systolic dimensions and thereby causes a lowering of the myocardial oxygen demand by diminishing the left ventricular tension. These findings support the work of other investigators that the chief pharmacologic action of glyceryl trinitrate is to decrease the oxygen requirements of the myocardium. The finer mechanisms of this action appear to be related to the effects on the microcirculation of heart muscle.

II. Cardiovascular Systems

The cardiovascular actions of the organic nitrates and nitrites are complex when these drugs are administered to anesthetized or unanesthetized animals or man. The hemodynamic results reflect the multiple influences on the pre- and post-capillary beds, the relaxation of relatively large arteries, cardiac output as modified by the position of the subject as body "pools" are changed, the degree of tolerance to the drugs, and disease states of the cardiovascular system. For these reasons attempts have been made to simplify the pharmacologic evaluation of these drugs by studies on isolated systems such as arterial strips and heart-lung preparations.

The actions on the heart are considered in connection with *in vivo* test systems to measure the effects of these drugs on the coronary circulation. It should be emphasized that these cardiovascular effects are elicited by the intact molecule of these drugs before undergoing hepatic enzymic changes. The metabolites are not vasodepressive and this explains why oral doses have a decreased effect on the cardiovascular system.

Injected intravenously or administered orally to the anesthetized dog all the clinically effective organic nitrates or nitrites cause a fall in systemic blood pressure. This depressor response is not a reliable indicator of the usefulness of these drugs as antianginal agents. Thus, erythritol tetranitrate, isomannide dinitrate, isosorbide dinitrate, styracitol tetranitrate, polygalitol tetranitrate, mannitan tetranitrate, sorbitan tetranitrate, and erythritan dinitrate all exhibit a depressor effect but only several of these compounds have proved to be of even limited value clinically (KRANTZ et al., 1939a, 1939b); GREGG (1950). It is now well recognized that most hypotensive drugs also cause a similar decrease in coronary artery resistance with a concomittant lowering of myocardial nutrition as a result of a decrease in flow in the arteriolar tree.

Some investigators have concluded that because the decrease in blood pressure elicited by the organic nitrates is of longer duration than the fleeting coronary vasodilation, the blood pressure fall must be the major cause of the beneficial effects. In addition, the lowering of systemic blood pressure decreases the afterload on the heart and the immediate oxygen requirements. Thus, GILLIS and MELVILLE (1970) were not able to demonstrate an increase in coronary flow in the dog open-chest preparation after sublingual doses of 0.22, 0.65, and 1.95 mg of glyceryl trinitrate. The higher doses produced a significant decrease in blood pressure (22 and 27 mm Hg). However, intravenous doses consistently produced a prolonged fall in blood pressure. Similar findings have been reported by many investigators MELVILLE et al. (1965); BERNSTEIN et al. (1966); GILLIS and MELVILLE (1970). VYDEN et al. (1970). In this connection it is of interest to note that the original suggestions of BRUNTON in 1867 and MURRELL in 1879 to use amyl nitrite and glyceryl trinitrate in anginal patients was based on the fall in blood pressure these drugs produce.

The non-specific vasodilator effects of the organic nitrates and nitrites are manifest on the blush areas of the skin, the meningeal and intracranial vessels, the intraocular vessels, and the venous circulation BOGAERT (1972). After a dose of nitroglycerin a subjective feeling of warmth in the clavicle area is noticed with an objective "flush." Amyl nitrite notoriously causes a throbbing in the temples after inhalation as a result of smooth muscle relaxation of the meningeal and intracranial vessels so that with each pulse the receptors in the meninges are stimulated via distension. The symptoms are usually a measure of individual tolerance to an organic nitrate. These are general vasodilator effects, but unlike many drugs used in hypertension, the organic nitrates and nitrites do not block the outflow of the sympathetic nervous system as a part of their pharmacologic action (ECKSTEIN et al., 1951; POPOVICH et al., 1956).

There are many reports in the pharmacologic literature that the organic nitrates and nitrites cause an increase in intraocular pressure presumably by dilation of intraocular vessels. For this reason textbooks caution against the use of these drugs by patients with glaucoma. WHITWORTH and GRANT (1964) reviewed these reports and were unable to find a single case that demonstrated a worsening of glaucoma by the use of these vasodilators. Early animal experiments with amyl nitrite demonstrated either an increase or a decrease in intraocular pressure in several species. More recent studies in human subjects and animals failed to produce evidence of significant changes in intraocular pressure after the administration of glyceryl trinitrate. WHITWORTH and GRANT (1964) studied 34 persons administered doses of glyceryl trinitrate or pentaerythrityl tetranitrate for changes in intraocular pressure. Some individuals had normal pressures, some intermediate, and some subjects had definite episodes of angle-closure glaucoma. In all persons the intraocular pressure either remained constant or decreased briefly and only slightly. These authors conclude that there is no pharmacologic or clinical evidence to restrict the use of these drugs in the presence of open-angle glaucoma.

BERNSTEIN et al. (1966) observed that the complex cardiovascular effects of glyceryl trinitrate can explain results obtained in various laboratories when different techniques are employed and when measurements are conducted at different times in the manifestation of the drug's actions. The early increased coronary flow detected after direct intracoronary injection, followed by a reduction in cardiac work, may be a reflection of the drug's action on the myocardial vessels before it reaches a sufficient concentration in the periphery to exert its effect on these blood vessels. This would explain the transient increase in coronary flow that is generally recorded in experimental animal preparations where the coronary flow is measured directly. The subsequent general decrease in systemic arterial pressure, the peripheral effect, is accompanied by a decrease in coronary flow. This secondary effect on the coronary circulation may predominate in some experimental animal models and may be the most noteworthy clinical finding in patients BERNSTEIN et al. (1966); BING et al. (1964); COHEN et al. (1965); GORLIN et al. (1959); HOLLANDER et al. (1963); ROSS et al. (1964).

It seems well established that the organic nitrates and nitrites decrease cardiac size (BRANDT et al., 1952; WILLIAMS et al., 1965); lower central venous filling pressure (BRACHFELD et al., 1959; GORLIN et al., 1959; ROWE et al., 1961), and reduce cardiac work (BERNSTEIN et al., 1966; BRACHFELD et al., 1959; GORLIN et al., 1959; ROWE et al., 1961). These studies have been reviewed by ROWE (1966).

The decrease in systemic blood pressure produced by glyceryl trinitrate is accompanied by peripheral venous pooling and includes an action on the splanchnic and pulmonary beds. FERRER et al. (1966) studied the extent to which these latter two areas are involved in the circulatory readjustments to the drug. Studies were conducted on 18 subjects with heart disease following the sublingual administration of doses of from 0.3 to 0.6 mg glyceryl trinitrate. Contrary to expectations, they found the drug produced an overall vasoconstriction on the splanchnic circulation with no evidence of venous pooling. However, there was vasodilation and pooling of blood in the pulmonary vascular bed. The splanchnic vasoconstriction is in contrast to the splanchnic vasodilation observed in anesthetized laboratory animals. The difference may be caused by the decreased reflex of animals under anesthesia. The reduced pulmonary artery pressure observed in normal animals and men coincides with the pulmonary vasodilation reported by JOHNSON et al. (1957) in patients with angina pectoris taking glyceryl trinitrate sublingually.

III. Pulmonary Circulation

Although there are conflicting reports in the literature, it now seems that most workers agree that glyceryl trinitrate and isosorbide dinitrate are vasodilators for the pulmonary vascular beds. The comprehensive studies of AVIADO et al. (1968a) demonstrated this action in the anesthetized dog for these two drugs. The pulmonary vascular resistance was calculated from direct measurements of pulmonary flow and pulmonary arterial pressure. These findings are in conformity with a similar reduction in pulmonary resistance in man after isosorbide dinitrate FREMONT (1961); DRESDALE et al. (1963) and glyceryl trinitrate JOHNSON et al. (1957, 1959); MULLER and RORVIK (1958).

In the perfused lung of the dog *in situ* glyceryl trinitrate and isosorbide dinitrate cause a reduction in perfusion pressure AVIADO et al. (1968a). The effect is more pronounced after continuous infusion of serotonin. In the dog heart-lung preparation these drugs cause an increase in coronary blood flow. In explanation of the failure of other workers to demonstrate pulmonary vasodilation in experimental animals AVIADO et al. (1968b) point out that the measurement of pulmonary arterial pressure alone cannot detect vasodilation because the augmentation in pulmonary blood flow can mask any reduction in pulmonary arterial pressure. In addition, these workers note that in the intact dog pulmonary blood flow is determined largely by the primary influence of the organic nitrates on the systemic venous return. The literature related to the studies on the musculotropic cardiopulmonary vasodilators, including the organic nitrates and nitrites, has been reviewed by AVIADO (1965) and AVIADO et al. (1968b). Because the physiologic goal is adequate oxygenation of the myocardium in coronary artery disease, greater attention should be directed to pharmacologically improving the pulmonary circulation to achieve this end ROUGHGARDEN and NEWMAN (1966). The organic nitrates and nitrites represent only a step in this direction.

IV. Metabolism of Cardiac Muscle

Searching for a mechanism of action of the organic nitrates and nitrites KRANTZ et al. (1951) investigated the actions of these drugs on the energy yielding enzyme systems of the vasculature. The ATPase activity of the aorta of the rabbit was partially but not completely inhibited by the rapidly-acting vasodilators amyl nitrite, glyceryl trinitrate and isobutylglycollate nitrate. Sodium nitrite did not inhibit this enzyme ATPase. In addition, the enzyme from the smooth muscle of the uterus or from skeletal muscle was not inhibited by any of these vasodilators.

The organic nitrates have also been shown to inhibit oxidative phosphorylation of liver mitochondria and the transphosphorylating enzymes of other arterial tissues (CARR et al., 1953). There may be a possible relationship between these effects and the actions of other coronary vasodilators. The vasodilator effects of dipyridamole (Persantin) have been ascribed to its metabolic actions on the heart by increasing the level of adenosine triphosphate (BRETSCHNEIDER et al., 1959). However, this drug does not improve exercise tolerance in anginal patients. The drug does not increase the "efficiency" of the work performed in heart-lung preparations as measured by oxygen uptake, as does pentaerythrityl tetranitrate in this test system (AVIADO et al., 1968). Dipyridamole does not increase collateral coronary flow as does glyceryl trinitrate according to FAM and MCGREGOR (1968) and therefore the two drugs differ in their site of action.

Chemical compounds that favorably influence the metabolism or biochemical events of cardiac muscle may prove clinically efficacious in chronic angina pectoris; however, it has been difficult to demonstrate discrete pharmacologic actions in model animal systems that explain the clinical effectiveness. The numerous antianginal drugs developed from animal studies that have disputed clinical value attest to these pharmacologic problems. Multiple sites of action reflecting positive findings in animals may indeed be involved because the clinical literature suggests a synergistic response when certain of these drugs are used concomitantly in therapy.

V. Actions of Other Smooth Muscles

The organic nitrates and nitrites relax all types of smooth muscle and their pharmacologic effects related to this activity have interesting but limited therapeutic uses. The nitrate and nitrite drugs decrease smooth muscle tone by a direct musculotropic action independent of autonomic innervation. The effects on smooth muscle are not mediated by any known neurotransmitter substance, e.g. serotonin, histamine, or acetylcholine, and no receptor mechanism or structure has been identified.

Bronchodilatation has been demonstrated in the guinea pig, dog, and rabbit after the intravenous injection of glyceryl trinitrate (BARLOW and BEAMS, 1933; CUNY and QUIVY, 1942). Sodium or amyl nitrite are known to relax the isolated bronchial smooth muscle preparation. The inhalation of pentaerythrityl tetranitrate dissolved in gamma-butyrolactone has been shown to reduce pulmonary resistance in the anesthetized dog by AVIADO et al. (1969) who reviewed the literature citations on the possible use of the nitrates and nitrites in the treatment of bronchial asthma. Glyceryl trinitrate sublingually and erythrityl tetranitrate orally have been reported to be of limited value in patients with bronchial asthma HIRSHLEIFER and ARORA (1961). Octyl nitrite (2-ethyl-n-hexyl-l-nitrite) with a vapor pressure of 3.3 mm at 25° has a long history of use in angiospastic disease KRANTZ et al. (1938); CARR et al. (1951). Perhaps a volatile and stable organic nitrite of this type would fulfill the requirements for an inhalation agent for use in the treatment of bronchial asthma. Apparently octyl nitrite has not been tried in this clinical condition.

VI. Significance of Normal Blood Levels of the Nitrate and Nitrite Ions

The ions of nitric and nitrous acid are not foreign to the blood of many species. RATH and KRANTZ (1942a) showed that the blood of the dog, monkey, steer, and man contains approximately 10 µg nitrite per 100 ml (1 in 10^7) and the blood of man and some animal species normally contains approximately 100 µg nitrate per 100 ml (1 in 10^6). The constancy of this level of blood nitrite has been a matter of speculation for years. An analysis of the blood nitrite concentration of 170 subjects of both sexes ranging in age from 9 to 91 years revealed a statistically significant diminution of blood nitrite with age. This was confirmed in an additional 32 subjects with an average age of 73 years. There was no apparent explanation for the lower nitrite level in older individuals. Prolonged fasting, or feeding amino acids, ammonium chloride, potassium nitrate or organic nitrate drugs to dogs did not change the blood nitrite level whereas a small dose of sodium nitrite caused a marked increase.

At the time these observations were made there was considerable interest in the conversion of inorganic nitrates to nitrite in the intestine by *E. coli* and the L. aerogenes microorganisms ZOBELL (1932). STIEGLITZ and PALMER (1934, 1937) reported nitrite present in the blood of normal human subjects and these workers speculated that the nitrite arose from bacterial action in the gut. In reviewing the various possible sources of nitrite, RATH and KRANTZ (1942a) observed that animal and plant tissues contain a number of enzymes capable of reducing inorganic nitrates to nitrites. Other workers had shown the liver of many species to be a rich source of these enzymes and it was suggested at that time that the liver is likely the chief site of this conversion in the body. These elementary findings have been confirmed and extended by the cogent investigations of NEEDLEMAN and his co-workers (NEEDLEMAN and HUNTER, 1965) (see chapter on organic nitrate biotransformation).

There does not appear to have been a follow-up on observations of normal levels of nitrate and nitrite in the blood of man. The concentration of these ions in the blood is not associated with the systolic, diastolic, or pulse pressures RATH and KRANTZ (1942a, b). The reason the organic nitrates and nitrites act as drugs may be related to the fact that NO_3 or NO_2 ions or even organic nitrate molecules either normally play a role in tissue metabolism or, acting at the cellular level, they sufficiently resemble a metabolic intermediate to bring about a modified tissue response CARR (1958).

Pharmacologically these facts are significant. For example, they place in perspective the levels of blood nitrite obtained after a depressor dose of sodium nitrite or an organic nitrate. In dogs, one minute after a dose of $NaNO_2$ intravenously that caused a 26% reduction in the carotid artery pressure, the blood nitrite level averaged 740 μg per 100 ml RATH and KRANTZ (1942b). It is noteworthy that 45 min later with the blood pressure still 25 percent below the original value, the blood nitrite level was only 68 μg per 100 ml. In these studies additional confirmation was obtained that the organic nitrates erythrityl tetranitrate, isomannide dinitrate, and glyceryl trinitrate in depressor intravenous doses did not increase the level of nitrite in the blood more than 9 μg per 100 ml, an insignificant amount. The evidence is now convincing that the action of the organic nitrate drugs is not related to hydrolysis and nitrite formation.

In the gut of the rat pentaerythritol tetranitrate has been shown to be hyrolyzed by intestinal bacteria to the tri-, di-, and mono-nitrates DICARLO et al. (1967). Greatest absorption of the ^{14}C-labeled drug occurred within two hours from the large intestine, presumably from bacterial action. It is not known if the organic nitrate drugs taken by mouth by patients undergo this form of bacterial decomposition or if it significantly influences the drug effects.

The recent interest in the carcinogenic, mutagenic, and teratogenic effects of the nitrosamines formed by species of enterobacteria in the acid conditions in the mammalian stomach should be noted in regard to organic nitrate and nitrite medication SCHELINE (1973). Recent experimental studies have demonstrated that nitrite can be formed from nitrate in the gastrointestinal tract by bacteria in the human stomach, in the rat cecum, and by isolated strains of human intestinal bacteria. SCHELINE (1973) has reviewed these studies and discussed their possible relationships to ingested foods and drugs. Investigators have not considered the significance of frequent and prolonged ingestion of the organic nitrate or nitrite drugs in relation to the possible effects via actions of intestinal microorganisms.

VII. Plasma Levels of Nitrates

As noted in the introduction, the bioavailability of different dosage forms of the organic nitrates, the site of administration, and the rate of metabolic destruction and excretion influence the pharmacologic potency and duration of action of these drugs. The obvious point of reference would be plasma or tissue levels as reflected in either dose-response effects in animals or clinical effectiveness in patients. Recently this has been attempted for a few selected agents in this series. The long-sought prolonged acting "coronary vasodilator" could be evaluated most objectively on the basis of blood plasma levels.

BOGAERT (1972) reviewed the reports on plasma levels of nitrates as related to their effectiveness and observed that there are no data on man to test for a correlation between glyceryl trinitrate concentrations and effects. The analytical methods are poor and have been criticized as not measuring glyceryl trinitrate (BERRY and ROACH, 1958; RITSCHEL and CLOTTEN, 1970). A more sensitive gas chromatographic method has been developed ROSSEEL and BOGAERT (1972). In animal experiments a dose-response curve could not be constructed to show a relationship between plasma levels of glyceryl trinitrate in the rabbit and the hypotensive effects (BOGAERT et al., 1970). There are two reports on plasma levels of pentaerythritol tetranitrate in man using radioactive labeled drug DAVIDSON et al. (1970, 1971).

References

ANDERSON, F. F., CRAVER, B. N.: A pyrex apparatus for the perfusion of the coronary circulation of mammalian hearts. J. Pharmacol. exp. Ther. **93**, 135—141 (1948).

ARBORELIUS, M., LECEROF, H., MALM, A., MALMBORG, R. O.: Acute effect of nitroglycerin on haemodynamics of angina pectoris. Brit. Heart J. **30**, 407—411 (1968).

AVIADO, D. M.: The lung circulation. Oxford: Pergamon Press 1965.

AVIADO, D. M., FOLLE, L. E., BELLET, S.: Cardiopulmonary effects of glyceryl trinitrate and isosorbide dinitrate. Cardiologia (Basel) **52**, 287—303 (1968a).

AVIADO, D. M., ITO, H., CHO, Y. W., BELLET, S.: Coronary vasodilators on myocardial oxygen consumption and ammonia production. Cardiologia (Basel) **53**, 27—46 (1968b).

AVIADO, D. M., KISHIMOTO, T., KNEIDINGER, H. J.: Bronchopulmonary effects of pentaerythrityl tetranitrate and isoproterenol. J. Pharmacol. exp. Ther. **165**, 274—285 (1969).

BARBOUR, H. G., PRINCE, A. L.: The perfused isolated rabbit heart. J. exp. Med. **21**, 330—338 (1915).

BARLOW, O. W., BEAMS, A. J.: A comparison of the bronchodilating action of several anti-asthmatic agents after anaphylactic and histamine shock in the guinea pig. J. Pharmacol. exp. Ther. **47**, 111—130 (1933).

BECKER, L. C., FORTUIN, N. J., PITT, B.: Effects of ischemia and antianginal drugs on the distribution of radioactive microspheres in the canine left ventricle. Circulation Res. **28**, 263—269 (1971).

BERNSTEIN, L., FRIESINGER, G. C., LICHTLEN, P. R., ROSS, R. S.: The effect of nitroglycerin on the systemic and coronary circulation in man and dogs. Circulation **33**, 107—116 (1966).

BERRY, J. W., ROACH, T. C.: An evaluation of blood nitrate levels. Circulation **17**, 1014—1046 (1958).

BING, R. J.: Cardiac metabolism. Physiol. Rev. **45**, 171—213 (1965).

BING, R. J., BENNISH, A., BLUEMCHEN, G., COEHEN, A., GALLAGHER, J. P., ZALESKI, E. J.: The determination of coronary flow equivalent with coincidence counting technique. Circulation **29**, 833—846 (1964).

BING, R. J., COWAN, C., BOTTCHER, D., CORSINI, G., DANIELS, C. G.: A new method of measuring coronary blood flow in man. J. Amer. med. Ass. **205**, 277—280 (1968).

BOGAERT, M. G.: Organic nitrates in angina pectoris. Arch. int. Pharmacodyn. Ther. **196**, 25—34 (1972).

BOGAERT, M. G., ROSSEEL, M. T., DESCHAEPDRYVER, A. F.: The metabolic fate of nitroglycerin (trinitrin) in relation to its vascular effects. Europ. J. Pharmacol. **12**, 224—230 (1970).

BRACHFELD, N., BOZER, J., GORLIN, R.: Action of nitroglycerin on the coronary circulation in normal and mild cardiac subjects. Circulation **19**, 697—704 (1959).

BRANDT, J. L., COCCESSE, A., DOCK, W.: Slitkymographic evidence that nitroglycerine decreases heart volume and stroke volume while increasing amplitude of ballistocardiographic waves. Amer. J. Med. **12**, 650—658 (1952).

BRETSCHNEIDER, H. J., FRANK, A., BERNARD, I., KOCHSEIK, K., SCHELER, F.: Die Wirkung eines Pyrimidopyrimidin-Derivates auf die Sauerstoffversorgung des Herzmuskels. Arzneimittel-Forsch. **9**, 49—59 (1959).

BRUNTON, T. L.: On the use of nitrite of amyl in angina pectoris. Lancet **1867 II**, 97—98.

CARR, C. J.: The pharmacology of the vasodilator nitrate-nitrite drugs. Int. Rec. Med. **171**, 121—129 (1958).

CARR, C. J., BELL, F. K., BRADYHOUSE, M. F., KRANTZ, J. C., JR.: Effect of vasodilators upon the dephosphorylating enzymes of dogs' coronary arteries. J. Pharmacol. exp. Ther. **108**, 385—392 (1953).

CARR, C. J., BURGISON, R. M., FASSELL, M. S., KRANTZ, J. C., JR.: Alkyl nitrites XVI. Comparative depressor responses of octyl nitrite and glyceryl trinitrate. Proc. Soc. exp. Biol. (N.Y.) **76**, 759—760 (1951).

CITTERS, R. L., VAN: Physiology and biophysics, p. 690. Theodore C. RUCH and HARRY D. PATTON, (Eds.). Philadelphia, Pa: W. B. Saunders Co. 1966.

COHEN, A., GALLAGHER, J. P., LUEBS, E. D., VARGA, Z., YAMANAKA, J., ZALESKI, E. J., BLUEMCHEN, C., BING, R. J.: The quantitative determination of coronary flow with a positron emitter (rubidium 84). Circulation **32**, 636—649 (1965).

CUNY, L., QUIVY, D.: Action vaso-dilatatrice de la trinitrine, etudieé par la pléthysmographie de la muqueuse nasale. C.R. Soc. Biol. (Paris) **136**, 283—284 (1942).

DARBY, T. D., ALDINGER, E. E.: Further studies of the effect on myocardial energy utilization elicited by nitroglycerin. Circulation Res. **8**, 100—108 (1960).

DAVIDSON, I. W. F., MILLER, H. S., DICARLO, F. J.: Absorption, excretion and metabolism of pentaerythritol tetranitrate by humans. J. Pharmacol. exp. Ther. **175**, 42—50 (1970).

DAVIDSON, I. W. F., MILLER, H. S., DICARLO, F. J.: Pharmacodynamics and biotransformation of pentaerythritol tetranitrate in man. J. Pharm. Sci. **60**, 274—277 (1971).

DEMARIA, A. N., VISMARA, L. A., AUDITORE, K., AMSTERDAM, E. A., ZELIS, R., MASON, D. T.: Effects of nitroglycerin on left ventricular cavity size and cardiac performance determined by ultrasound in man. Amer. Soc. Clin. Pharmacol. Ther. 1974 meeting abstract. Clin. Pharmacol. Ther. **15**, 204 (1974).

DICARLO, F. J., COUTINKO, C. B., CREW, M. C.: Sites of absorption of pentaerythritol tetranitrate. Arch. Int. Pharmacodyn. Ther. **167**, 163—170 (1967).

DOMENECH, R. J., HOFFMAN, J. I. E., NOBLE, M. I. M., SAUNDERS, K. B., HENSON, J. R., SUBIJANTO, S.: Total and regional coronary blood flow measured by radioactive microspheres in consicious and anesthetized dogs. Circulation Res. **25**, 581—596 (1969).

DRESDALE, D. T., YUCEOGLU, Y. Z., REYES, A., JR., LUNGER, M., NASSAR, A. M.: Hemodynamic effects of isosorbide dinitrate in patients with rheumatic heart disease and pulmonary hypertension. A preliminary study. Angiology **14**, 349—357 (1963).

ECKENHOFF, J. E., HAFKENSCHIEL, J. H.: Effect of nikethamide on coronary blood flow and cardiac oxygen metabolism. J. Pharmacol. exp. Ther. **91**, 362—369 (1947).

ECKENHOFF, J. E., HAFKENSCHIEL, J. H., HARMEL, M. H., GOODALE, W. T., LUBIN, M., BING, R. J., KETY, S. S.: Measurement of coronary blood flow by the nitrous oxide method. Amer. J. Physiol. **152**, 356—364 (1948).

ECKSTEIN, R. W., NEWBERRY, W. B., MCEACHEN, J. A., SMITH, G.: Studies of the anti-adrenergic effects of nitroglycerin on the dog heart. Circulation **4**, 534—540 (1951).

ESSEX, H. E., HERRICK, J. F., BALDES, E. J., MANN, F. C.: Blood flow in the circumflex branch of the left coronary artery of the intact dog. Amer. J. Physiol. **117**, 271—279 (1936).

FAM, W. M., MCGREGOR, M.: Effect of nitroglycerin and dipyridamole on regional coronary resistance. Circulation Res. **22**, 649—659 (1968).

FERRER, M. I., BRADLEY, S. E., WHEELER, H. O., ENSON, Y., PREISIG, R., BRICKER, P. W., CONROY, R. J., HARVEY, R. M.: Some effects of nitroglycerin upon the splanchnic pulmonary, and systemic circulations. Circulation **33**, 357—373 (1966).

FORTUIN, N. J., KAIHARA, S., BECKER, L. C., PITT, B.: Regional myocardial blood flow in the dog studied with radioactive microspheres. Cardiovasc. Res. **5**, 331—336 (1971).

FREMONT, R. E.: The actions of organic nitrates on the cardiopulmonary and peripheral circulations. Angiology **12**, 391—400 (1961).

GILLIS, R. A., MELVILLE, K. I.: Coronary flow changes and cardiac adrenergic blockade during nitroglycerin infusions. Europ. J. Pharmacol. **13**, 15—22 (1970).

GOLDSTEIN, R. E., STINSON, E. B., EPSTEIN, S. E.: Effects of nitroglycerin on coronary collateral function in patients with coronary occlusive disease. Abstracts. Amer. J. Cardiol. **31**, 135 (1973).
GORLIN, R., BRACHFELD, N., MACLEOD, C., BOPP, P.: Effect of nitroglycerin on the coronary circulation in patients with coronary artery disease or increased left ventricular work. Circulation **19**, 705—718 (1959).
GREGG, D. E.: The coronary circulation in health and disease. Philadelphia, Pa.: Lea and Febiger 1950.
GREGG, D. E., LONGINO, F. H., GREEN, P. A., CZERWONKA, L. J.: A comparison of coronary flow determination of the nitrous oxide method and by a direct method using the rotameter. Circulation **3**, 89—94 (1951).
HADDY, F. J.: Physiology and pharmacology of the coronary circulation and myocardium, particularly in relation to coronary artery disease. Amer. J. Med. **47**, 274—286 (1969).
HIRSHLEIFER, I., ARORA, Y.: Nitrites in the treatment of bronchial asthma. Dis. Chest **36**, 275—283 (1961).
HOLLANDER, W., MADOFF, I. M., CHOBANIAN, A. V.: Local myocardial blood flow as indicated by the disappearance of NaI^{131} from the heart muscle: Studies at rest, during exercise, and following nitrite administration. J. Pharmacol. exp. Ther. **139**, 53—59 (1963).
JOHNSON, J. B., FAIRLEY, A., CARTER, C.: Effects of sublingual nitroglycerin on pulmonary arterial pressure in patients with left ventricular failure. Ann. intern. Med. **50**, 34—42 (1959).
JOHNSON, J. B., GROSS, J. F., HALE, E.: Effects of sublingual administration of nitroglycerin on pulmonary-artery pressure in patients with failure of the left ventricule. New Engl. J. Med. **257**, 1114—1117 (1957).
KAIHARA, S., VAN HEERDEN, P. D., MIGITA, T., WAGNER, H. N.: Measurement of distribution of cardiac output. J. Appl. Physiol. **25**, 696—700 (1968).
KHOURI, E. M., GREGG, D. E.: Minature electromagnetic flow meter applicable to coronary arteries. J. Appl. Physiol. **18**, 224—227 (1963).
KOLIN, A.: (1960) Circulatory system. Methods; blood flow determination by electromagnetic method. In: GLASSER, O. (Ed.): Medical Physics, Vol. III, pp. 141—155. Chicago, III.: Year Book Publ. Inc. 1960.
KOLIN, A.: Cardiovascular research. VI. World Congress of Cardiology, London Sept. 1970.
KRANTZ, J. C., JR., CARR, C. J., BRYANT, H. H.: Alkyl nitrites. XIV. The effect of nitrites and nitrates on arterial triphosphatase. J. Pharmacol. exp. Ther. **102**, 16—21 (1951).
KRANTZ, J. C., JR., CARR, C. J., FORMAN, S. E.: The pharmacology of 2-ethylhexyl nitrite. J. Pharmacol. exp. Ther. **64**, 302—306 (1938).
KRANTZ, J. C., JR., CARR, C. J., FORMAN, S. E.: Alkyl nitrites. V. The pharmacology of the high molecular weight alkyl nitrites. Proc. Soc. exp. Biol. (N.Y.) **42**, 472—474 (1939a).
KRANTZ, J. C., JR., CARR, C. J., FORMAN, S. E., ELLIS, F. W.: Alkyl nitrates. III. A pharmacologic study of a new series of organic nitrates. J. Pharmacol. exp. Ther. **67**, 187—190 (1939b).
KRANTZ, J. C., JR., LU, G. G., BELL, F. K., CASCORBI, H. F.: Nitrites. XIX. Studies of the mechanism of action of glyceryl trinitrate. Biochem. Pharmacol. **11**, 1095—1099 (1962).
LANGENDORFF, O.: Pflügers Arch. ges. Physiol. **61**, 291 (1895). Cited by CHARLIER, 1971.
LEIGHNINGER, D. S., RUEGER, R., BECK, C. S.: Effect of glyceryl trinitrate (nitroglycerin) on arterial blood supply to ischemic myocardium. Amer. J. Cardiol. **3**, 638—646 (1959).
LEVY, J. V.: Effect of organic nitrates on myocardial oxygen consumption *in vitro*. Brit. J. Pharmacol. **38**, 743—748 (1970).
MASON, D. T., ZELIS, R., AMSTERDAM, E. A.: Actions of the nitrites on the peripheral circulation and myocardial oxygen consumption: significance in the relief of angina pectoris. Dis. Chest **59**, 296—305 (1971).
MELVILLE, K. I., GILLIS, R. A., SEKELJ, P.: Coronary flow, blood pressure and heart dose-response changes after nitroglycerin administration. Canad. J. Physiol. Pharmacol. **43**, 9—18 (1965).
MORAWITZ, P., ZAHN, K.: Dtsch. Arch. klin. Med. **116**, 364—370 (1914). Cited by KRANTZ et al. (1939a).
MULLER, O., RORVIK, K.: Hemodynamic consequences of coronary heart disease. Brit. Heart J. **20**, 302—310 (1958).
MURRELL, W.: Nitro-glycerine as a remedy for angina pectoris. Lancet **1879 I**, 80—81, 113—115, 151—152, 225—227.

NEEDLEMAN, P., HUNTER, F. E., JR.: The transformation of glyceryl trinitrate and other nitrates by glutathione-organic nitrate reductase. Mol. Pharmacol. **1**, 77—86 (1965).

PARKER, J. O., LEDWICK, J. R., WEST, R. O., CASE, R. B.: Reversible cardiac failure during angina pectoris. Circulation **39**, 745—757 (1969).

PARKER, J. O., WEST, F. R. O., GIORGI, S.: The effect of nitroglycerin on coronary blood flow and the hemodynamic response to exercise in coronary artery disease. Amer. J. Cardiol. **27**, 59—65 (1971).

POPOVICH, N. R., ROBERTS, F. F., CRISLIP, R. L., MENGES, H., JR.: Ineffectiveness of nitroglycerine as an antiadrenergic agent on the cat heart. Circulation Res. **4**, 727—730 (1956).

RATH, M., KRANTZ, J. C., JR.: Nitrites. VIII. Blood-nitrite content of man and other species. J. Pharmacol. exp. Ther. **76**, 27—32 (1942a).

RATH, M., KRANTZ, J. C., JR.: Nitrites. IX. A further study of the action of organic nitrates. J. Pharmacol. exp. Ther. **76**, 33—38 (1942b).

RITSCHEL, W. A., CLOTTEN, R.: Entwicklung einer peroralen nitroglycerinprophyllin-retard-form. Arzneimittel-Forsch. **20**, 1180—1187 (1970).

ROBINSON, B. F.: Mode of action of nitroglycerin in angina pectoris. Brit. Heart J. **30**, 295—302 (1968).

ROSS, R. S., UEDA, K., LICHTLEN, P. R., REES, J. R.: Measurement of myocardial blood flow in animals and man by selective injection of radioactive gas into the coronary arteries. Circulation Res. **15**, 28—41 (1964).

ROSSEEL, M. T., BOGAERT, M. G.: Gas chromatography of the nitrate esters of glycerol, isosorbide and isomannide. J. Chromatog. **65**, 364—367 (1972).

ROUGHGARDEN, J. W., NEWMAN, E. V.: Circulatory changes during the pain of angina pectoris. Amer. J. Med. **41**, 935—945 (1966).

ROWE, G. G.: The nitrous oxide method for determining coronary flow in man. Amer. Heart J. **58**, 268—281 (1959).

ROWE, G. G.: Effects of drugs on the coronary circulation of man. Clin. Pharmacol. Ther. **7**, 547—557 (1966).

ROWE, G. G., CASTILLO, C. A., AFONSO, S., CRUMPTON, C. W.: Coronary flow measured by the nitrous oxide method. Amer. Heart J. **67**, 457—468 (1964).

ROWE, G. G., CHELIUS, C. J., ALFONSO, S., GURTNER, H. P., CRUMPTON, C. W.: Systemic and coronary hemodynamic effects of erythrol tetranitrate. J. clin. Invest. **40**, 1217—1222 (1961).

SCHELINE, R. R.: Metabolism of foreign compounds by gastrointestinal microorganisms. Pharmacol. Rev. **25**, 451—523 (1973).

SEVELIUS, G., JOHNSON, P. C.: Myocardial blood flow determined by surface counting and ratio formula. J. Lab. clin. Med. **54**, 669—679 (1959).

STIEGLITZ, E. J., PALMER, A. E.: A colormetric method for the determination of nitrite in blood. J. Pharmacol. exp. Ther. **51**, 398—410 (1934).

STIEGLITZ, E. J., PALMER, A. E.: Nitrite in normal human blood. Arch. intern. Med. **59**, 620—624 (1937).

TAWAB, S. A., CARR, C. J., KRANTZ, C. J.: The pharmacology of thiocyanobenzoic acids. J. Pharmacol. exp. Ther. **96**, 416—421 (1949).

TAYLOR, S. H.: Reversible left-ventricular failure in angina pectoris. Lancet **31**, 902—907 (1970).

TRUITT, E. B., JR.: A note on the modification of the Anderson-Craver perfusion apparatus for interchanging perfusion fluids. J. Amer. Pharm. Ass. **44**, 382 (1955).

VOEGTLIN, C., MACHT, D. I.: The action of nitrites and drugs on the digitalis group on the isolated coronary artery. J. Pharmacol. exp. Ther. **5**, 77—86 (1913).

VYDEN, J. K., CARVALHO, M., BOSZORMENYI, E.: Effect of glyceryl trinitrate (nitroglycerin) on the systemic and coronary circulation of the dog. Amer. J. Cardiol. **25**, 53—58 (1970).

WEST, J. W., GUZMAN, S. V.: Coronary dilation and constriction visualized by selective arteriography. Circulation Res. **7**, 527—536 (1959).

WHITWORTH, C. G., GRANT, M. M.: Use of nitrate and nitrite vasodilators by glaucomatous patients. Arch. Ophthal. **71**, 492—496 (1964).

WILLIAMS, J. F., GLICK, G., BRUNWALD, W.: Studies on cardiac dimensions in intact anesthesized man. Circulation **32**, 767—771 (1965).

WINBURY, M. M.: Experimental approaches to the development of antianginal drugs. Advanc. Pharmacol. **3**, 1—82 (1964).

Winbury, M. M.: Problems in laboratory evaluation of antianginal agents, p. 26. Amsterdam: North Holland Pub. Co. 1967.
Winbury, M. M.: Redistribution of left ventricular blood flow produced by nitroglycerin. Circulation Res. Suppl. No. 1. **1**, 140—147 (1971).
Winbury, M. M., Gobel, L. P.: Effect of nitrites on nutritional circulation of heart and hindlimb. Amer. J. Physiol. **212**, 1062—1066 (1967).
Winbury, M. M., Hawe, B. B., Weiss, H. R.: Effect of nitroglycerine and dipyridamole on epicardial and endocardial oxygen tension — further evidence for redistributic of myocardial blood flow. J. Pharmacol. exp. Ther. **176**, 184—199 (1971).
ZoBell, C. E.: Factors influencing the reduction of nitrates and nitrites by bacteria in semisolid media. J. Bacteriol. **24**, 273—281 (1932).

CHAPTER 5

Biotransformation of Organic Nitrates

PHILIP NEEDLEMAN

With 19 Figures

I. Isolation and Characterization of Organic Nitrate Reductase

A. Initial Demonstrations of the Degradation of Organic Nitrate

The investigation of organic nitrate biotransformation began with the observation by HAY (1883) and by CRANDALL (1929, 1933) that inorganic nitrite appears after incubation of glyceryl trinitrate (GTN) with blood. CRANDALL et al. (1929) demonstrated that GTN rapidly disappeared from the circulation after intravenous administration to dogs and inorganic nitrite could be qualitatively detected. YAGODA and VON OETTINGEN (1944) incubated GTN, erythrityl tetranitrate (ETN), and pentaerythrityl tetranitrate (PETN) with dog blood and demonstrated the formation of inorganic nitrite.

B. Role of Liver and Glutathione in the Transformation of Organic Nitrates

OBERST and SNYDER (1948) reported inorganic nitrite was formed when the nitrate esters, GTN, 1-glucosan trinitrate, and mannitol hexanitrate (MHN) were incubated with rabbit liver homogenates. They believed that two systems were involved in the transformation of organic nitrates. The first, occurring principally in the liver was inactivated by heating to 100° for 45 min. The second system which was heat-stable was present in liver, muscle, and blood.

HEPPEL and HILMOE (1950) found that GTN and erythrityl tetranitrate (ETN) undergo a spontaneous (non-enzymatic) reaction with reduced glutathione (GSH) to form inorganic nitrite and oxidized glutathione. They concluded that the heat-stable factor in the degradation of the organic nitrates was GSH. The reduction of GTN and ETN by GSH was found to be catalyzed by a liver enzyme. They performed a balance study and noted that 2 μM GSH were oxidized for every micromole of nitrite formed during the incubation of GTN with hog liver enzyme. The equivalency of the reaction was supported by NEEDLEMAN and HUNTER (1965) who coupled the GTN transformation reaction to glutathione reductase. Glutathione reductase catalyzed the reduction of oxidized glutathione by TPNH and the coupled reaction should proceed as follows:

$$\mathrm{GTN} + 2\mathrm{GSH} \longrightarrow \mathrm{GSSG} + \mathrm{NO_2^-} + \text{other products}$$

$$2\mathrm{GSH} + \mathrm{TPN} \xleftarrow[\text{reductase}]{\text{glutathione}} \mathrm{GSSG} + \mathrm{TPNH}\,.$$

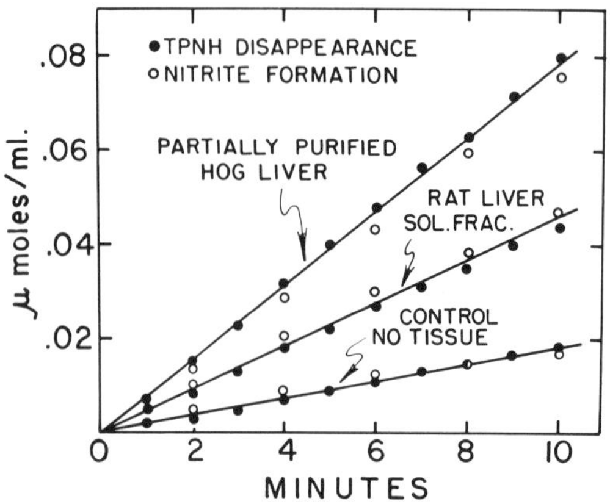

Fig. 1. Comparison of the rates of TPNH disappearance and nitrite formation during GTN transformation. Control, no tissue (i.e. GTN and GSH incubated in buffer only); partially purified hog liver, 50 μg protein; rat liver soluble fraction, 1.0 mg protein (NEEDLEMAN and HUNTER, 1965; with permission from Academic Press, Inc.)

A comparison of the rate and stoichiometry of TPNH disappearance and nitrite formation was made (Fig. 1). Three incubation systems were employed so that the comparisons could be made in systems with the nonenzymatic reaction (GTN + GSH), with liver soluble fraction and with partially purified enzyme. In all three cases the TPNH consumption equaled the nitrite formation (NEEDLEMAN and HUNTER, 1965).

The relationship of liver glutathione to GTN metabolism was studied in isolated perfused rat livers (NEEDLEMAN and HARKEY, 1971). Such perfusion experiments permitted evaluation of total liver GTN degradation (not merely the GSH-dependent reaction) as well as simultaneous consideration of the effect of GTN on some endogenous liver metabolites. In addition, by perfusing the livers without blood, the complication of nonenzymatic degradation due to the presence of GSH in erythrocytes was removed. Rat livers were perfused without recirculation with a fixed concentration of GTN. The liver preparations were unable to maintain a constant rate of GTN metabolism. The lowest percentage metabolism was observed with the highest GTN concentration, whereas, the highest percentage disappearance occurred with the lowest level. In contrast to these percentage differences, the total amount of GTN metabolized was nearly independent of the perfusion concentration, thereby implying the depletion of some endogenous component. Treatment of rats with bromobenzene a substance known to deplete hepatic glutathione, before liver perfusion caused a marked inhibition (90% decrease) of GTN degradation compared to controls (NEEDLEMAN and HARKEY, 1971). The loss of liver GSH was greatly accelerated when the livers were perfused with increasing concentrations of GTN. Fifty min of perfusion with 4.5 mM GTN led to an 85 percent decrease in liver GSH. Bromobenzene pretreatment caused a 70% decrease in GSH. This small reserve of GSH was nearly completely depleted (95%) by perfusion with GTN. The bromobenzene treatment drastically inhibited GTN metabolism. Perfusion without drug for 50 min did not alter the hepatic ATP levels. When isolated rat livers were perfused with

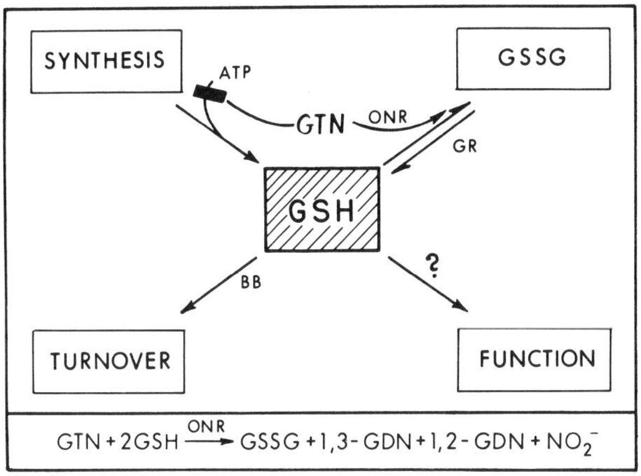

Fig. 2. Schematic diagram of the interrelationship between GTN transformation and endogenous liver GSH. Abbreviations: ONR, organic nitrate reductase; GR, glutathione reductase; BB, bromobenzene. (NEEDLEMAN and HARKEY, 1971; with permission from Pergamon Press)

GTN, a concentration-dependent depletion of ATP was observed. The synthesis and breakdown of GSH in liver is a rapid process. A unifying hypothesis developed to explain this collection of data is illustrated in Fig. 2. The isolated rat liver is perfused with GTN, which oxidizes GSH and degrades the GTN. The GSSG is reduced rapidly by glutathione-reductase and TPNH. With increasing concentration of GTN in the perfusion medium, the isolated rat liver was found to be incapable of maintaining a constant rate of GTN degradation. The high concentration of GTN caused a decrease in ATP resulting from inhibition of mitochondrial phosphorylation (NEEDLEMAN and HUNTER, 1965; HUNTER et al., 1953). The low ATP in turn would interfere with the synthesis of GSH, whereas the degradation process rapidly continues, resulting in a net depletion of liver GSH. The level of GSH becomes limiting and the perfused liver possesses a decreased ability to degrade GTN continuously. Bromobenzene, on the other hand, does not interfere with GSH synthesis but rather it enhances GSH depletion by conjugation.

It is possible that blood or organs other than the liver enzymatically degrade a significant portion of administered GTN. The contribution of hepatic inactivation of organic nitrates was evaluated in totally eviscerated rats (LANG et al., 1972). After intravenous administration of ^{14}C-GTN in control animals, there was a rapid disappearance of this compound from the blood. The biological half-time was less than 1 min (Fig. 3a). There was a simultaneous rapid appearance of GTN metabolites in the blood (Fig. 3b), which reached peak concentrations at 2—5 min. The time course of disappearance of ^{14}C-GTN from the blood of eviscerated animals proceeded much more slowly than in controls with an apparent half-time of 7 to 8 min. Furthermore, there was no increase in the initial low concentrations of GTN metabolites in the blood with time (Fig. 3b). These data establish that the degradation *in vivo* of GTN is carried out primarily in the liver (LANG et al., 1972). BOGAERT et al. (1969) administered GTN to rabbits whose livers were excluded from the blood circulation

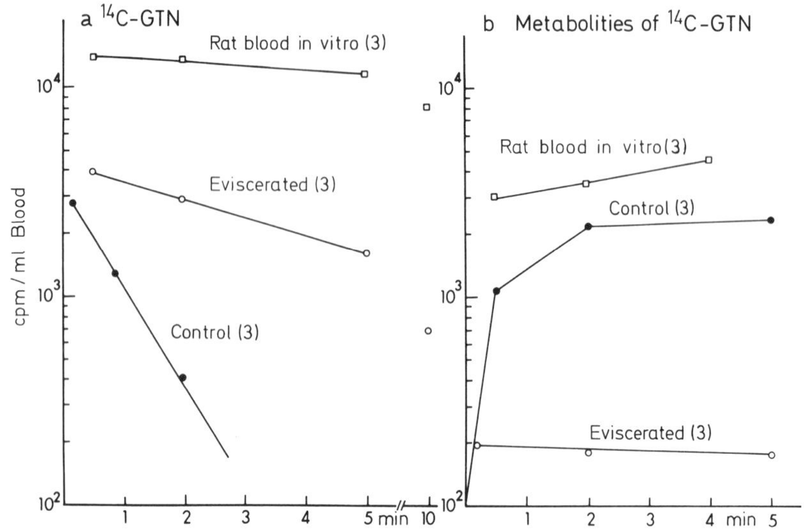

Fig. 3. (a) Time course of disappearance of ^{14}C-GTN from the blood. GTN-1,3-^{14}C (0.2 μc in 0.2 mg of unlabeled carrier GTN) was administered through a jugular vein cannula to a heparinized, pentobarbital anesthetized rat. Carotid blood samples were withdrawn and immediately injected into petroleum ether (which quantitatively extracts all parent GTN) and rapidly mixed, evaporated and counted. (b) Time course of appearance of GTN metabolites in the blood. The GTN free blood (after petroleum ether extraction) was extracted with absolute ethanol (which quantitatively removes the GTN metabolites), evaporated, and counted. (LANG et al., 1972; with the permission of Pergamon Press)

by clamping the hepatic artery and hepatic and portal veins and noted a greatly prolonged peak in nitrate blood levels. The slow rate of degradation of GTN in rat blood *in vitro* has been reported by DICARLO and MELGAR (1970). They state that denitration of GTN by rat blood serum has a half-time of about 20 min. This slow rate of denitration *in vitro* coupled with the apparent lack od degradation in eviscerated rats would indicate that blood plays only a small role in the disappearance rates of GTN from the circulation of intact animals. These results are consistent with the notion that the liver is essential for the *in vivo* degradation of GTN.

C. Subcellular Localization of Hepatic Glutathione-Organic Nitrate Reductase

HUNTER and FORD (1965) observed that MHN was a more powerful uncoupler of oxidative phosphorylation in rat liver mitochondria than was GTN. They observed a GSH-dependent denitration of MHN, ETN, and GTN in rat liver mitochondria preparations. The appearance of inorganic nitrite was most rapid with MHN and slowest with GTN, thus, rapid removal by the mitochondrial reaction cannot explain why GTN is less potent than MHN as an uncoupler. NEEDLEMAN and KRANTZ (1965) performed a differential centrifugation of rat liver homogenates prepared in isotonic sucrose and demonstrated that the primary site of the GTN-metabolizing enzyme was in the $100000 \times g$ soluble fraction rather than in the mitochondrial pellet. The low level of mitochondrial activity was probably attributable to contamination with the 100000 × g supernatant fraction.

D. Purification and Kinetic Properties of Hepatic Organic Nitrate Reductase

HEPPEL and HILMOE (1950) purified an enzyme from hog liver acetone powder. They employed ammonium sulfate and alcohol fractionation as well as adsorption on calcium phosphate gel and achieved a 100 fold increase in specific activity compared to the acetone powder extract. This partially purified enzyme was inhibited by cupric sulfate, stimulated by cyanide, and was unaffected by dialysis or the lack of oxygen. The pH optimum was between 7 and 8. The optimal substrate concentrations for the enzyme-catalyzed denitration were 5×10^{-3} M GSH and 3×10^{-3} M GTN. With excess GTN, the rate was proportional to GSH concentration between 2.5×10^{-4} and 1.6×10^{-5} M.

POSADAS DEL RIO (1970) has partially purified organic nitrate reductase from fresh liver extracts rather than acetone powder. Ammonium sulfate and alcohol fractionation, and DEAE-Sephadex chromatography were employed. The effluents from the DEAE-Sephadex column showed two distinct peaks of enzymatic activity with different relative activities toward organic nitrates. For the first peak isolated from rat liver the relative activities for GTN: ETN: MHN were 1:4:18. The ratios obtained for the second peak were 5:8:18. For partially purified rat liver organic nitrate reductase the Km for GSH was 1.5×10^{-5} M with GTN, 5×10^{-5} with ETN, and 3.7×10^{-5} with MHN. Guinea pig liver enzyme yielded two peaks with activity ratios of 1:5:33 and 16:78:100 respectively (POSADAS DEL RIO, 1970). POSADAS DEL RIO and HUNTER (1973) reported molecular weight values from a calibrated Sephadex colum, of 14000 and 43700 for the two different enzyme peaks.

E. Substrates for Organic Nitrate Reductase

NEEDLEMAN and HUNTER (1965) developed a rapid, sensitive, enzymatic assay based on the reaction of organic nitrates with GSH to yield GSSG. The spectrophotometric or fluorometric method measured TPNH disappearance as the GSSG is catalytically reduced by glutathione reductase. Rat liver 100000 × g supernatant fraction was partially purified by the method of HEPPEL and HILMOE (1950) and a comparison of the maximum velocities (from Lineweaver-Burk plots) of a number of aliphatic nitrates was performed (Table 1). Linear-chain polynitrate esters, such as MHN, ETN, and GTN were rapidly transformed by the liver soluble enzyme in the presence of GSH. On the other hand, branched-chain alcohol nitrates, such as pentaerythritol tetranitrate (PETN), pentaerythritol trinitrate (PETRIN), and trimethylol ethane trinitrate,were slowly transformed by liver nitrate reductase. Replacement of the nitrate group by hydrogen in a linear ester decreased the rate of the enzymic reaction as noted when ETN was compared to 1,2,4-butanetriol trinitrate, or BTTN to 1,4-butanediol dinitrate. Introduction of an ether linkage into a linear chain nitrate compound further decreased the rate of enzymic transformation, as in the case of di- and triethylene glycol dinitrate. Replacement of a nitrate ester group with a free hydroxyl decreased the velocity of enzymic degradation, since GTN was transformed much more rapidly than GDN, and GDN more rapidly than GMN. In

Table 1. Comparison of the maximum velocities of alkyl nitrate as substrates for GSH-organic nitrate reductase (NEEDLEMAN and HUNTER, 1965)

Alkyl nitrates	Organic nitrate reductase V_{max} mmoles/kg protein/min
Mannitol hexanitrate (MHN)	830
Erythritol tetranitrate (ETN)	358
Glyceryl trinitrate (GTN)	120
Isosorbide dinitrate (ISD)	21.5
1,2,4-Butanetriol trinitrate	12.5
Trimethylol ethane trinitrate	11.1
Pentaerythritol trinitrate (PETRIN)	9.1
1,2-Glyceryl dinitrate (GDN)	5.0
1,4-Butanediol dinitrate	3.1
Polyglycidyl nitrate	2.6
1,3-Glyceryl dinitrate (GDN)	2.5
Triethylene glycol dinitrate	1.7
Diethylene glycol dinitrate	1.2
1-Glyceryl mononitrate (GMN)	0.7

addition, if the nitrate group was replaced by hydrogen in a linear ester the rate of the enzymic reaction decreased. The branched-chain compound PETN represented an exception to these generalizations. This might be the result of the very low solubility of PETN in the experimental system. Anhydride formation, as in isosorbide dinitrate, markedly decreased enzymic hydrolyis (Table 1).

F. Induction and Inhibition of Organic Nitrate Reductase

NEEDLEMAN and KRANTZ (1965) pretreated rats with phenobarbital for 4 days and noted an enhanced rate of GTN metabolism by rat liver homogenates. The enhancement of the 10000 × g supernatant fraction enzyme was surprising since the ability of phenobarbital to increase the rate of drug metabolism is generally attributed to activation of the liver microsomal enzymes which metabolize foreign compounds. BOGAERT et al. (1969a, 1969b) found that phenobarbital pretreatment of rabbits accelerated excretion of metabolites and decreased the peak plasma nitrate ion values after GTN administration.

Chronic administration *in vivo* of phenobarbital (1 mg/ml in drinking water for two weeks) to rats accelerated the rate of GTN metabolism by their isolated perfused livers (NEEDLEMAN and HARKEY, 1971). The amount of GTN metabolized in 50 min by the livers from phenobarbital-pretreated rats was 95 ± 9 mmoles/kg net weight of liver which represents a 42% increase over controls. The total amount of GTN metabolized was also greater because phenobarbital induced a 25% increase in liver weight. Pretreatment with phenobarbital produced no significant changes in endogenous liver GSH or ATP levels. Tolerance to the cardiovascular effects of GTN were induced by repeated administration of GTN and there was no difference in the degradation of GTN by perfused livers from tolerant or control rats. Bromobenzene pretreatment caused a marked inhibition of

GTN degradation with only 6 ± 0.2 mmoles/kg of GTN metabolized or a 90% decrease compared to controls. The effect of the various pretreatments was borne out by measuring inorganic nitrite as the end product of GTN degradation. The highest rate of nitrite formation occurred with phenobarbital pretreatment, whereas there was virtually no denitration of GTN by livers from bromobenzene-treated animals. Finally, there was no significant difference in the rate of NO_2-formation between controls and livers removed from GTN-tolerant animals (NEEDLEMAN and HARKEY, 1971).

LEE and BELPAIRE (1972) pretreated rats with phenobarbital for 3 days and noted an increased rate of GTN metabolism by the soluble fraction of liver homogenates. They reported that in phenobarbital induced rats the increased formation of inorganic nitrite during GTN metabolism was accompanied by an accelerated TPNH disappearance rate, and increased activity of both glucose-6-phosphate dehydrogenase and glutathione reductase. The protein synthesis inhibitors, DL-ethionine or actinomycin D completely inhibited the enhancement of nitrate metabolism caused by phenobarbital (LEE and BELPAIRE, 1972). BOGAERT et al. (1971), showed the phenobarbital pretreatment in man decreased the severity of the headache and nausea when 5 mg of GTN was administered.

BOGAERT et al. (1970) reported that SKF-525A pretreatment inhibited organic nitrate metabolism in dogs and rabbits. They reported that SKF-525A increased the plasma levels of GTN, however, without affecting the vascular effects. In contrast, LEE and BELPAIRE (1972) could not demonstrate inhibition of nitrate metabolism whether the SKF-525A was administered *in vivo* or added directly to the rat liver enzyme. NEEDLEMAN et al. (1971) found that *in vivo* administration of either phenobarbital or SKF-525A to rats did not significantly alter the *in vivo* oxidation of GTN to carbon dioxide.

G. Degradation of Organic Nitrates by Plasma

DI CARLO et al. (1969, 1970) studied GTN biotransformation by rat blood serum. The denitration proceeded at a slow rate with a half-time of about 20 min. The pH optimum for the reaction was at pH 7.8 with a maximum activity at 50 to 57° C. Unlike hepatic organic nitrate reductase, the serum enzyme did not require GSH. The reaction was inhibited by p-chloromercuribenzoate, iodoacetamide, and silver nitrate indicating that sulfhydryl groups were essential for activity. DI CARLO et al. (1965) had demonstrated that pentaerythritol tetranitrate was degraded by human blood and that the enzyme system appeared to be concentrated in the erythrocytes.

JOHNSON et al. (1972) incubated organic nitrates in rat blood and found that GTN and isosorbide dinitrate (ISD) were slowly metabolized by blood with a half-time of 15 to 20 min; whereas, mannitol hexanitrate (MHN) was rapidly degraded with a one minute half-time. The slow rate of degradation *in vitro* coupled with the apparent lack of denitration in eviscerated rats (LANG et al., 1972; NEEDLEMAN et al., 1971), indicate that blood plays only a minor role in the disappearance of GTN and other organic nitrates from the circulation of intact animals, with the possible exception of MHN.

POSADAS DEL RIO and HUNTER (1972) reported that blood serum from guinea pig, rat and rabbit, and bovine serum albumin reacted very slowly with GTN, ETN, and

PETN, whereas, MHN was rapidly denitrated. These reactions were independent of GSH, but in contrast to DI CARLO and MELGAR (1970), the degradation of MHN by rabbit serum or bovine serum albumin was not inhibited by p-hydroxymercuribenzoate, iodoacetamide, or N-ethylmaleimide.

H. Comparison of Glutathione-Organic Nitrate Reductase to Other Enzymes with Similar Properties

TSURUTA and HASEGAWA (1970) described an enzyme isolated from either plasma or liver that catalyzes the degradation of ethylene glycol dinitrate into inorganic nitrate and ethlyene glycol mononitrate. The enzyme catalyzes the denitration of ethylene glycol dinitrate (nitroglycol) in the absence of GSH cofactor, at a pH 6.3 optimum, with a Km of 3.0 mM. This inorganic nitrate forming enzyme appears to be quite different than the hepatic organic nitrate reductase originally reported by HEPPEL and HILMOE (1950).

FOUTS and BRODIE (1956) described a GSH independent, microsomal, flavoprotein nitroreductase in rabbit kidney and liver which reduced aromatic nitro compounds to the corresponding amines. OTSUKA (1961) investigated two enzymes in hog liver, nitro- and nitroso-reductase, that were found to be specific for the nitro to nitroso and nitroso to amine steps respectively. OMURA (1959) isolated a cattle spleen enzyme and a mouse liver enzyme which acted as an inorganic nitrate reductase which reduced inorganic nitrate to nitrite. Inorganic nitrate reductases have been isolated from bacteria as well as plants and have been shown to be flavoproteins that utilize pyridine nucleotides as electron donors (GARRET and NASON, 1969).

Many compounds foreign to the body are excreted as mercapturic acids. BOOTH et al. (1961) purified a GSH dependent rat liver enzyme which catalyzed the formation of glutathione-S-conjugates by replacement of halogen of aromatic compounds. COMBES and STAKELUM (1961) identified a GSH dependent enzyme in the soluble supernatant fraction of rat liver that catalyzes the conjugation of sulfobromophthalein sodium. JOHNSON (1963) studied an enzyme which conjugates glutathione with aliphatic halogen compounds. This enzyme was inactivated by dialysis whereas organic nitrate reductase was enhanced by dialysis (HEPPEL and HILMOE, 1950; NEEDLEMAN and KRANTZ, 1965). GROVER and SIMS (1964) studied an enzyme in which sulfobromophthalein was a competitive substrate in the reaction between 1,2-dichloro-4-nitrobenzene with GSH. The enzymatic activity of this enzyme was diminished by pretreating rats with phenobarbital, thereby, contrasting with organic nitrate reductase which was induced by phenobarbital (Section I.F.).

Various investigators, studying the metabolism of halogenated nitrobenzenes, have shown the displacement of nitro groups rather than halide groups. BRAY et al. (1953) demonstrated in rabbits the loss of the nitro group from 2,3,5,6-tetrachloronitrobenzene. BETTS et al. (1957) noted that in the formation of mercapturic acids from polychloronitrobenzenes, the nitro group was replaced by a cysteinyl or N-acetylcysteyl radical. AL-KASSAB et al. (1963) presented evidence to show that the enzyme in the supernatant fractions of rat liver, which catalyzed the replacement of halogen, will also displace the nitro group of polychloronitrobenzene with GSH. In all cases, one nitrite ion was liberated for each GSH conjugated.

Organic nitrates and GSH undergo a redox reaction and no permanent mercapturic acid conjugation product is formed, thus organic nitrate reductase appears to differ from the enzymes that have been shown to conjugate organic compounds with GSH.

The natural substrate for glutathione-organic nitrate reductase (E.C. 1.8.6.1, Glutathione:polynitrate reductase) is unknown. There are no naturally occurring aliphatic organic nitrate esters. One possibility is that the liver enzyme catalyzes transhydrogenation reactions between disulfide peptides, with reduced GSH serving as the hydrogen donor. Such hepatic SH-SS interchange reactions have previously been reported (RACKER, 1955; DE LORENZO et al., 1966; and KOHNO et al., 1968). However, the GSH dependent reduction of the disulfide linkage in insulin appears to be liver microsomal enzyme instead of a liver soluble fraction enzyme (ANSORGE et al., 1973).

II. Isolation and Characterization of Organic Nitrate Metabolites

A. Metabolic Pathway in the Degradation of Glyceryl Trinitrate, Isosorbide Dinitrate, Mannitol Hexanitrate, and Erythrityl Tetranitrate

1. Metabolism by Liver Homogenates

a) Glyceryl Trinitrate. OBERST and SNYDER (1948) reported that glyceryl trinitrate (GTN) was metabolized to inorganic nitrite by rabbit liver homogenates. HEPPEL and HILMOE (1950) observed that GTN and ETN reacted with reduced glutathione (GSH) to form oxidized glutathione and inorganic nitrite; the rate of nitrite formation was enhanced by a hog liver enzyme. HUNTER and FORD (1955) accounted for less than one nitrite ion per molecule of GTN metabolized. The position of the liberated nitrite was unknown, and no consideration of other metabolic products had been undertaken.

NEEDLEMAN and KRANTZ (1965) demonstrated that the transformation of GTN in the presence of GSH produced two organic nitrate products which are less lipid soluble than is the parent molecule. Organic solvent extraction of tissue or enzyme incubations, blood, urine, or intact organs was employed to isolate the parent organic nitrates as well as the nitrate metabolites which were then separated by thin-layer chromatography (NEEDLEMAN and KRANTZ, 1965; NEEDLEMAN and HUNTER, 1965). Chromatographically, there were no differences in the GTN metabolites produced by, (a) the non-enzymatic reaction between GTN and GSH, (b) the liver enzyme catalyzed reaction of GTN and GSH, (c) the urinary excretion products after GTN administration to adult rats, and (d) synthetic 1,3- and 1,2-glyceryl dinitrate (GDN) (NEEDLEMAN and KRANTZ, 1965).

The time course for the hepatic degradation of GTN was associated with a similar rate for the formation of 1,3- and 1,2-GDN. The non-enzymic reaction of GTN and GSH produced a slow linear decrease of GTN and a linear production of 1,3- and 1,2-GDN. During this 2 hrs incubation only traces of glyceryl mononitrate were found (NEEDLEMAN and HUNTER, 1965). After 1 hr of incubation, 40% of the original GTN remained and 69% of the total remaining organic nitrate was present as 1,2- and 1,3-GDN. Since the reaction was started with 4 mM GTN, this indicated that 2.4 mmoles per liter of reaction mixture was transformed. During the 1 hr incubation,

1.7 mmoles of inorganic nitrite was formed per liter of reaction mixture. Thus, 0.71 nitrite ion was recovered per GTN transformed, which was in agreement with the earlier finding of Hunter and Ford (1955) that less than one nitrite was found per molecule of GTN metabolized. The total of the nitrate groups found in the 1,3-GDN and 1,2-GDN and appearing as inorganic nitrite accounted for about 90% of the nitrate groups in the GTN that had undergone enzymic reaction (Needleman and Hunter, 1965). Therefore, the major route of GTN degradation by the liver enzyme appeared to be denitration with formation of the glyceryl dinitrates and inorganic nitrite. The enzymic rate of GTN degradation and metabolite formation approached zero after 1 hr which could be the result of product inhibition, exhaustion of the reactants, or inactivation of the enzyme. No inhibition of the GTN transformation was exhibited following the addition of a mixture of 1,3- and 1,2-GDN of inorganic nitrite to the enzymic incubation nor was the time course of GTN transformation altered by the addition of supplementary GSH. Preincubation of the enzyme with either substrate for 30 min did not substantially alter the reaction when the second substrate was added (Needleman and Hunter, 1965).

A comparison of the maximum velocities of the enzymic transformation of various glyceryl nitrates, indicated that the trinitrate ester was metabolized more than 20 times faster than the dinitrates, which were in turn metabolized more rapidly than the mononitrate by liver organic nitrate reductase. The slow rate of GDN degradation indicated by the low V_{max} (Table 1) was consistent with the finding of Needleman and Krantz (1965) that the dinitrates of glycerol appeared as the primary urinary metabolites after GTN administration to rats. The fact that GMN was practically unaltered was in agreement with the finding of Heppel and Hilmoe (1950) that no glycerol was found after GTN degradation. The metabolism of 1,2-GDN proceeded somewhat more rapidly than 1,3-GDN. This difference may account for the unequal levels of these metabolites accumulating in the enzymic experiments. Lee (1973) confirmed that the enzymatic (hepatic) denitration of GDN is much slower than that of GTN and that the denitration of GMN is even slower than that of the GDN. Liver homogenates of GTN produced larger quantities of 1,3-GDN than of 1,2-GDN, whereas, 1,2-GDN was the primary metabolite recovered after incubating GTN with cat, rabbit, or dog liver homogenates.

In summary, Needleman and Krantz (1965) and Needleman and Hunter (1965) demonstrated that the major route for glyceryl trinitrate transformation appeared to be denitration in the presence of reduced glutathione (GSH). One molecule of glyceryl trinitrate reacted with two GSH to release one inorganic nitrite ion from either the 2- or 3-position to form 1,3- or 1,2-glyceryl dinitrate. There was no product inhibition of the glyceryl trinitrate degradation reaction. The denitration of glyceryl dinitrate proceeded at only 2 to 5% of the rate for glyceryl trinitrate. Glyceryl mononitrate was practically unaltered by the liver enzyme.

b) Liver Homogenate Degradation of Other Nitrates. Chromatographic analysis of the degradation of the principal organic nitrate vasodilators used therapeutically was performed after incubation with hepatic glutathione-organic nitrate reductase (Needleman and Hunter, 1965). These nitrate esters (GTN, MHN, PETN, ETN, and ISD) oxidized GSH and released inorganic nitrite in the presence of the enzyme. With a chromatographic solvent system consisting of benzene: ethyl acetate: acetic acid 80:20:5 the greater the esterification the higher the migration on the plate. Thus, the completely nitrated parent compounds moved farther (i.e. higher Rf) than the denitration products, a pattern that reflected the increased water solubility on replacing the nitrate ester with a hydroxyl. These chromatograms showed only organic nitrates because the material applied represented the ether extracts of aqueous incubations and the color was developed with diphenylamine. The compound nearest the top of the chromatogram was always the parent compounds. The GTN spot was followed by 1,3-GDN and 1,2-GDN, respectively. With mannitol hexanitrate (MHN) four definite metabolites and a trace of another were present after 4 hrs. The transformation velocity of MHN, as measured by the fluorometric method, was about seven times faster than GTN (Section I.E., Table 1). Pentaerythrityl tetranitrate (PETN) showed large amounts of unchanged parent molecule and small amounts of three metabolites, an observation that is in agreement with the low rate of enzymic transformation. According to DI CARLO et al., (1965), these metabolites are the tri-, di-, and mononitrates. Erythrityl tetranitrate (ETN) was metabolized three times faster than GTN (Table 1) with the appearance of large amounts of four organic nitrate metabolites at 4 hrs. Isosorbide dinitrate was very slowly metabolized (Table 1). This is reflected by the large amounts of the unchanged parent compound as well as one major nitrate metabolite (NEEDLEMAN and HUNTER, 1965).

2. Liver Perfusion Experiments

a) Glyceryl Trinitrate. NEEDLEMAN and HARKEY (1971) continuously recirculated GTN-1, 3-^{14}C through an isolated perfused rat liver for 10 min. The disappearance of the parent compound was extremly rapid with a half-time of approximately 1 min and 90% loss by 5 min. The glyceryl dinitrates rose rapidly to a plateau between 2 and 10 min. After an initial lag period, the glyceryl mononitrate concentration rose slowly but steadily throughout the perfusion period. The total of the GDN and GMN accounted for the GTN metabolized. At 0.5, 2, 5, and 10 min, the inorganic nitrite concentration in the media from livers perfused with 1 mM GTN was 0.10 ± 0.02, 0.48 ± 0.06, 0.74 ± 0.06, and 0.88 ± 0.08 mM ($n = 6$) respectively (NEEDLEMAN and HARKEY, 1971). The rate of GTN degradation by the isolated perfused rat liver was consistent with the maximal velocity achieved with hepatic glutathione-organic nitrate reductase (NEEDLEMAN and HUNTER, 1965; NEEDLEMAN and HARKEY, 1971).

b) Erythrityl Tetranitrate, Isosorbide Dinitrate and Pentaerythrityl Trinitrate. JOHNSON et al. (1972) compared the rate of degradation by isolated perfused (with 100 ml of recirculating media) rat livers of various organic nitrates (1 mM) and determined the effects of these drugs on endogenous GSH and adenosine triphosphate (ATP). The disappearance of ETN was extremely rapid and exponential with a half-time of approximately one minute. The flow rate of the liver perfusion was 50 ml/min; hence, it would take approximately one minute for the liver to be presented with one-half of the perfusing fluid. Thus, the ETN was being degraded as fast as it was being presented to the liver. The other nitrates tested were metabolized at slower rates characterized by the following half-times: GTN, 2 min; ISD, 5 min; and PETRIN, seven minutes. The common metabolite formed in the degra-

Table 2. Comparison between organic nitrate metabolism and effects on endogenous ATP and GSH. Controls represent livers perfused without drug for 50 min. Column 1 lists the organic nitrate and in parentheses indicates the number of rat livers tested with nonrecirculating liver perfusion (concentration of organic nitrate, 1×10^{-3} M). Values in Column 2 were obtained by analyzing the effluent media for disappearance of parent organic nitrate. Aliquots were taken at various intervals over the 30-min perfusion period. Columns 3 and 4 indicate the mean ± S.E. for endogenous liver ATP and total GSH. (JOHNSON et al., 1972)

Compound	Total liver clearance[a]	ATP[a]	Total GSH[a]	V_{max}[b] GSH–ONR[c]	For loss of respiratory-control of rat liver mitochondria μmole/l
MHN				7.0	27
ETN (4)	85	0.99 ± 0.14	0.76 ± 0.06	3.6	270
GTN (4)	46	1.33 ± 0.05	0.97 ± 0.05	1.0	530
ISD (6)	34	1.38 ± 0.08	0.95 ± 0.04	0.22	1500
PETRIN (6)	30	1.33 ± 0.06	0.94 ± 0.05	0.09	4200
Control (7)		1.84 ± 0.05	2.44 ± 0.09		

[a] Millimoles per kilogram wet weight after 30 min of perfusion (for controls, after 50 min perfusion).
[b] NEEDLEMAN and HARKEY, 1971.
[c] Moles per kilogram wet weight per hour.
[d] NEEDLEMAN and HUNTER, 1966.

dations of all these organic nitrate esters was inorganic nitrite. The inorganic nitrite concentrations in perfusion media increased as the parent organic nitrate concentration decreased. Approximately 1 mole of NO_2^- was liberated per mole of either ETN, GTN or PETRIN metabolized. On the other hand, ISD liberated 2 mole of NO_2^- per mole of ISD metabolized in the liver perfusion. Inorganic nitrite itself was not degraded when perfused through the liver.

Perfusion without Recirculation. GTN perfused through rat liver was previously shown to cause a reduction of endogenous GSH and ATP (NEEDLEMAN and HARKEY, 1971). The decrease in ATP was apparently the result of the inhibitory effect of GTN on mitochondrial phosphorylation. A comparison of the effects of perfusing rat livers with non-recirculated media containing 1 mM concentration of various organic nitrates is shown in Table 2. The total amount of organic nitrate metabolized in the perfusion correlated closely to the previously measured V_{max} with liver glutathione-organic nitrate reductase (Table 1). The nitrate degradation was associated with a moderate depletion of the endogenous stores of total GSH and ATP measured in $HClO_4$ extracts of the perfused livers (Table 2). The largest changes were noted with ETN perfusion where there was a 50% reduction in ATP and a 67% fall in GSH (JOHNSON et al., 1972). The fall in endogenous levels of GSH and ATP was accompanied by a decreased ability of perfused rat livers to degrade organic nitrates. There was an inverse relationship between the rate of liver organic nitrate degradation and the concentrations required for complete loss of respiratory control in rat liver mitochondria. The high concentrations of organic nitrates interfere with mitochondrial phosphorylation and eventually decreased the level of GSH which requires ATP in its synthesis (NEEDLEMAN and HARKEY, 1971).

3. Absorption and Distribution of GTN

DI CARLO et al. (1968) demonstrated the ^{14}C-GTN was rapidly absorbed after oral administration to rats. More than half of the radioactivity was removed from the gastrointestinal tract 30 min after treatment. The major tissue concentrations of absorbed radioactivity were found in the liver and carcass, whereas, the heart, lung, kidney, and spleen took up only small quantities of ^{14}C-counts. Neither the plasma nor tissue radioactivity was identified. The urinary metabolites were characterized and included: 1,2-glyceryl dinitrate, 1,3-glyceryl dinitrate, glyceryl mononitrate and glycerol.

4. Plasma Levels, Binding, and Metabolism of GTN

DI CARLO and MELGAR (1969c, 1970) studied the binding of organic nitrates to rat blood plasma. About 60% of the GTN was bound to rat plasma proteins. During the course of the binding experiments the GTN was metabolized to 1,3- and 1,2-glyceryl dinitrate (GDN) in the ratio of 2:1 respectively. These metabolites were also bound by plasma with 1,2-GDN (60%) being bound more extensively than the 1,3-GDN (33%). The properties of plasma organic nitrate reductase are described in Section I.G.

BOGAERT et al. (1969b, 1970) measured inorganic nitrate blood levels after GTN administration. They found an unusual time course of plasma nitrate levels and there was no relationship between blood levels and the vascular effects of GTN. These workers administered 1 mg/kg of GTN to rabbits and dogs and found that the transient blood pressure depression did not parallel the plasma nitrate levels which reached a maximum at 10 to 20 min after intravenous injection. Indeed, after oral administration of GTN to rabbits they found high plasma levels of inorganic nitrate but the blood pressure was unaffected. The most likely interpretation of their results is that they were not distinguishing between the plasma levels of the parent compound and its less active metabolites.

5. Conversion of ^{14}C-Glyceryl Trinitrate to ^{14}C–CO_2

The liver enzyme glutathione-organic nitrate reductase can rapidly denitrate GTN to 1,3- and 1,2-GDN (NEEDLEMAN and KRANTZ, 1965). Denitration of the GDNs proceeded at only 2 to 5% of the rate for GTN. Glyceryl mononitrate (GMN) was practically unaffected by the liver enzyme (NEEDLEMAN and HUNTER, 1965). DI CARLO et al. (1968) treated rats (orally) with ^{14}C-labeled GTN or glycerol. The elimination of radioactive CO_2 showed a 2 hr lag phase after GTN that was not detected after glycerol. By 24 hr about one-third of the GTN was exhaled as carbon dioxide compared to half of the administered glycerol.

NEEDLEMAN et al. (1971) also studied the *in vivo* oxidation of glycerol and GTN in rats. Glycerol oxidation to $^{14}CO_2$ proceeded rapidly in normal as well as eviscerated rats. The oxidation of GTN to CO_2 in untreated rats was extremely slow. At 4 hrs, when 50% of the glycerol would have been converted, only 5% of the GTN was accounted for as CO_2. Only 17% of the label was exhaled as CO_2 by 24 hrs. A small fraction of GTN must be degraded to glycerol since DI CARLO et al. (1969d) have reported that about 1% of the radioactivity from ^{14}C-GTN (administered as a single oral dose to rats) could be recovered from the liver as lipid, glycogen, protein, RNA, and DNA.

The influence of several factors that alter *in vitro* GTN metabolism (Section I.F.) were evaluated for their influence on GTN oxidation *in vivo* (NEEDLEMAN et al., 1971). Pretreatment of rats with phenobarbital or SKF-525A had no effect on GTN oxidation nor was there an enhancement of CO_2 released in GTN-tolerant animals. Bromobenzene pretreatment, which previously has been shown to deplete liver glutathione and to inhibit GTN degradation in liver perfusion experiments (NEEDLEMAN and HARKEY, 1971) caused a moderate reduction in net GTN conversion. Eviscerated rats with or without nephrectomy were unable to oxidize GTN to CO_2; thus, removal of the viscera interfered at some point in the GTN biotransformation system. Since eviscerated rats readily oxidize glycerol, the interruption in the GTN degradative pathway must lie somewhere in the denitration sequence (NEEDLEMAN et al., 1971).

In an effort to determine the tissue site of CO_2 formation, GTN-^{14}C (0.10-μc, 0.65 μmole of GTN) was incubated for 1 hr with tissue homogenates of brain, heart, intestine, kidney, liver, lung, skeletal muscle, spleen, stomach and blood. No $^{14}CO_2$ production was detected with any of the homogenates (NEEDLEMAN et al., 1971). Aliquots of the incubation media were taken for inorganic nitrite (NO_2^-) determination. Liver homogenates formed 0.693 μmole of NO_2^-, blood formed 0.315 μmole and the remaining tissue formed 0.2 μmole of NO_2^- from GTN. On the other hand, homogenates or minces of kidney, brain, liver and muscle were capable of oxidizing labelled glycerol to $^{14}CO_2$ (NEEDLEMAN et al., 1971). Thus, if labelled glycerol had been formed as a result of GTN degradation in brain, liver, kidney or muscle, it would have been converted to readily detectable $^{14}CO_2$. Finally, when GTN was incubated with GSH in the presence of liver homogenates, no glycerol could be detected (NEEDLEMAN et al., 1971). Similarly, HEPPEL, and HILMOE (1950) were unable to detect the generation of glycerol associated with the glutathione-dependent denitration of GTN by liver. Thus, there did not appear to be an active enzyme system in liver (or the other tissues tested) that was capable of catalyzing the complete denitration of GTN metabolites to glycerol. This notion was supported by several pieces of evidence: (1) liver homogenates readily were demonstrated to metabolize GTN to GDN and GMN and little if any inorganic nitrite formation occurred in other tissues; (2) isolated perfused rat livers were capable of rapidly degrading high concentrations of GTN (NEEDLEMAN and HARKEY, 1971); (3) glycerol could not be detected in liver homogenates after incubation with GTN; (4) ^{14}C-GTN was not converted by liver (or other tissues) to $^{14}CO_2$, whereas glycerol could be oxidized by these tissues; and (5) evisceration of rats inhibited $^{14}CO_2$ formation after the administration of GTN-^{14}C whereas glycerol was still readily oxidized to CO_2. Another possibility would be that GTN or its metabolites were secreted into the intestinal tract (possibly in the bile) and that some bacteria have a nitrate reductase capable of degrading GMN. This probably was not the case because oral pretreatment of rats with neomycin (500 mg/kg) once daily for three days did not alter the rate or quantity of $^{14}CO_2$ exhaled from ^{14}C-GTN treated rats. The site and mechanism of *in vivo* CO_2 formation is unknown.

6. Blood Clearance of GTN, Isosorbide Dinitrate, and Mannitol Hexanitrate, from Intact Animals

JOHNSON et al. (1972) found that after administration (i.v.) of ^{14}C-GTN and ^{14}C-ISD (Fig. 4) to rats, there was a rapid initial fall in the blood level of the parent compounds with a $t_{1/2}$ of about one minute. Disappearance of the parent compound from the blood involved a number of processes which might include mixing of the drug with blood, tissue distribution and binding, enzymatic and non-enzymatic degradation and excretion. The initial disappearance rate of GTN and ISD was much more rapid than that of ^{14}C-mannitol (extracellular marker) (Fig. 4). On the other hand, the GTN and ISD blood clearance curves proceeded at essentially the same rate as rose bengal (used as an index of function of the hepatic polygonal cells). The half-time to reach the peak blood level of the nitrate metabolites was about 30 sec for GTN and about 60 sec for ISD. The GTN and ISD curves were interpreted to mean that GTN and ISD are rapidly taken up by tissues and rapidly metabolized by liver as shown by rapid metabolite appearance (Fig. 4). The tailing-off portion of the curve appeared to represent diffusion of drug back into blood from the tissue. BOGAERT et al. (1970) demonstrated that the rapid fall in blood levels of GTN after i.v. administration to rabbits was the result of rapid uptake by tissues (especially the liver). After the initial fall of the blood nitrate level they noted a secondary increase in

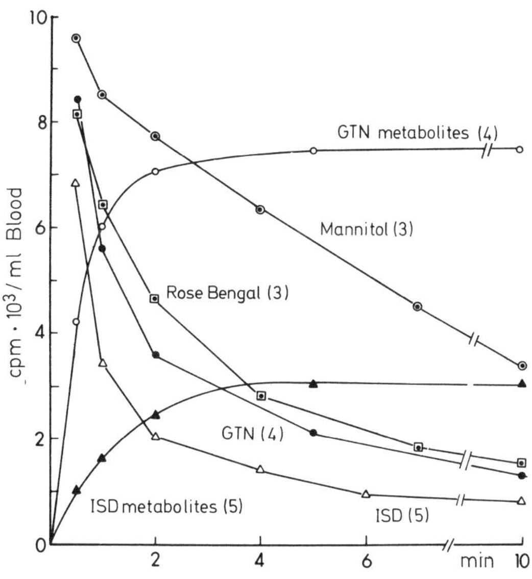

Fig. 4. Blood clearance of various isotopic compounds in rats. The following compounds were injected into the jugular veins of pentobarbital-anesthetized rats: GTN-1,3-^{14}C, 1 μC, 0.5 mg/kg; ISD-^{14}C uniformly labeled, 0.8 μC, 0.5 mg/kg; mannitol-1-^{14}C, 1 μC, 0.5 mg/kg; rose bengal-^{131}I, 0.5 μC. (JOHNSON et al., 1972; with permission from the Williams and Wilkins Co.)

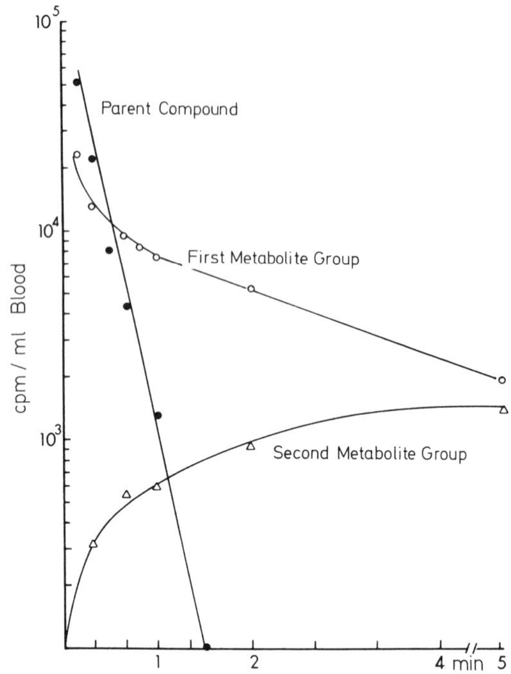

Fig. 5. The time course of MHN disappearance and metabolite appearance. Rats were injected with MHN-1-^{14}C (1 μC, 1 mg/kg) in the jugular vein. Arterial blood samples were drawn and extracted with ethyl acetate, dried, cold carrier added, and the mixture was chromatographed on silica gel plates with benzene-ethyl acetate-acetic acid (4:1:0.1). (JOHNSON et al., 1972; with permission from the Williams and Wilkins Co.)

blood levels that was associated with decreasing tissue drug levels. DI CARLO et al. (1968) also noted a high concentration of radioactivity in liver in rats after oral ^{14}C-GTN treatment and they noted a redistribution of label back into the blood with time.

The *in vivo* clearance of MHN from the blood of rats was extremely rapid (Fig. 5; JOHNSON et al., 1972). The $t_{1/2}$ for disappearance of the parent compound is about 10 sec and none is detectable at 90 sec. Even in the first blood sample there is a very high level of the first metabolite group (about 40% of the level of the parent MHN) presumably in which only one or two nitrate groups are de-esterified. None of the second metabolite group was detectable at 10 sec, and only about 1% of the radioactivity in the blood was in this group at 20 sec even though the level of the parent compound was falling off rapidly. The appearance curve of the second metabolite group was more closely associated in time with the disappearance curve of the first metabolite group than with the disappearance curve of the unchanged MHN. This implied that the denitration occurred sequentially (JOHNSON et al., 1972). MHN has been shown to be an excellent substrate for liver organic nitrate reductase (NEEDLEMAN and HUNTER, 1965, Section I.E.). In addition, the significant blood metabolism (Section I.G.) of MHN further accelerates the blood clearance rate and probably accounts for the absence of a tailing-off of the disappearance curve. It was concluded that the rapid disappearance of the organic nitrates from blood represented the sum

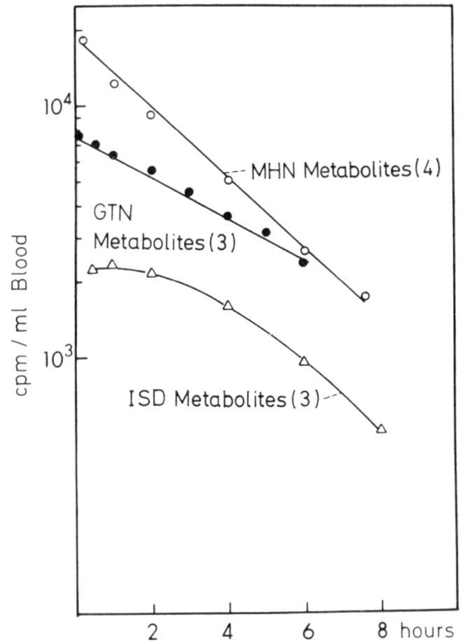

Fig. 6. The long-term blood clearance of metabolites of organic nitrates after jugular vein administration. The following compounds were injected: GTN-1,3-^{14}C (1 μC, 0.5 mg/kg), MHN-1-^{14}C (2.5 μC, 2.5 mg/kg), and ISD-^{14}C (uniformly labeled, 0.8 μC, 0.5 mg/kg). The blood samples (0.25 ml) were extracted with ethanol and counted. Thin-layer chromatography indicated that no parent organic nitrates were present by 15 min after jugular vein administration. (NEEDLEMAN et al., 1972; with permission from the Williams and Wilkins Co.)

of distribution, non-hepatic metabolism (for MHN) and hepatic metabolism which was limited only by the rate at which the drug was presented to the liver via the blood.

The rates of disappearance of the organic nitrate metabolites from the blood, after i.v. administration to rats, were slower than their appearance rate by several orders of magnitude (NEEDLEMAN et al., 1972) (Fig. 6). Metabolites of GTN and MHN disappeared with first-order rates, whereas the ISD metabolites followed a more complicated clearance curve. The approximate half-times for metabolite clearance from rat blood *(in vivo)* for MHN was 2 hrs, for ISD (after the first 2 hrs) was 2.5 hrs, and for GTN was almost 4 hrs (Fig. 6).

SISENWINE and RUELIUS (1971) characterized the blood clearance of ^{14}C-isosorbide dinitrate (ISD) after administration in dogs. The plasma levels following intravenous administration of ^{14}C-ISD are shown in Fig. 7. The peak concentration of unchanged ISD was obtained at 2 min and then disappeared rapidly with a half-time of about 5 min. The major plasma metabolite 5-isosorbide mononitrate (ISMN) peaked at 15 min and disappeared at a much slower rate than the parent compound ($t_{1/2}$ about 2 hrs). Thus, the data of SISENWINE and RUELIUS (1971) and NEEDLEMAN et al. (1972) are in close agreement regarding the blood clearance pattern for ISD and its metabolites after i.v. administration to dog or rats. The plasma clearance of 2-isosorbide mononitrate paralleled that for the 5-isomer but at only approximately

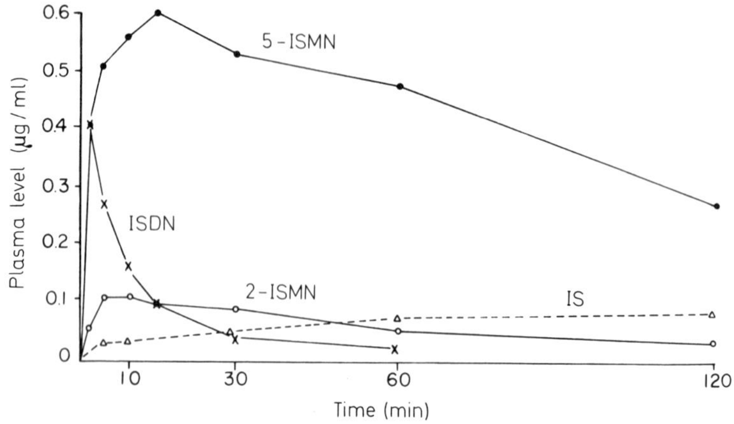

Fig. 7. Plasma levels of ^{14}C-isosorbide dinitrate and metabolites after a 1.0 mg/kg intravenous dose. IS, isosorbide; ISDN, isosorbide dinitrate; ISMN, isosorbide mononitrate. (SISENWINE and RUELIUS, 1971; with the permission of the authors and Williams and Wilkins)

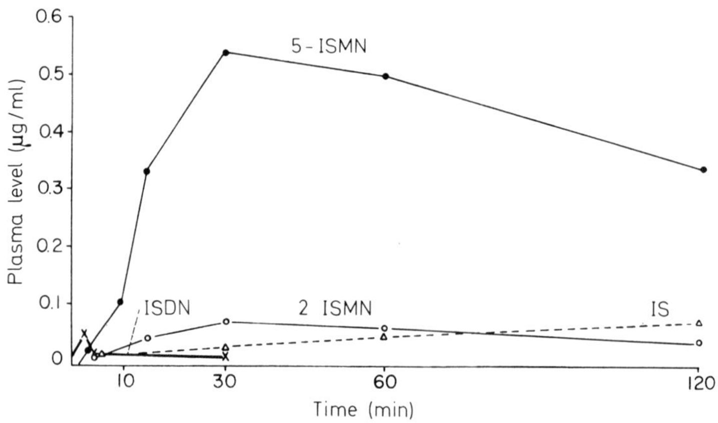

Fig. 8. Plasma levels of ^{14}C-isosorbide dinitrate and metabolites after a 1.0 mg/kg oral dose. IS, isosorbide; ISDN, isosorbide dinitrate; ISMN, isosorbide mononitrate. (SISENWINE and RUELIUS, 1971; with the permission of the authors and Williams and Wilkins)

1/7 the concentration. SHERBER et al. (1970) used gas chromatography (sensitive to as little as 0.01 µg ISD) and noted a similar rapid rate of disappearance of intact ISD from rabbit blood after i.v. administration.

SISENWINE and RUELIUS (1971) observed a quantitatively different blood clearance pattern after oral administration of ISD. Only minute quantities (0.02 µg/ml) of unchanged material briefly appeared in the circulation (Fig. 8). The major metabolite 5-ISMN reached its peak concentration at a later time (30 min) but also disappeared at a $t_{1/2}$ of about 2 hrs. 2-ISMN was again found to parallel 5-ISMN but at a much lower concentration. Free isosorbide was present after both i.v. or oral administration.

7. Urinary Excretion

a) GTN Metabolites — Urinary Excretion. NEEDLEMAN and KRANTZ (1965) identified the urinary metabolites to be 1,3-GDN, 1,2-GDN, and trace amounts of GMN after oral treatment of rats with GTN. DI CARLO et al. (1968) administered ^{14}C-GTN orally and accounted for 21% of the original radioactivity in the urine. At 4 hrs they found: no unchanged GTN, 2% of the administered dose as 1,3- and 1,2-GDN, 4% as GMN, and 7% as glycerol. They accounted for 20% in the feces and another 20% was elimination as exhaled CO_2. BOGAERT et al. (1969a) identified 1,3-GDN and GMN in rabbit urine after the i.v. administration of GTN. They reported that phenobarbital increased the rate and amount of metabolite excretion whereas with SKF-525A pretreatment there were no metabolites excreted in the urine after GTN. After i.v. administration of 1,3-GDN, 1,3-GDN and GMN were found in the urine, whereas after 1,2-GDN treatment (i.v.) only GMN was detected. NEEDLEMAN et al. (1971) administered ^{14}C-GTN intravenously and recovered 50% of the administered radioactivity in the pooled 24 hr urine. The major urinary metabolite was GMN

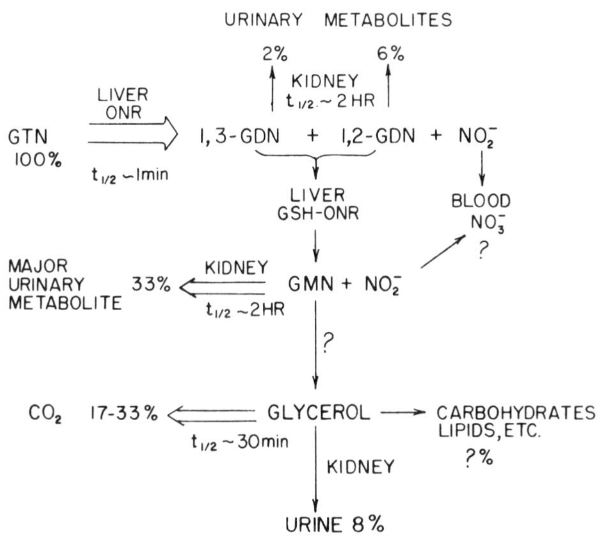

Fig. 9. Schematic representation of the *in vivo* metabolism, clearance, and excretion of glycerol nitrates following the administration of ^{14}C-GTN to rats. The percentage indicates the original ^{14}C-radio-activity administered as GTN. The urinary metabolites were from pooled 24 hr samples (NEEDLEMAN, et al., 1971). The exhaled CO_2 data represents the total for 24 hrs (DI CARLO et al., 1968; NEEDLEMAN et al., 1971). The blood disappearance and urine appearance data was taken from JOHNSON et al. (1972) and NEEDLEMAN et al. (1972). All the half times ($t_{1/2}$) were from *in vivo* experiments

(65%) and the total of the GMN and the water-soluble metabolites (presumably including glycerol) made up 80% of the excreted label. Four percent of the urinary radioactivity was 1,3-GDN and an additional 12% was in the form of 1,2-GDN. The pattern of urinary metabolites from GTN was not changed in animals that were pretreated with phenobarbital, SKF-525A, bromobenzene, or GTN (NEEDLEMAN et al., 1970).

b) GTN Degradation and Elimination Sequence. The metabolic pathway for the degradation and elimination of GTN is summarized in Fig. 9. Administration of GTN to rats was associated with an extremely transient blood level of the unchanged parent compound ($t_{1/2}$ 1 min; JOHNSON et al., 1972). The GTN appears to be rapidly degraded by GSH-organic nitrate reductase (ONR) to 1,3- and 1,2-GDN (NEEDLEMAN and KRANTZ, 1965; NEEDLEMAN and HUNTER, 1965). GDN in turn was degraded to GMN by the same liver enzyme but at a much slower rate than the intact nitrate ester (NEEDLEMAN and HUNTER, 1965). The blood metabolite level consisted of 1,3-GDN, 1,2-GDN, and GMN. The blood disappearance rate was quite slow ($t_{1/2}$ 2 hrs) and was regulated by the rate at which the metabolites were excreted by the kidney into the urine (NEEDLEMAN et al., 1972) A portion of the labeled compound was converted to CO_2 which was then exhaled, thus less than 100% of the original label appeared in the urine (DI CARLO et al., 1968; NEEDLEMAN et al., 1971). The oxidation of GTN to CO_2 necessitates the formation of glycerol, the mechanism and tissue site of glycerol formation remains unknown (NEEDLEMAN et al., 1971) however, any glycerol that was formed could be phosphorylated by glycerokinase and thereby enter the glycolytic pathway. DI CARLO et al. (1969) recovered labeled lipid, glycogen, protein and nucleic acids in liver following the administration of ^{14}C-GTN. Finally, the fate of the formed inorganic nitrite has not been extensively studied. HEPPEL and PORTERFIELD (1949) demonstrated that rat liver and kidney homogenates catalyzed the oxidation of inorganic nitrite to inorganic nitrate. In this reaction hydrogen peroxide from an oxidase was utilized by catalase for the coupled oxidation of inorganic nitrite.

c) Other Organic Nitrates. The *in vivo* transformation of the vasodilator organic nitrates was determined by ether extraction of the pooled urine of rats treated (10 mg, i.p.) with these compounds (NEEDLEMAN and HUNTER, 1965). The chromatogram of the urine extracts showed that some of the parent molecule of each compound appears in the urine along with an assortment of metabolites. The major metabolites of GTN were 1,3-GDN and 1,2-GDN, with a trace of GMN. The urine from MHN-treated rats showed one definite and traces of two other metabolites, an indication that the denitration of the metabolites continued *in vivo*. PETN was excreted with three metabolites. ETN was excreted with four major metabolites and a trace of another. ISD was excreted primarily as one metabolite, with traces of the parent compound and of a second metabolite. The qualitative pattern of urinary metabolites was strikingly similar to the pattern of nitrate metabolites extracted from *in vitro* incubation of nitrates and liver homogenates. The enzymatic denitration of organic nitrates lead to the generation of water soluble metabolites which were readily eliminated in the urine. Thus, the *in vivo* mechanism of organic nitrate detoxication appears to be dependent upon the enzymic denitration observed with hepatic glutathione-organic nitrate reductase.

NEEDLEMAN et al. (1972) studied the quantitative pattern of the urinary excretion of nitrates metabolites following intravenous administration of ^{14}C-labeled organic nitrates. The rates of appearance of urinary metabolites directly reflected the rates of blood clearance (Fig.6) of organic nitrate metabolites. The accumulated sum of the ISD and MHN urinary metabolites approached 100% of the administered label by 24 hrs, whereas, urinary excretion of GTN did not (NEEDLEMAN et al., 1972). Approximately 20% of administered GTN has been accounted for as carbon dioxide (DICARLO et al., 1968; NEEDLEMAN et al., 1971). The urinary radioactivity represented nitrate metabolites that were poor substrates for further degradation. This was supported by the observation that bilateral nephrectomy of rats results in constant blood levels of metabolites (NEEDLEMAN et al., 1972).

d) Isosorbide Dinitrate Degradation and Elimination. NEEDLEMAN and HUNTER (1965) demonstrated the denitration of isosorbide dinitrate (ISD) by hepatic glutathione-organic nitrate reductase. Polar isosorbide nitrate metabolites were extracted from rat urine after ISD administration (NEEDLEMAN and HUNTER, 1965; NEEDLEMAN et al., 1972) but these metabolites were not identified. DIETZ (1967) qualitatively identified 2- and 5-isosorbide mononitrate (ISMN) in dog and human urine after the oral administration of ISD.

SISENWINE and RUELIUS (1971) treated dogs with ^{14}C-ISD (orally or i.v.) and studied blood clearance (Section II.A.6.) and urinary excretion. Thin layer chromatography exhibited a similar urinary metabolite pattern in dogs by either route of administration. 80% of the administered radioactivity was found in the pooled 24 hrs urine. No unchanged ISD was found in the urine nor was 2-ISMN. The 5-ISMN and isosorbide (IS) were found to contribute about 5% and 16% of the radioactivity found in the pooled 24 hr urine. They also found other polar metabolites which they presumed to be glucuronides. The polar metabolites did not appear to be the result of direct conjugation of isosorbide, since ^{14}C-isosorbide was recovered unchanged from the urine after oral administration (SISENWINE and RUELIUS, 1971).

REED et al. (1971) further characterized the urinary metabolites after the oral administration of ^{14}C-ISD to dogs. No unchanged ISD was excreted. Twenty to thirty percent of the carbon skeleton of ISD was excreted as neutral metabolites principally isosorbide (IS), 5-ISMN (or isosorbide-5-endomononitrate), 2-ISMN (or isosorbide-2-exomononitrate), and isoidide. The remainder primarily consisted of the ether glucuronide of 5-ISMN and ether monoglucuronides of IS.

The metabolic pathway for the degradation and elimination of ISD is summarized in Fig. 10 (SISENWINE and RUELIUS, 1971). Administration of ISD was associated with an extremely transient blood level of unchanged parent compound (rat $t_{1/2}$ 1 min, JOHNSON et al., 1972; dog $t_{1/2}$ 7 min, SISENWINE and RUELIUS, 1971). There were only negligible blood levels of unchanged ISD following oral treatment (SISENWINE and RUELIUS, 1971). The initial biotransformation occurred by denitration in the presence of hepatic glutathione-organic nitrate reductase (NEEDLEMAN and HUNTER, 1965; JOHNSON et al., 1972). The 5-ISMN was present in much higher concentrations in the blood than the 2-ISMN thereby indicating a stereospecificity in the biotransformation (SISENWINE and RUELIUS, 1971). The mononitrates disappeared from the plasma more slowly than the parent ISD. Low levels of IS also

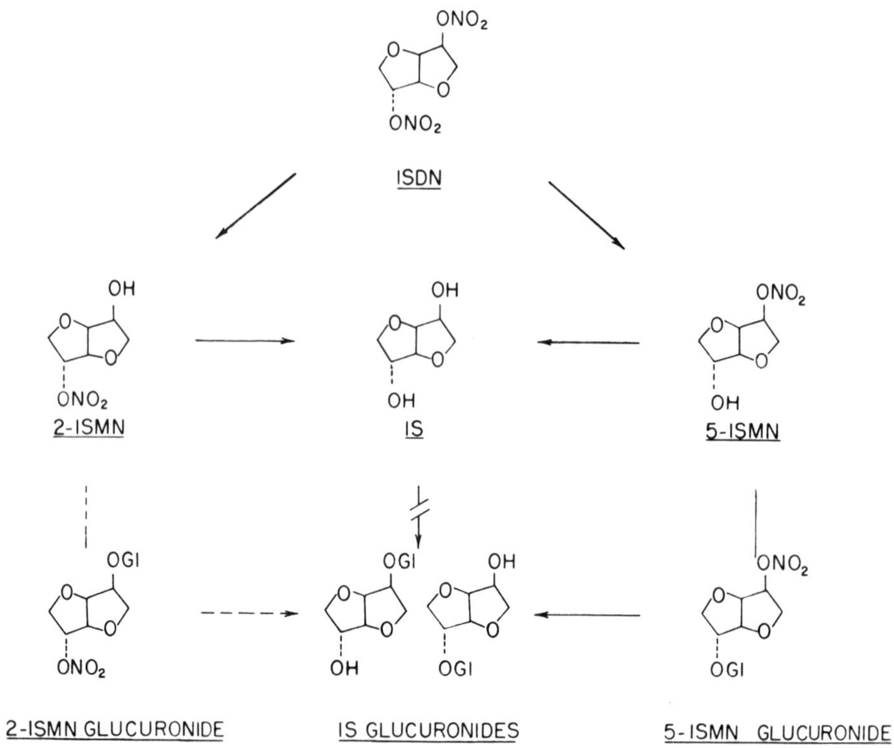

Fig. 10. Metabolic biotransformation of isosorbide dinitrate. (SISENWINE and RUELIUS, 1971; with the permission of the authors and Williams and Wilkins)

appeared in the plasma. Unlike GTN, the disappearance of the metabolites of ISD not only was determined by renal filtration but also required conjugation leading to the formation of glucuronides of 5-ISMN and of IS (REED et al., 1971) (Fig. 10).

ROSSEEL and BOGAERT (1973) treated rats orally with the dinitrates of isosorbide, and its stereoisomers isomannide, and isoidide. They found only trace amounts of the parent compounds in the urine, but qualitatively identified the mononitrates, the denitrated alcohols, and large amounts of conjugated mononitrates. They found evidence for inversion from the endo- to the exo-position, since after the administration of isosorbide dinitrate, isoiodide mononitrate and isoidide were found in the urine. Similarly, after isomannide dinitrate treatment 5-isosorbide mononitrate and isosorbide were found.

B. Metabolic Pathway in the Degradation of Pentaerythritol-Tetranitrate and Trinitrate

1. Absorption, Distribution, and Excretion of Pentaerythritol Tetranitrate (PETN)

DI CARLO et al. (1965c) orally administered radioactive PE and PETN to mice. The PE was rapidly absorbed and excreted unchanged in the urine, whereas PETN was absorbed slowly and excreted as PE. DI CARLO et al. (1967a, b) demonstrated in rats that PE and its mono-, di-, and trinitrates, rather than PETN, accounted for the major radioactivity in the blood after oral treatment with ^{14}C-PETN. They also showed evidence that absorption of PETN from the large intestine was enhanced due to degradation of PETN into more rapidly absorbed metabolites. About 7 to 8% of ^{14}C-PETN was absorbed from the gastrointestinal tract during the first hour, 14% after 2 hrs, 24% after 4 hrs, and 60% after 18 hrs. 10% of the dose was eliminated in the feces by the end of 18 hrs. At 1 hr, there was little PE-dinitrate in the blood, but it increased to 28% of the radioactivity by 4 hrs. PE-mononitrate was the only nitrate present at 18 hrs. "PETN and PE-trinitrate were not detected in blood at any time interval studied" (DI CARLO et al., 1967b).

DI CARLO et al. (1965a) incubated ^{14}C-PETN with human blood and chromatographically assayed the metabolites. The red blood cells were more effective than plasma in enzymatically degrading PETN in a stepwise fashion to yield PE-trinitrate, PE-dinitrate, PE-mononitrate, and possibly PE. Rat blood plasma and erythrocytes showed a strong binding affinity for PETN and PE-trinitrate, whereas PE-dinitrate and PE-mononitrate were poorly bound by plasma or red cells (DI CARLO et al., 1965b).

The first urine collection (at 2 hrs) after the oral administration of ^{14}C-PETN to rats, contained PE-mononitrate as the main metabolite being 52% of the administered dose, PE-dinitrate was 33%, and PE was 16% (DI CARLO et al., 1967b). By 18 hrs there was no PE-dinitrate, 27% of the radioactivity was PE-mononitrate and 73% was PE. There was no detectable PETN or PE-trinitrate in the urine.

2. Absorption, Distribution, and Excretion of PE-Trinitrate

The lack of aqueous solubility of PETN has generated interest in studying the properties of the more soluble PE-trinitrate. PE-trinitrate was partially metabolized by hepatic glutathione organic nitrate reductase (NEEDLEMAN and HUNTER, 1965) and by perfused rat livers (NEEDLEMAN and HARKEY, 1971). DI CARLO et al. (1969a) compared the relative rates of absorption, plasma levels, and urinary excretion of GTN, PETN, and PE-trinitrate after oral administration of high doses (10 mg/kg) to rats (Fig. 11). PE-trinitrate was found to be absorbed much faster than PETN but at a comparable rate to GTN. The approximate half-time for blood clearance rate for GTN (metabolites) was 2 to 2.5 hrs, and for the PE-trinitrate was 2 to 3 hrs, which was consistent with the similar urinary clearance rate for both of these nitrates (DI CARLO et al., 1969a). On the other hand, they reported the unusual finding that there was no change in plasma levels of radioactivity after PETN administration, and only a slow rate of urinary clearance of the label.

By 18 hrs, 50% of the radioactivity after oral PE-trinitrate treatment appeared in the urine as PE (62%), PE-mononitrate (23%) and PE-dinitrate (16%) (DI CARLO et al., 1969a). There was no (i.e. $< 1\%$) PE-trinitrate present in the blood. Even at the earliest time sample (1 hr), there was only a trace amount (4%) of the PE-dinitrate, some PE-mononitrate (28%) and predominantly PE (67%). Thus, as with PETN (Section II, B. 1.), following oral administration of PE-trinitrate there was little or no unchanged parent compound present in the circulation. Similar

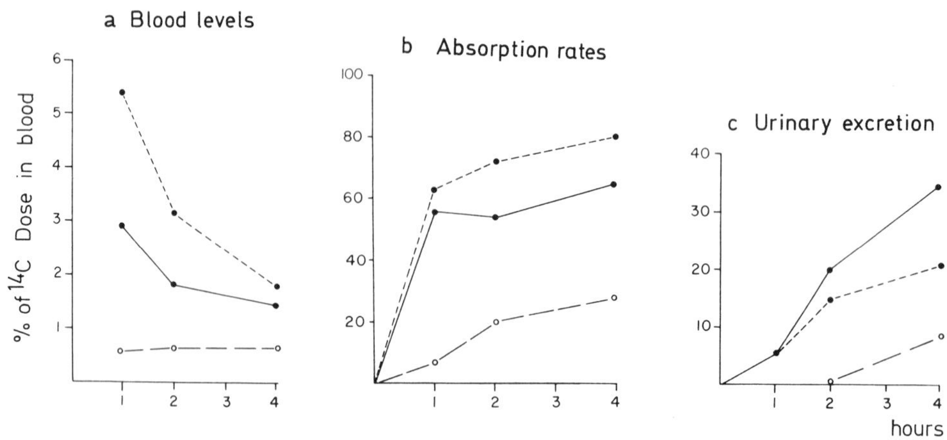

Fig. 11a—c. Comparison of rates of change of radioactivity in rats after the oral administration of organic nitrates (10 mg/kg) PE-trinitrate, ×; GTN, ●: and PETN, ○. (Presented with permission from DICARLO et al., 1969a and with the consent of Pergamon Press)

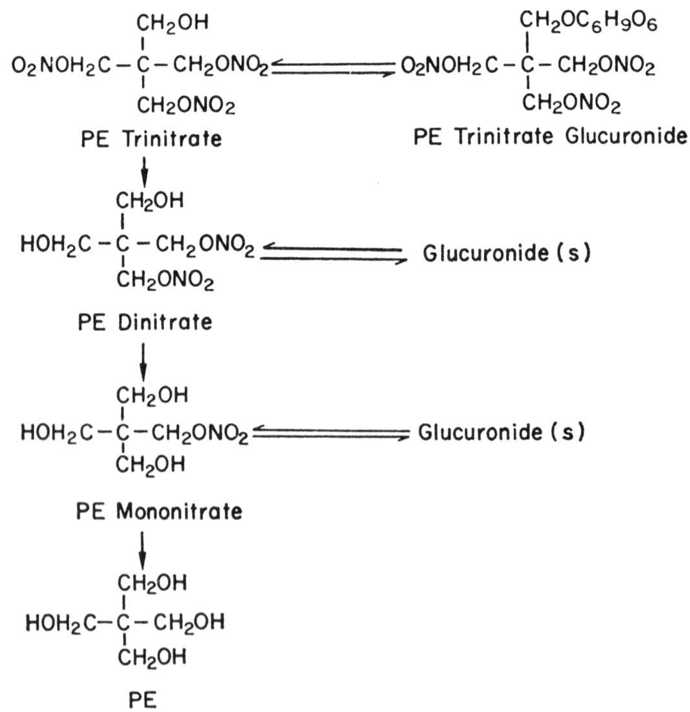

Fig. 12. Pathways of PE trinitrate biotransformation. (Reproduced with permission from CREW et al., 1971 and Pergamon Press)

results were obtained when PE-trinitrate was administered orally to dogs (DI CARLO et al., 1969b).

CREW et al. (1971) demonstrated bilary excretion of PE-trinitrate metabolites when ^{14}C-PE-trinitrate was administered intravenously (51% of dose at 4 hrs) or orally (31%). This difference was found to be due to PE-dinitrate-glucuronide, whereas, the PE-trinitrate-glucuronide was the same 10% of the dose in 4 hrs after i.v. or oral treatment. The contribution of the enterohepatic circulation was indicated by the observation that bile collection caused a 60% reduction in the radioactivity that appeared in the urine of ^{14}C-PE trinitrate treated rats. Thus, the bilary glucuronides were reabsorbed from the intestine of intact animals (CREW et al., 1971). They proposed that absorption was preceded by hydrolysis with intestinal β-glucuronidase. The metabolic degradation sequence is schematically presented in Fig. 12 (CREW et al., 1971).

C. Degradation of Other Organic Nitrate Esters

1. Ethylene Glycol Dinitrate (EGDN)

CLARK and LITCHFIELD (1967) incubated EGDN with rat blood at 37° and demonstrated that breakdown of the parent compound was complete within 2 hrs resulting in the generation of ethylene glycol mononitrate (EGMN). Inorganic nitrite was initially produced and was itself metabolized to nitrate. EGMN was resistant to *in vitro* destruction by rat blood which degraded only 4% of the material in 4 hr.

Injection of high concentrations of EGDN subcutaneously in rats produced peak blood levels of the parent compound in 30 min and fell to zero by 8 hr, whereas EGMN was rapidly produced reaching a peak at about 3 hr and falling to zero in 12 hr (CLARK *and* LITCHFIELD, 1967). Inorganic nitrite was maximal at 1 to 2 hr, falling to zero in 12 hr,whereas inorganic nitrate rose slowly to its peak at 3 to 5 hr. Sixty percent of the administered drug appeared in the urine by 24 hr. There was no EGDN, a trace of EGMN (1.5% of the administered dose), no inorganic nitrite (<0.1%) and mostly inorganic nitrate (58%) was present in the urine. Thus, the EGDN appears to be denitrated to EGMN which in turn was completely degraded in the body before urinary excretion.

2. Propylene Glycol 1,2-Dinitrate (PGDN)

CLARK and LITCHFIELD (1969) demonstrated that the metabolism of PGDN *in vitro* (rat blood) or *in vivo* (rats, s.c.) resulted in the formation of the 1- and 2-isomers of propylene glycol mononitrate, inorganic nitrite, and inorganic nitrate. The mononitrates are further metabolized *in vivo* with the result that only small amounts were excreted and the major urinary metabolite was inorganic nitrate (56% of the original PGDN).

3. 1-Chloro-2,3-Propanediol Dinitrate (CPD)

DIETZ (1967) orally treated dogs with CPD and isolated two metabolites from the urine. The metabolites were tentatively identified at 1-chloropropyl-3-glucuronide-2-

nitrate and 1-chloropropyl-2-glucuronide-3-nitrate. Presumably the initial degradation was hepatic denitration and subsequent formation of the glucuronide prior to urinary excretion.

III. Relationship between Organic Nitrate Metabolism and Biological Activity

A. Temporal Relationship between Plasma Levels of the Parent Compound and Its Metabolites and Biological Activity

1. Vasodilatation After Portal and Jugular Vein Injections

Jugular vein administration of organic nitrates in anesthetized rats resulted in a transient vasodepression, usually of a 1 to 4 min duration, depending upon the dose

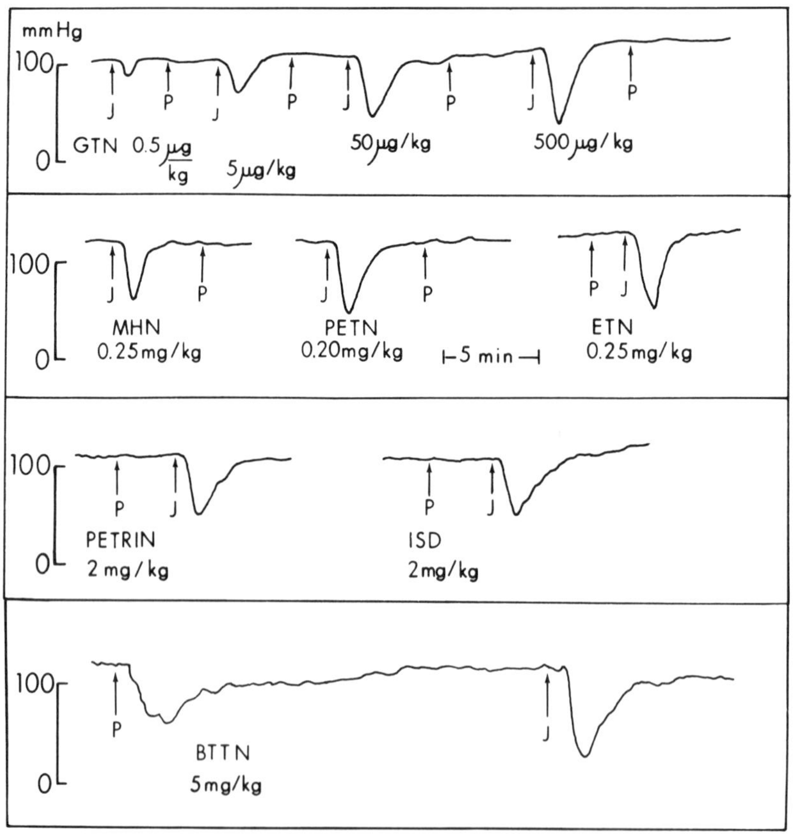

Fig. 13. The comparison between jugular vein (J) and portal vein (P) injections of organic nitrates on blood pressure responsiveness. PETRIN, pentaerythritol trinitrate; BTTN, 1,2,4-butanetriol trinitrate. (NEEDLEMAN et al., 1972; with permission from Williams and Wilkins)

(NEEDLEMAN et al., 1972). There was essentially no difference in the duration of the fall in blood pressure produced by GTN or by MHN, pentaerythritol tetranitrate (PETN), ISD, or ETN (Fig. 13). Jugular vein administration of log doses of GTN produced a typical dose-response curve, whereas injection of the same amount of drug into the portal vein produced no blood pressure fall. This experiment demonstrated that the liver has the capacity in a single passage to prevent organic nitrate-induced vasodepression. The only exception found was 1,2,4-butanetriol trinitrate. Low doses (1.25 mg/kg or less) injected in the portal vein produced no response, but higher doses (2.5 and 5 mg/kg) exceeded the liver capacity and a vasodepression was produced (Fig. 13). This compound which has some potential as an antianginal agent was found previously to be more slowly degraded by glutathione-organic nitrate reductase than the other drugs tested (NEEDLEMAN and HUNTER, 1965).

COMMARATO et al. (1973) compared the vasodilation produced by GTN or PE-trinitrate when injected either intravenously or into the portal vein (pv). In rats i.v. administered GTN was a 100 times more potent than the comparable p.v. treatment and similarly PE-trinitrate was 50 times more potent when administered i.v. instead of p.v. They observed similar results in cats and dogs. These workers reported that extremely high doses of GTN or PE-trinitrate given by intraduodenal or oral administration caused a vasodepression, but they were only able to show a very transient (~ 1 to 2 min) decrease in coronary vessel resistance with the PE-trinitrate. On the other hand, in previous work reported by this laboratory they were unable to demonstrate blood levels of intact parent compound (i.e. either PE-tetranitrate or PE-trinitrate) nor substantial amounts of the initial metabolite (PE-dinitrate) after oral administration of either PE-tetranitrate or PE-trinitrate (DAVIDSON et al., 1971). Finally, the oral administration of very high doses of organic nitrates in an effort to overcome hepatic degradation capacity would be expected to exaggerate side effects and to induce tolerance to the administered agent and cross tolerance to GTN (SCHELLING and LASAGNA, 1967).

2. Blood Clearance and Biological Effectiveness

NEEDLEMAN et al. (1972) collected carotid artery blood samples at 10 sec intervals after jugular vein administration of radioactive organic nitrate to rats. The extremely rapid disappearance of the intact parent compounds necessitated rapid sampling. The initial fall in blood concentration of the parent compound was at a half-time rate of 10 to 14 sec for GTN, ISD, and MHN. The disappearance of MHN was a first order process and was more than 99% complete by 90 sec. The clearance of GTN and ISD was biphasic and proceeded with a half-time of about one minute in the slower portion of the curves. Blood was cleared of more than 80% of the parent nitrate by one minute. By 10 min only 5% of the radioactivity found at 10 sec remained and by 15 min there was no detectable unchanged GTN or ISD in the blood. The rates of disappearance of the metabolites were slower than their appearance several orders of magnitude (Fig. 6). The approximate half-times for metabolite clearance from the blood for MHN was 2 hrs, for ISD was 2.5 hrs, and for GTN was almost 4 hrs (Fig. 6). (NEEDLEMAN et al., 1972). The blood clearance data following intravenous administration of labeled organic nitrates explicitly indicate that the

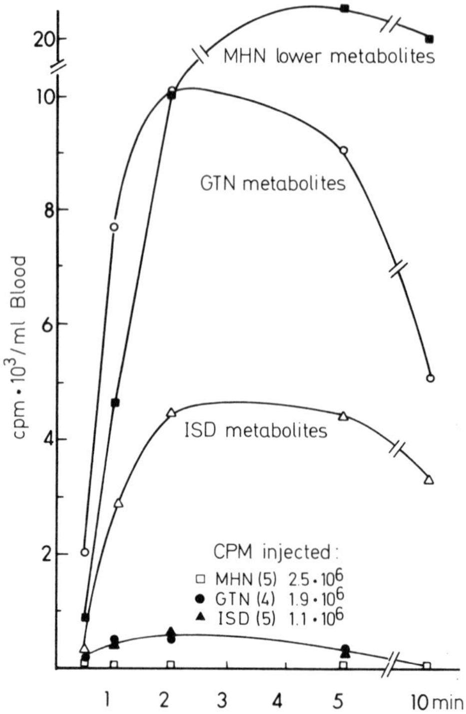

Fig. 14. The blood clearance of organic nitrates and their metabolites after portal vein injection in rats. The following compounds were administered: MHN-1-^{14}C (1 μC, 1 mg/kg), GTN-1, 3-^{14}C (1 μC, 0.5 mg/kg) and ISD-^{14}C (uniformly labeled, 0.5 μC, 0.25 mg/kg). (NEEDLEMAN et al., 1972; with permission from Williams and Wilkins)

transient duration (1 to 4 min) of the biological response (vasodepression) correlated directly with the transient circulation time (80% removed by 1 min) for the parent compound. The vasodepression (1 to 4 min) was completely out of phase with the circulation time for the nitrate metabolites ($t_{1/2}$ 2 hrs) (NEEDLEMAN et al., 1972).

The radioactive organic nitrates were injected as a bolus directly into the portal vein to determine if hepatic inactivation was the result of binding or of rapid biotransformation (Fig. 14; NEEDLEMAN et al., 1972). The results demonstrated that little or none of the intact parent compound passes through the liver after portal vein injection. There was, therefore, no circulating intact nitrates and there was no blood pressure depression (Figs. 13 and 14). The organic nitrate metabolites had little effect on systemic blood pressure, since following portal administration of labeled nitrates there was an immediate appearance of high blood levels of metabolites without production of a vasodilation. These portal vein experiments indicate that *in vivo* the liver could inactivate even a bolus injection of organic nitrates, which represented an extreme condition, since normally the drugs reached the hepatic circulation after dilution in the blood and tissue and were present at a lower concentration.

3. Plasma Levels After Oral Administration

a) Experimental Animals. SISENWINE and RUELIUS (1971) treated dogs with ^{14}C-ISD and observed only transient blood levels of intact ISD (Fig. 7) after intravenous administration, and they found essentially no parent compound after oral administration (Fig. 8). On the other hand, in both cases there were high blood concentrations of 5-ISMN for long periods of time. DI CARLO et al. (1967a, 1967b) observed similar results in that they found no intact nitrates in the blood following oral administration of PETN or PE-trinitrate. NEEDLEMAN et al. (1972) orally administered MHN or GTN to rats and noted rapid absorption with little or no intact organic nitrates appearing in the blood, but with high levels of metabolites. They also demonstrated that no intact GTN was absorbed into the lymph after the oral administration, thus eliminating this possible route of avoiding hepatic inactivation. BOGAERT et al. (1970) observed that oral administration of GTN to rabbits did not lower blood pressure. This finding is consistent with the observation that intact organic nitrate is required for vasodilation and that after oral administration of nitrates no unchanged parent compound reaches the circulation to produce a vasodilation.

b) Humans. BOGAERT and ROSSEEL (1972) developed a sensitive gas chromatographic method for following plasma levels of organic nitrates. They administered GTN to humans sublingually (3 min under the tongue) and noted peak plasma levels of the parent compound in the first blood sample at 4 min and clearance rate in which at least half of the intact GTN disappeared in 1 to 3 min. A transient tachycardia was associated with the transient duration of circulating GTN. ROSSEEL and BOGAERT (1973) treated 5 human volunteers with ISD sublingually and found (gas chromatography) peak blood levels of intact ISD by 6 min. The blood clearance rate on the parent compound was rapid with 60% disappearance occurring by 15 min or less.

DAVIDSON et al. (1971) treated 15 male volunteers with ^{14}C-PETN (20 or 40 mg tablet). The pattern of metabolites in blood or urine of humans was exactly the same as in experimental animals. By 48 hr, 60% of the 20 mg dose and 32% of the 40 mg dose appeared in the urine. PE and PE-mononitrate were the major urinary metabolites accounting for 98% of the radioactivity. A substantial portion of the administered drug was excreted in the feces, corresponding to 32 and 41% of the 20 and 40 mg doses. The half-time for renal elimination of the PETN metabolites (either 20 or 40 mg dose) was 8 hrs for PE, and about 7 hrs for PE-mononitrate. Peak blood levels occurred from 4 to 8 hrs. *PETN and PE-trinitrate were not detected in blood* (Fig. 15). The major circulating metabolite was PE with lower levels of PE-mononitrate and trace amounts of PE dinitrate (DAVIDSON et al., 1971). There was no qualitative or quantitative difference in the excretion patterns and blood levels exhibited by coronary artery disease patients ($n = 5$) and controls ($n = 10$). PARKER et al. (1973) have shown that PE-dinitrate, PE-mononitrate, and PE have little or no peripheral or coronary vasodilator activity and cannot account for the biological activity of the parent compound.

PE-trinitrate is more soluble than the largely insoluble PETN, therefore, the trinitrate has vasodilator potential. ^{14}C-PE-trinitrate was administered to humans

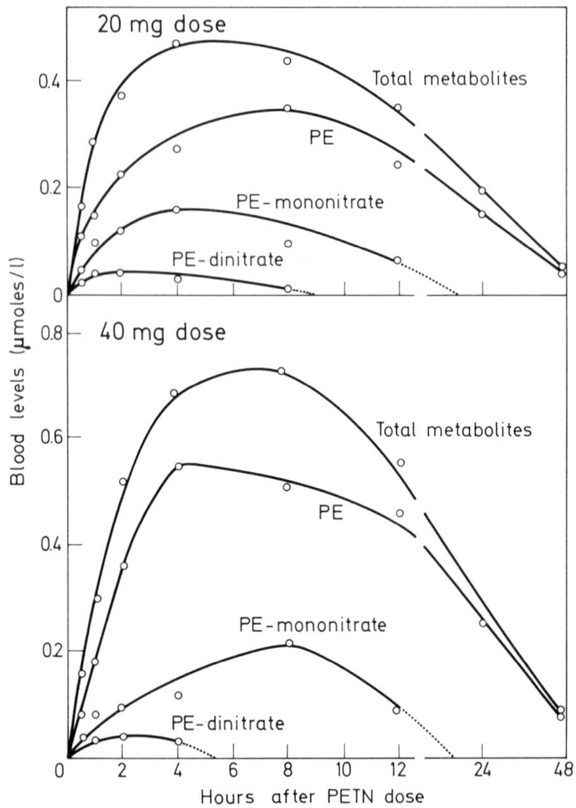

Fig. 15. Mean human blood levels of total radioactivity and of drug metabolites after 20- and 40-mg oral doses of ^{14}C-pentaerythritol tetranitrate (From DAVIDSON et al., 1971; with permission from Am. Pharmaceutical Assoc.)

by either the oral or sublingual route (DAVIDSON et al., 1970, 1971). The improved solubility characteristics were reflected in that only 2% was recovered in the feces. No PE-trinitrate, and essentially no PE-dinitrate were in the urine. The principal urinary metabolites were PE (30%) and PE-mononitrate (69%) and the half-time of renal elimination was 10 and 7 hrs, respectively. The mononitrate was the principal urinary metabolite whereas PE represented the major blood form. No intact PE-trinitrate appeared in the blood (Fig. 16). The PE-dinitrate was present for only 2 to 3 hrs.

The qualitative and quantitative pattern of biotransformation of organic nitrates in humans is the same as in experimental animals. The primary route of degradation of organic nitrates was enzymatic denitration by hepatic glutathione-organic nitrate reductase. NEEDLEMAN et al. (1972) showed that fresh human liver biopsy samples had the same maximum enzyme velocity (0.13 mmole/kg liver/20 min) for glutathione-dependent denitration as does rat liver (0.13 mmoles/kg liver/20 min) which

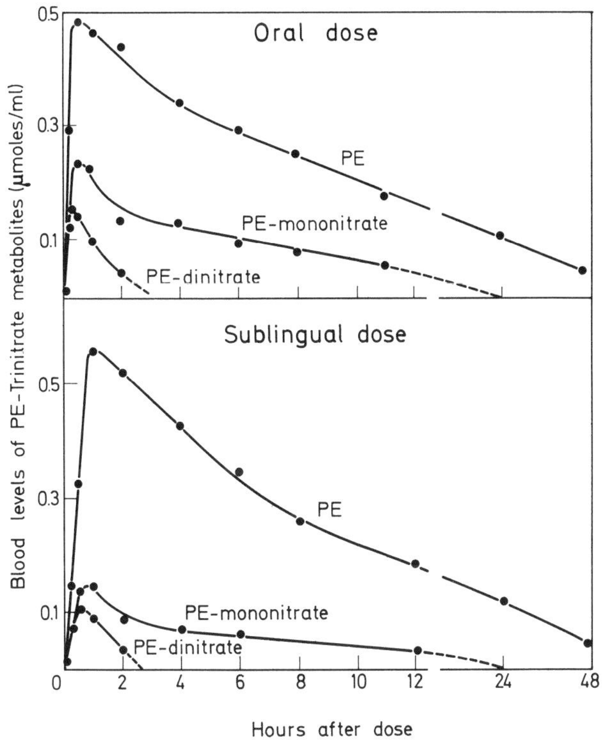

Fig. 16. Mean blood levels of drug metabolites after oral and sublingual administration of 10 mg of PE-trinitrate to 5 subjects. (DAVIDSON et al., 1971; with permission from C. V. Mosby)

was the model species for most of the nitrate biotransformation studies. Since these enzyme comparisons were on a liver weight basis, humans actually have a total of at least 200 times more enzyme available than rats.

B. Biological Activity of Metabolites

1. Glyceryl Trinitrate

NEEDLEMAN et al. (1969) compared the potency of a number of organic nitrates as blood pressure depressants in dogs. The compounds were compared by evaluating the dosage required to produce a 10 to 20% vasodepression. GTN (25 μg/kg) was at least 10 to 14 times more potent than its denitration products the glyceryl dinitrates. The highly water soluble breakdown product of GTN metabolism, GMN (>1000 μg/kg), lacked vasodilator activity, whereas, inorganic nitrite required very high doses (more than 40 times the GTN dose) to depress blood pressure. Inorganic nitrate (>6000 μg/kg) was found to be completely inactive as a vasodilator. PETN (20 μg/kg) and butanetiol trinitrate (45 μg/kg) were more potent than their lower nitrates. In general, the more active vasodepressor compounds were the nitrates with high oil/water partition coefficients. The less lipid-soluble compounds required progressively higher doses to elicit an equivalent fall in blood pressure (NEEDLEMAN et al., 1969).

BOGAERT et al. (1968) compared the cardiovascular effects of GTN, 1,3-GDN, and 1,2-GDN. They found little difference in effectiveness between the glyceryl dinitrates. The GDN dose response curves were parallel to that of GTN. GDN was only 2% as active as GTN in lowering guinea pig blood pressure, 0.2% in relaxing rabbit aorta strips, and 5% as active as GTN in decreasing dog hindleg resistance.

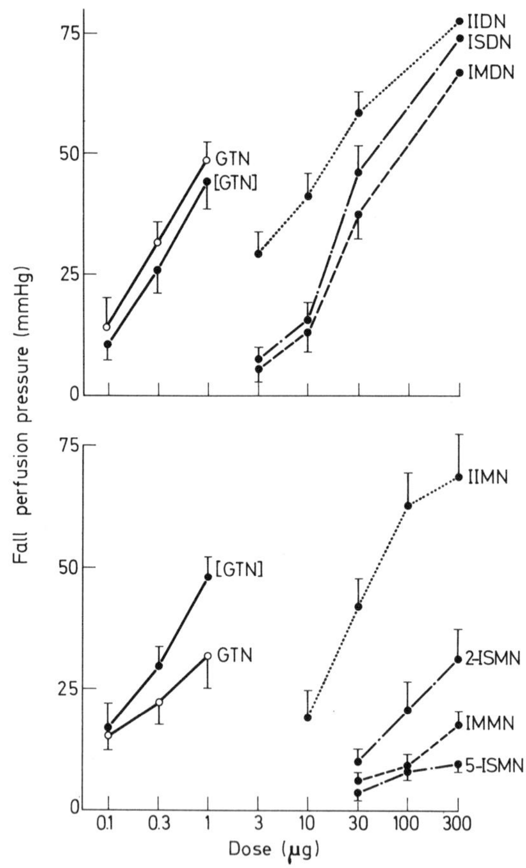

Fig. 17. Injection of different nitrates into the perfused hindleg of the dog. Upper graph: dinitrates of isoidide (IIDN), isosorbide (ISDN) and isomannide (IMDN) and nitroglycerin (GTN) in a group of 6 dogs; all doses were given to all animals except for the 300 μg dose of the dinitrates which was given to 2 dogs only. Lower graph: mononitrates of isoidide (IIMN) and isomannide (IMMN), 2-isosorbide mononitrate (2-ISMN) and 5-isosorbide mononitrate (5-ISMN) and nitroglycerin (GTN) in 6 dogs; all doses were given to all animals. In both graphs, GTN stands for the randomized injections and [GTN] stands for the preliminary dose response curve. (BOGAERT and ROSSEEL, 1972; with permission from the authors and Springer-Verlag)

2. Isosorbide Dinitrate

WENDT (1972) compared the cardiovascular potency of GTN, ISD, 5-ISMN, and 2-ISMN. In order to produce a 10 ml/min change in blood flow in the circumflex coronary artery in dogs the following doses were required: GTN — 1 μg; ISD — 100 μg; 2-ISMN — 300 μg; 5-ISMN — 3000 μg. The order of potency required to reduce pressure by 10 mm Hg in the perfused dog hindlimb was: GTN — 0.1 μg; ISD — 2 μg; 2-ISMN — 10 μg; and 5-ISMN — 200 μg (WENDT, 1972).

BOGAERT and ROSSEEL (1972) compared the vasodilator potency of isomeric organic nitrates on the perfused dog hindleg (Fig. 17). In each case the denitration metabolite of isosorbide dinitrate (ISDN), isoidide dinitrate (IIDN), and isomannide dinitrate (IMDN) were less potent than the parent compound. The 2-ISMN was only 1/6 as potent a vasodilator of the dog hindlimb as the intact ISDN, whereas the 5-ISMN was only 1/60 the potency (BOGAERT and ROSSEEL, 1972; Fig. 17).

SISENWINE and RUELIUS (1971) clearly demonstrated that 5-ISMN is the predominant circulating metabolite in the blood after either oral or intravenous administration of ISD (Fig. 8 and 9). Much lower concentrations of the 2-ISMN metabolite were present. 5-ISMN has been clearly shown by WENDT (1972) and BOGAERT and ROSSEEL (1972) to be only 1/30 to 1/60 as potent as ISD. These observations strongly support the evidence that the intact parent nitrate ester is the biologically active species and that denitration inactivates the compound.

3. Pentaerythritol Trinitrate

PARKER et al. (1973) demonstrated that the vasodilator action of PE-trinitrate was not due to its metabolites. They demonstrated that PE-trinitrate was 1/5 as potent as GTN as a coronary vasodilator and as a systemic vasodepressor. PE-dinitrate was only 1/50 as potent as the PE-trinitrate, PE-monoitrate was 1/100 the potency of PE-trinitrate and PE was completely inactive.

IV. Summary and Conclusions

The biotransformation of organic nitrate esters is implemented by a redox reaction and is manifested by the conversion of a potent lipid soluble vasodilator compound into water soluble metabolites which have much lower biological potency and which are readily excreted in the urine. Studies involving (1) the isolated partially purified liver enzyme from rats, guinea pigs, hogs, and humans, (2) isolated perfused rat livers, (3) eviscerated rats, (4) rat, rabbit, dog, and human blood distribution studies, and (5) rat, rabbit, dog, and human urinary excretion profiles; all have indicated that destruction of organic nitrates is rapidly and specifically catalyzed by hepatic glutathione-organic nitrate reductase.

The blood clearance data explicitly indicate that the parent nitrate ester (after intravenous administration) has a transient lifetime, whereas, the nitrate metabolites circulate for hours. The duration of the vasodilator effectiveness of organic nitrates was in direct temporal correlation with blood levels of the intact ester and was

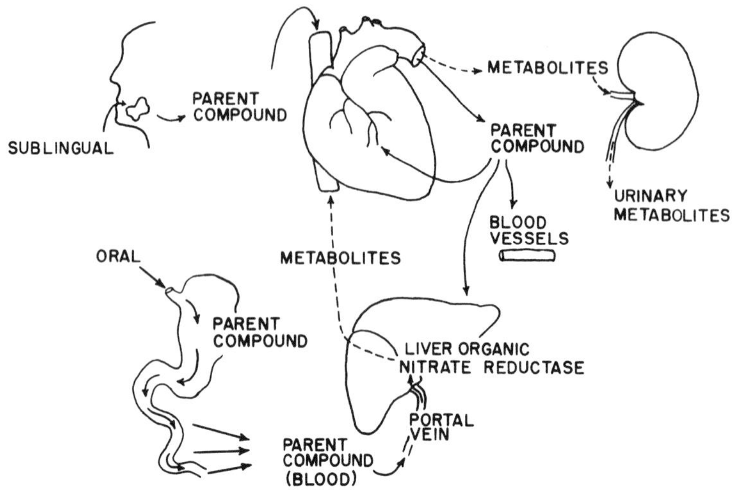

Fig. 18. Comparison of the distribution and fate of organic nitrates administered orally or sublingually. After oral administration intact (parent) organic nitrate is absorbed from the gastrointestinal tract and is delivered through the portal vein blood to the liver where it is metabolized by glutathione organic nitrate reductase. The inactive metabolites are excreted in the urine. Sublingual administration permits exposure of the coronary and peripheral vascular smooth muscle to intact (parent) organic nitrate ester prior to liver inactivation

completely out of phase with the metabolites. Thus, the parent compound appears to be the active species.

The thrust of nitrate metabolism experiments in rats, dogs, and humans is that after oral administration of various organic nitrates, essentially none of the parent compound is present in the circulation to relax vascular smooth muscle. Thus, following oral administration, the nitrates are absorbed into the portal circulation and are, rapidly and completely degraded by the liver (glutathione-organic nitrate reductase) before reaching the systemic circulation and therefore can have little chance of producing vasodilation (schematically presented in Fig. 18). Consistent with these results are the large and growing numbers of clinical studies which indicate that orally administered organic nitrates are ineffective (see Chapter by ARONOW). According to Modell (1970), "The history of failure with so-called long-acting nitrates is an unbroken one". One would anticipate that long-term effects of a "long-lasting" vasodilator would be associated with sustained blood levels of the active compound. This has not proven to be the case. After oral administration or shortly after i.v. administration of intact nitrates, the predominant circulating species has been metabolites. The primary circulating metabolites of GTN or ISD are much too low in potency to account for the biological effect. The only other metabolite thus far tested was mannitol pentanitrate (BLUM et al., 1971) which had very weak vasodilator activity in dogs. The circulating metabolites although unassociated with the time course of the nitrate induced vasodilation would still be involved in provoking side effects. BOGAERT et al. (1971) noted severe headaches after GTN treatment of human

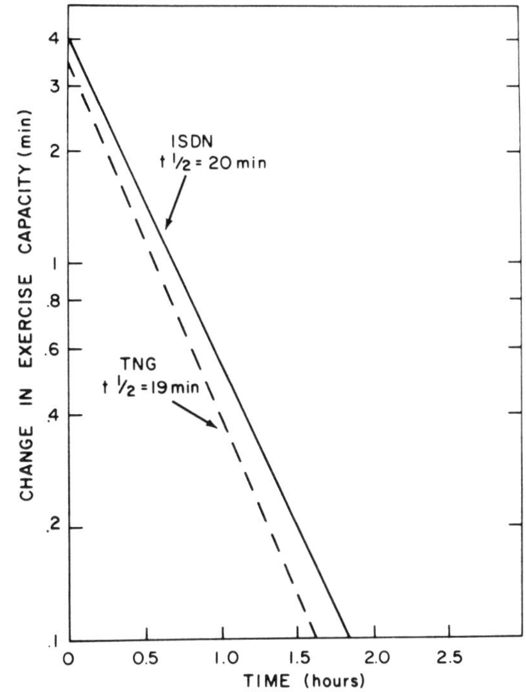

Fig. 19. Comparison of the influence of ISDN and of nitroglycerin on exercise capacity assessed at varying times after treatment. Doses of ISDN and nitroglycerin (TNG) matched to produce similar circulatory effects at rest resulted in similar increment in exercise capacity initially. This increment tended to disappear at approximately the same rate for both drugs. (GOLDSTEIN et al. 1971; with permission of the author and the Amer. Heart Assoc.)

volunteers which were out of time phase with biological effects, and the headaches were not accompanied by any change in blood pressure or heart rate.

The sublingual administration of organic nitrates still represents a rational approach to the acute relief of an angina pectoris attack. RISEMAN et al. (1958) showed that ETN, MHN and triethanolamine trinitrate were effective when administered sublingually instead of orally. Buccal absorption of drug initially avoids hepatic destruction, and since only about 15% of the cardiac output is delivered to the liver, a transient but effective circulation level of intact organic nitrate would occur. Little difference in the duration of action of various organic nitrates taken by the sublingual route should be anticipated because the hepatic organic nitrate reductase is highly active in humans. Such a comparison was carried out by GOLDSTEIN et al. (1971) who adjusted the sublingual dosage of ISD and GTN to be equipotent regarding circulatory changes in triple product and in exercise tolerance. Under these conditions there was no significant difference in the duration of action of these nitrates in the patients tested (Fig. 19). Hepatic destruction of organic nitrates following sublingual administration should only be dependent upon the rate at which they are delivered to the liver. It is conceivable that different patients could vary in their time course of response to sublingual nitrates. The amount of drug delivered to the liver could be influenced by such conditions as differential volumes of distribution for the various organic nitrates or radically altered (by stress, exercise, or angina) hepatic blood flow. There are no current data that assess these factors.

Acknowledgement: The research performed by the author was supported by U.S.P.H.S. grant from NIH, HE-11771.

References

AL-KASSAB, S., BOYLAND, E., WILLIAMS, K.: An enzyme from rat liver catalyzing conjugations with glutathione. 2. Replacement of nitro groups. Biochem. J. **87**, 4—9 (1963).

ANSORGE, S., BOHLEY, R., KIRSCHKE, H., LANGNER, J., WIEDERANDERS, B., HANSON, H.: Metabolism of insulin and glucagon. Glutathione-insulin transhydrogenase from microsomes of rat liver. Europ. J. Biochem. **32**, 27—35 (1973).

BETTS, J. J., BRAY, H. G., JAMES, S. P., THORPE, W. V.: The metabolism of the trichloronitrobenzenes in the rabbit. Biochem. J. **66**, 610—621 (1957).

BLUM, S. W., QUINN, J. B., HOWE, B. B., HEFNER, M. A., WINBURY, M. M.: Pharmacologic and biochemical evaluation of organic nitrates: Attempted correlation of activities. J. Pharmacol. exp. Ther. **176**, 684—691 (1971).

BOGAERT, M. G., ROSSEEL, M. T.: Plasma levels in man of nitroglycerin after buccal administration. J. Pharm. Pharmacol. **24**, 737—738 (1972a).

BOGAERT, M. G., ROSSEEL, M. T.: Vascular effects of the dinitrate and mononitrate esters of isosorbide, isomannide, and isoidide. Arch. Pharmacol. **275**, 339—342 (1972b).

BOGAERT, M. G., ROSSEEL, M. T., BELPAIRE, F. M.: Metabolism of nitroglycerin in man. Influence of phenobarbital. Arch. int. Pharmacodyn. Ther. **192**, 198—199 (1971).

BOGAERT, M. G., ROSSEEL, M. T., SCHAEPDRYVER, A. F. DE: Cardiovascular effects of glyceryl dinitrates as compared to glyceryl trinitrate. Arch. int. Pharmacodyn. **176**, 458—460 (1968).

BOGAERT, M. G., ROSSEEL, M. T., SCHAEPDRYVER, A. F., DE: Excretion in urine of metabolites of glyceryl trinitrate in rabbits. Arch. int. Pharmadocyn. Ther. **179**, 480—489 (1969a).

BOGAERT, M. G., ROSSEEL, M. T., SCHAEPDRYVER, A. F., DE: Biotransformation of glyceryl trinitrate in rabbits. Arch. int. Pharmacodyn. Ther. **177**, 487—491 (1969b).

BOGAERT, M. G., ROSSEEL, M. T., SCHAEPDRYVER, A. F., DE: Metabolic fate of nitroglycerin in relation to its vascular effects. Europ. J. Pharmacol. **12**, 224—230 (1970).

BOOTH, J., BOYLAND, E., SIMS, P.: An enzyme from rat liver catalyzing conjugations with glutathione. Biochem. J. **79**, 516—524 (1961).

BRAY, H. G., HYBS, Z., JAMES, S. P., THORPE, W. V.: The metabolism of 2,3,5,6- and 2,3,4,5-tetrachloronitrobenzene in the rabbit and the reduction of aromatic nitro compounds in the intestine. Biochem. J. **53**, 266—273 (1953).

CLARK, D. G., LITCHFIELD, M. H.: Metabolism of ethylene glycol dinitrate and its influence on the blood pressure of the rat. Brit. J. Industr. Med. **24**, 320—325 (1967).

CLARK, D. G., LITCHFIELD, M. H.: The toxicity, metabolism, and pharmacologic properties of propylene glycol 1,2-dinitrate. Toxicol. Appl. Pharmacol. **15**, 175—184 (1969).

COMBES, B., STAKELUM, G. S.: A liver enzyme that conjugates sulfobromophthalein sodium with glutathione. J. clin. Invest. **40**, 981—990 (1961).

COMMARATO, M. A., WINBURY, M. M., KAPLAN, H. R.: Glyceryl trinitrate and pentrinitrol (pentaerythritol trinitrate): Comparative cardiovascular effects in dog, cat and rat by different routes of administration. J. Pharmacol. exp. Ther. **187**, 300—307 (1973).

CRANDALL, L. A., JR.: The fate of glyceryl trinitrate in the tolerant and non-tolerant animal. J. Pharmacol. exp. Ther. **48**, 127—140 (1933).

CRANDALL, L. A., JR., LEAKE, C. D., LOEVENHART, A. S., MUEHLBERGER, C. W.: The rate of elimination of glyceryl trinitrate from the blood stream after intravenous administration in dogs. J. Pharmacol. exp. Ther. **37**, 283—296 (1929).

Crew, M. C., Gala, R. L., Haynes, L. J., DiCarlo, F. J.: Biliary excretion and biotransformation of pentaerythritol trinitrate in rats. Biochem. Pharmacol. **20**, 3077—3089 (1971).

Davidson, I. W. F., Miller, H. S., Jr., DiCarlo, F. J.: Absorption, excretion and metabolism of pentaerythritol tetranitrate by humans. J. Pharmacol. exp. Ther. **175**, 42—50 (1970).

Davidson, I. W. F., Miller, H. S., Jr., DiCarlo, F. J.: Pharmacodynamics and biotransformation of pentaerythritol tetranitrate in man. J. Pharm. Sci. **60**, 274—277 (1971).

Davidson, I. W. F., Rollins, F. O., DiCarlo, F. J., Miller, H. S., Jr.: The pharmacodynamics and biotransformation of pentaerythritol trinitrate in man. Clin. Pharmacol. Ther. **12**, 972—981 (1971).

DeLorenzo, F., Goldberger, R. F., Steers, E., Jr., Givol, D., Anfinsen, C. B.: Purification and properties of an enzyme from beef liver which catalyzes sulfhydryl-disulfide interchange in proteins. J. biol. Chem. **241**, 1562—1567 (1966).

DiCarlo, F. J., Coutinko, C. B., Crew, M. C.: Sites of absorption of pentaerythritol tetranitrate. Arch. int. Pharmacodyn. **167**, 163—170 (1967a).

DiCarlo, F. J., Coutinko, C. B., Sklow, N. J., Haynes, L. J., Crew, M. C.: Binding of pentaerythritol tetranitrate and its metabolites by rat blood plasma and erythrocytes. Proc. Soc. exp. Biol. (N.Y.) **120**, 705—709 (1965b).

DiCarlo, F. J., Crew, M. C., Coutinko, C. B., Haynes, L. J., Sklow, N. J.: The absorption and biotransformation of pentaerythritol tetranitrate-1,2-^{14}C by rats. Biochem. Pharmacol. **16**, 309—316 (1967b).

DiCarlo, F. J., Crew, M. C., Haynes, L. J., Melgar, M. D., Gala, R. L.: The absorption and biotransformation of glyceryl trinitrate-1,3-^{14}C by rats. Biochem. Pharmacol. **17**, 2179—2183 (1968).

DiCarlo, F. J., Crew, M. C., Haynes, L. J., Wilson, M.: Pentaerythritol trinitrate metabolism by the rat. Biochem. Pharmacol. **18**, 1985—1990 (1969a).

DiCarlo, F. J., Crew, M. C., Sklow, N. J., Coutinko, C. B., Nonkin, P., Simon, F., Bernstein, A.: Metabolism of pentaerythritol tetranitrate by patients with coronary artery disease. J. Pharmacol. exp. Ther. **153**, 254—258 (1966).

DiCarlo, F. J., Hartigan, J. M., Coutinko. C. B., Phillips, G. E.: Absorption, distribution and excretion of pentaerythritol and pentaerythritol tetranitrate by mice. Proc. Soc. exp. Biol. (N.Y.) **118**, 311—315 (1965c).

Di Carlo, F. J., Hartigan, J. M., Jr., Phillips, G. E.: Enzymatic degradation of pentaerythritol tetranitrate by human blood. Proc. Soc. exp. Biol. (N.Y.) **118**, 514—516 (1965a).

DiCarlo, F. J., Melgar, M. D.: Binding and metabolism of nitroglycerin by rat blood plasma. Proc. Soc. exp. Biol. (N.Y.) **131**, 406—408 (1969c).

DiCarlo, F. J., Melgar, M. D.: Nitroglycerin biotransformation by rat blood serum. Biochem. Pharmacol. **19**, 1371—1379 (1970).

DiCarlo, F. J., Melgar, M. D., Haynes, L. J., Gala, R. L., Crew, M. C.: Metabolism of pentaerythritol trinitrate and pentaerythritol by dogs. J. Pharmacol. exp. Ther. **168**, 235—239 (1969b).

DiCarlo, F. J., Viau, J., Melgar, M. D.: Incorporation of radioactivity from ^{14}C-nitroglycerin into rat liver glycogen, lipid, protein, ribonucleic acid, and deoxy-ribonucleic acid. Biochem. Pharmacol. **18**, 965—970 (1969d).

Dietz, A. J., Jr.: Biotransformation studies on l-chloro-2,3-propanediol dinitrate. J. Pharm. Sci. **56**, 1664—1665 (1967b).

Fouts, J. R., Brodie, B. B.: The enzymatic reduction of chloramphenicol, p-nitrobenzoic acid and other aromatic nitro compounds in mammals. J. Pharmacol. exp. Ther. **119**, 197—206 (1956).

Garret, R. H., Nason, A.: Further purification and properties of neurospora nitrate reductase. J. biol. Chem. **244**, 2870—2882 (1969).

Goldstein, R. E., Douglas, M. D., Rosing, M. D., Redwood, D. R., Beiser, G. D., Epstein, S. E.: Clinical and circulatory effects of isosorbide dinitrate: comparison with nitroglycerin. Circulation **43**, 629—640 (1971).

Grover, P. L., Sims, P.: Conjugations with glutathione. Distribution of glutathione-S-aryltransferase in vertebrate species. Biochem. J. **90**, 603—606 (1964).

Hay, M.: The chemical nature and physiological action of nitroglycerin. Practitioner **30**, 422—433 (1883).

Heppel, L. A., Hilmoe, R. J.: Metabolism of inorganic nitrite and nitrate esters. II. The enzymatic reduction of nitroglycerin and erythritol tetranitrate by glutathione J. biol. Chem. **183**, 129—138 (1950).
Heppel, L. A., Porterfield, V. T.: Metabolism of inorganic nitrite and nitrate esters. I. The coupled oxidation of nitrite by peroxide-forming systems and catalase. J. biol. Chem. **178**, 549—556 (1949).
Hunter, F. E., Jr., Ford, L.: Nitrite formation by enzymatic reaction of mannitol hexanitrate with glutathione. J. Pharmacol. exp. Ther. **113**, 186—191 (1955).
Hunter, F. E., Jr., Kahana, S., Ford, S.: Effect of inorganic and organic nitrites and nitrates on aerobic phosphorylation in liver mitochondria. Fed. Proc. **12**, 221 (1953).
Johnson, E. M., Jr., Harkey, A. B., Blehm, D. J., Needleman, P.: Clearance and metabolism of organic nitrates. J. Pharmacol. exp. Ther. **182**, 56—62 (1972).
Johnson, M. K.: A distinct enzyme of rat liver and kidney coupling glutathione with some aliphatic halogen compounds. Biochem. J. **87**, 4—9 (1963).
Kohno, K., Noda, K., Mizobe, M., Utsumi, I.: Enzymatic reduction of disulfide-type thiamine derivatives. Biochem. Pharmacol. **18**, 1685—1692 (1969).
Lang, S., Johnson, E. M., Jr., Needleman, P.: Metabolism of and vascular responses to glyceryl trinitrate in the eviscerated rat. Biochem. Pharmacol. **21**, 422—424 (1972).
Lee, N. H.: The metabolism of glyceryl trinitrate by liver and blood from different species. Biochem. Pharmacol. **22**, 3122—3124 (1973).
Lee, N. H., Belpaire, F. M.: Study of the increased glyceryl trinitrate metabolism after pretreatment with phenobarbital in rat liver. Biochem. Pharmacol. **21**, 3171—3177 (1972).
Lee, N. H., Belpaire, F. M.: Biotransformation of nitroglycerin by organic nitrate reductase. Arch. int. Pharmacodyn. Ther. **196**, 165—167 (1972).
Modell, W., (Ed.): Drugs of Choice, 1970—1971, p. 376. St. Louis, Mo.: C. V. Mosby Comp. 1970.
Needleman, P., Blehm, D. J., Harkey, A. B., Johnson, E. M., Jr., Lang, S.: The metabolic pathway in the degradation of glyceryl trinitrate. J. Pharmacol. exp. Ther. **179**, 347—353 (1971).
Needleman, P., Blehm, D. J., Rotskoff, K. S.: Relationship between glutathione-dependent denitration and the vasodilator effectiveness of organic nitrates. J. Pharmacol. exp. Ther. **165**, 286—288 (1969).
Needleman, P., Harkey, A. B.: Role of endogenous glutathione in the metabolism of glyceryl trinitrate by isolated perfused rat liver. Biochem. Pharmacol. **20**, 1867—1876 (1971 b).
Needleman, P., Hunter, F. E., Jr.: The transformation of glyceryl trinitrate and other nitrates by glutathione-organic nitrate reductase. Molec. Pharmacol. **1**, 77—86 (1965 a).
Needleman, P., Hunter, F. E., Jr.: Effects of organic nitrates on mitochondrial respiration and swelling: Possible correlations with the mechanism of pharmacologic action. Molec. Pharmacol. **2**, 134—143 (1966).
Needleman, P., Krantz, J. C., Jr.: The biotransformation of nitroglycerin. Biochem. Pharmacol. **14**, 1225—1230 (1965 b).
Needleman, P., Lang, S., Johnson, E. M., Jr.: Organic nitrates: Relationship between biotransformation and rational angina pectoris therapy. J. Pharmacol. exp. Ther. **181**, 489—497 (1972).
Oberst, F. W., Snyder, F. H.: Studies on nitrate esters. 1. Nitrite-producing systems in rabbit tissues. J. Pharmacol. exp. Ther. **93**, 444—450 (1948).
Omura, H.: Intracellular behavior of the nitrate reductase of animal tissues. Enzymologia **20**, 271—290 (1959).
Otsuka, S.: Studies on nitro-reducing enzymes of swine liver. Properties and cofactor requirements of nitro- and nitroso reductases. J. Biochem. (Tokyo) **50**, 85—94 (1961).
Parker, J. C., Chang, Y., Davidson, I. W. F.: Coronary vasodilator activity of pentaerythritol trinitrate and its metabolites assayed in the dog. Fed. Proc. **32**, 794 (1973).
Posadas del Rio, F.: Glutathione organic nitrate ester reductase-evidence for two or more enzymes. Fed. Proc. **29**, 412 (1970).
Posadas del Rio, F., Hunter, F. E., Jr.: GSH-organic nitrate ester reductase-purification and properties. Fed. Proc. **32**, 733 (1973).
Racker, E.: Glutathione-homocysteine transhydrogenase. J. biol. Chem. **217**, 867—874 (1955).

REED, D. E., MAY, J. F., HART, L. G., McCURDY, D. H.: Identification of urinary metabolites of isosorbide dinitrate in dogs. Arch. int. pharmacodyn **191**, 318—336 (1971).
RISEMAN, J. E. F., ALTMAN, G. E., KORETSKY, S.: Nitroglycerin and other nitrites in the treatment of angina pectoris. Circulation **17**, 22—39 (1958).
ROSSEEL, M. T., BOGAERT, M. G.: Isosorbide, isomannide, and isoidide dinitrate: Urinary excretion in the rat. Biochem. Pharmacol. **22**, 67—72 (1973).
ROSSEEL, M. T., BOGAERT, M. G.: GLC determination of nitroglycerin and isosorbide dinitrate in human plasma. J. Pharm. Sci. **62**, 754—758 (1973).
SCHELLING, J., LASAGNA, L.: A study of cross-tolerance to circulatory effects of organic nitrates. Clin. Pharmacol. Ther. **8**, 256—260 (1967).
SHERBER, D. A., MARCUS, M., KLEINBERG, S.: Rapid clearance of isosorbide dinitrate from rabbit blood. Determination by gas chromatography. Biochem. Pharmacol. **19**, 607—612 (1970).
SISENWINE, S. F., RUELIUS, H. W.: Plasma concentrations and urinary excretion of isosorbide dinitrate and its metabolites in the dog. J. Pharmacol. exp. Ther. **176**, 296—301 (1971).
TSURUTA, H., HASEGAWA, H.: Studies on nitroglycol poisoning on some properties of an enzyme which decomposes nitroglycol into inorganic nitrate. Ind. Health **8**, 99—118 (1970).
WENDT, R. L.: Systemic and coronary vascular effects of the 2- and the 5-mononitrate esters of isosorbide. J. Pharmacol. exp. Ther. **180**, 732—742 (1972).
YAGODA, H., OETTINGEN, W. F. VON: Determination of nitrite in biological fluids and the decomposition of aliphatic nitric esters *in vivo* and *in vitro*, Toxicology and Potential Dangers of Pentaerythritol Tetranitrate, Publ. Health Bull. No. **282**, 8 (1944).

CHAPTER 6

The Pharmacological and Biochemical Interaction of Organic Nitrates with Sulfhydryls: Possible Correlations with the Mechanism for Tolerance Development, Vasodilation, and Mitochondrial and Enzyme Reactions

PHILIP NEEDLEMAN and EUGENE M. JOHNSON, JR.

With 5 Figures

I. Sulfhydryl Reactivity of Organic Nitrates — Introduction

The known reactivity of organic nitrate vasodilators with reduced glutathione in the presence or absence of liver organic nitrate reductase (HEPPEL and HILMOE, 1950; NEEDLEMAN and KRANTZ, 1965; NEEDLEMAN and HUNTER, 1965) stimulated an investigation of the mechanism of the pharmacologic action of nitrates and the mechanism of tolerance which appear to involve either direct or enzymatic reactions with sulfhydryl groups. Sulfhydryl-containing compounds play a role in determining mitochondrial structure and are essential for oxidative phosphorylation. Organic nitrates have been demonstrated to uncouple oxidative phosphorylation by liver and heart mitochondria (NEEDLEMAN and HUNTER, 1966; BOIME and HUNTER, 1971). Nitrates also have been shown to inhibit monoamine oxidase (MAO), a mitochondrial enzyme containing many sulfhydryl groups (OGAWA and GUDBJARNASON, 1968; KALIN and KYLIN, 1969). The apparent mechanism of MAO-inhibition by nitrates is the result of a concentration-dependent oxidation of SH-groups (JAKSCHIK and NEEDLEMAN, 1973). Organic nitrates that are potent vasodilator compounds in dogs are substances that are readily denitrated in the presence of the endogenous SH compound, reduced glutathione, and nitrate reductase (NEEDLEMAN et al., 1969); furthermore, there is a positive correlation between the induction of organic nitrate tolerance and the oxidation of critical tissue sulfhydryl groups in vascular smooth muscle (NEEDLEMAN and JOHNSON, 1973).

II. Organic Nitrate-Tolerance

A. Induction of Tolerance

1. In Intact Animals and Man

Repeated exposure of humans to organic nitrates leads to a decreased responsiveness to the pharmacologic effects of these agents. Tolerance and cross-tolerance between nitrates develops in humans within a few days and is fairly well-established in 2 or 3 weeks (STEWART, 1905; CRANDALL et al., 1931; SCHWARTZ, 1946; SCHELLING and LASAGNA, 1967; ZELIS and MASON, 1969). Tolerance to glyceryl-trinitrate (GTN, has been produced in dogs (CRANDALL, 1933; BOGAERT and DE SCHAEPDRYVER,

Table 1. Experimental conditions employed for the induction of nitrate tolerance *in vivo*. The following abbreviations were employed in the table: GTN-glyceryl trinitrate; EGDN-ethylene glycol dinitrate; ISD-isosorbide dinitrate; PETN-pentaerythritol tetranitrate; $NaNO_2$-sodium nitrite; ETN-erythritol tetranitrate; s.c.-subcutaneous

Organic nitrate	Species	Treatment protocol	Shift in biological response	Reference
$NaNO_2$	Rabbit	30 mg/kg, s.c., 3 times daily for 7 days	Decreased vasodepressor response to either $NaNO_2$ or GTN. *Editors note*: never confirmed by other workers.	MYERS and AUSTIN (1929)
GTN, ETN, EGDN, methyl nitrate, amyl nitrite	a) Human b) Dog	a) Total amount needed to develop headache tolerance: GTN-52.5 mg; ETN-45 mg; EGDN-170 mg	a) Tolerance towards headache effects of the various nitrates b) Decreased vasodepressor response	a) CRANDALL et al. (1931) b) CRANDALL (1933)
PETN	Human	10 mg, 4 times daily for 2 weeks and 20 mg, 3 times daily for 2 weeks	Decreased vasodepressor response to 0.3 mg GTN (sublingual)	SCHELLING and LASAGNA (1967)
GTN	Rabbit	1 mg/kg every 30 min from 8 AM to 8 PM for 4 days	10-fold shift in blood pressure dose-response curve to GTN	BOGAERT (1968)
GTN	Dog	1 mg/kg, 20 times a day, s.c. for 4 days	50-fold shift in blood pressure dose-response curve to GTN	BOGAERT and DESCHAEPDRYVER (1968)
EGDN	Rat	65 mg/kg, s.c. daily, 5 days/week for 10 weeks	Inhibition of vasodepression produced by EGDN, 65 mg/kg dose	CLARK and LITCHFIELD (1969)
ISD	Human	120 mg/day for 6 weeks	ISD blocked the GTN-induced increase in calf venous volume	ZELIS and MASON (1969)
GTN	Rat	a) 10 mg/kg, 3 times daily for 7 days b) 25 mg/kg, 3 times daily for 7 days c) 100 mg/kg, 3 times daily for 7 days	a) 10-fold shift in blood pressure dose-response curve to GTN b) 100-fold shift in blood pressure dose-response curve to GTN c) > 1000-fold shift in blood pressure dose-response curve to GTN	NEEDLEMAN (1970) NEEDLEMAN (1973)
GTN	Dog	a) acute tolerance by infusion of 1 mg/kg over one hour b) chronic tolerance: 1 mg/kg, s.c., 20 times a day for 4 days	a) 5-fold shift in GTN vasodepressor dose b) 20–50-fold shift in GTN vasodepressor dose	RUSH et al. (1971)
EGDN	Rat	65 mg/kg, s.c., daily, 5 days/week for 8 weeks	Decreased corticosterone release by histamine	CLARK (1972)

1968; RUSH et al., 1971) rabbits (MYERS and AUSTIN, 1929; BOGAERT, 1968) and rats (NEEDLEMAN, 1970; NEEDLEMAN and JOHNSON, 1973). Similarly, tolerance to ethylene glycol dinitrate developed after repeated exposure of the drug in rats (CLARK and LITCHFIELD, 1969), rabbits (GROSS et al., 1942; HASEGAWA and SATO, 1963) and man (EBRIGHT, 1941; FORSSMAN et al., 1958; MCGUINESS and HARRI, 1961). On the other hand, EPSTEIN et al. (1971) reported no change in human responsiveness to isosorbide dinitrate after chronic administration of the drug. The regimens employed for the induction and maintenance of organic nitrate tolerance in experimental animals and man are shown in Table 1.

Tolerance to GTN proved to be a dose- and time-dependent phenomenon. Chronic treatment with 10 mg of GTN per kg, three times a day, desensitized rats to challenge doses of GTN in 4 days, and the response was maximal by 8 days (NEEDLEMAN, 1970). Tolerance to GTN was manifested by a shift in the dose-response curve for blood pressure depression. To elicit a 20% fall of mean blood pressure, a 10-fold increase in the GTN challenging dosage was required in the GTN-treated group (0.03 mg/kg), as compared with the controls (0.003 mg/kg). Administration of GTN at 100 mg/kg (s.c.) three times a day shifted the dose-response curve until by 7 days the vasodepressor response to GTN was completely abolished even at the highest dosage tested (1 mg/kg given i.v.). Although the rats no longer responded to GTN, their initial mean blood pressures were the same as the controls and they were just as responsive to the vasodepressor effect of histamine. The tolerance was completely reversed after 2 weeks of withdrawal from GTN treatment (NEEDLEMAN, 1970).

2. Nitrate-Tolerance at the Level of the Blood Vessel

The thoracic aortas of GTN-treated rats were tested to determine if tolerance was a phenomenon that could be demonstrated in the isolated organ. To produce a 20% relaxation of epinephrine-contracted blood vessels, the control aortas required 0.03 mg of GTN per kg (challenging concentration of GTN in the tissue chamber), whereas aortas removed from GTN-treated rats (100 mg/kg three times daily for 2 days) required 2.5 mg/liter (NEEDLEMAN, 1970). Comparable results were obtained in rats by HERMAN and BOGAERT (1971). Aortic strips removed from control and GTN-treated rabbits (200 mg/kg, three times daily for 3 days) showed similar results (NEEDLEMAN, 1970), as did rabbit aortas removed from animals treated with GTN, 1 mg/kg, 24 times a day for 4 days (BOGAERT, 1968).

B. Biotransformation of Organic Nitrate during Induction and Maintenance of Nitrate Tolerance

One of the possible causes of drug (nitrate) desensitization is a diminished concentration of free (active) drug in contact with its cellular receptor; this may be the result of such events as: enhanced biotransformation, enhanced excretion, decreased passage of drug across membrane barriers, or increased drug binding to inactive sites.

A number of experiments have now been accumulated which indicate that tolerance to the vascular effect of GTN is not the result of biotransformation: (1) there was no change in the quantity and pattern of urinary metabolites after the administration of GTN to tolerant animals (NEEDLEMAN et al., 1971; (2) there was no enhancement of the glutathione-organic nitrate reductase (ONR) activity in the livers of GTN-tolerant rats (ONR from rats treated with 100 mg/kg, s.c., 3 times daily for 6 days was 14.3 moles/kg protein/hr.), as compared to the ONR-activity from control rats (13.6) (NEEDLEMAN, unpublished data); (3) there was no change in the rate of degradation of GTN when perfused through rat livers isolated from tolerant rats, as compared to control animals (NEEDLEMAN and HARKEY, 1971); (4) there was no difference in the rate or quantity of degradation of organic nitrates by the blood from tolerant and non-tolerant dogs; (CLARK and LITCHFIELD, 1969); (5) evisceration of rats eliminated degradation of GTN *in vivo* without altering the decreased blood pressure responsiveness to GTN in tolerant animals (LANG et al., 1972); and (6) there was no difference between tolerant rats and controls in the rate of $^{14}CO_2$-formation after the administration of ^{14}C-GTN (NEEDLEMAN et al., 1971).

No intact ^{14}C-GTN was detected in tolerant rats at a time when there was about a 10-fold shift in the vasodepressor effect (16 hr after the last loading dose). The glyceryl dinitrates and glyceryl mononitrates (but no GTN) were found in liver, lung, and in the gastrointestinal tract. Trace amounts of nitrate metabolites were also detected in skin and brain. No measurable organic nitrates were found in the blood at the time of sacrifice (NEEDLEMAN, 1970).

C. Dissociation of Sympathetic Compensation from Tolerance to Glyceryl Trinitrate

CLARK and LITCHFIELD (1969) suggested that tolerance develops because of an alteration of sympathetic compensatory mechanisms to the vasodilation caused by chronic administration of organic nitrates. CLARK (1970) observed a supersensitivity to epinephrine (blood pressure elevation and induction of arrythmias) 24 hr after cessation of treatment of rats with ethylene glycol dinitrate (EGDN). He observed no changes in response to tyramine. On the other hand, VIGLIANI et al. (1968) observed that the tachycardia caused by tyramine was "much greater and longer" in EGDN-tolerant rats.

The following observations demonstrated that changes in sympathetic function were not responsible for the induction or maintenance of GTN tolerance: (1) accelerated sympathetic tone induced by cold exposure did not change blood pressure sensitivity to GTN in rats; (2) GTN-tolerant rats had no change in blood pressure sensitivity to direct (epinephrine)- or indirect (tyramine)-acting sympathomimetics; (3) inhibition of catecholamine synthesis (by alpha-methyl-tyrosine) did not alter either induction or maintenance of tolerance to nitrate; (4) GTN-tolerance did not alter normal carotid body compensatory reflexes; and (5) little or no cross-tolerance was observed between GTN and other vasodilators such as papaverine or histamine (JOHNSON et al., 1973). In support of this conclusion, it was observed (RUSH et al., 1971) that impairment of sympathetic function by guanethidine or general anesthesia during pretreatment with GTN had no effect on development of the tolerance.

D. Mechanism of the Development of Tolerance to Organic Nitrates

Organic nitrate tolerance is not the result of increased biotransformation or increased sympathetic compensatory responses. It has been demonstrated that blood

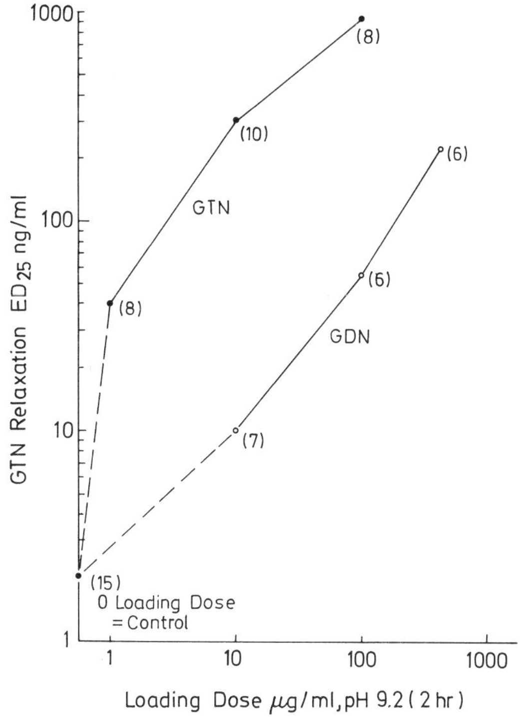

Fig. 1. Tolerance induced by varying levels of GTN and GDN. Strips were incubated for 2 hrs (37° C) at pH 9.2. (NEEDLEMAN and JOHNSON, 1973 with permission from Williams and Wilkins)

vessels taken from tolerant animals are less responsive to glyceryl trinitrate (GTN) *in vitro*. These observations have led to the conclusion that organic nitrate tolerance involves a qualitative or quantitative change in the interaction of this class of chemical compound with its specific vascular receptor.

An hypothesis of the mechanism involved in the induction of tolerance to nitrates was proposed in which GTN oxidizes a critical sulfhydryl group in the GTN "receptor." The disulfide form of the receptor apparently has a much lower affinity for the drug (NEEDLEMAN and JOHNSON, 1973).

1. Induction of Tolerance *in vitro*

Incubation of rabbit aortic strips for 2 hrs at pH 7.4 in the presence of GTN (100 μg/ml) caused only a 10-fold shift in the GTN dose-response curve, whereas incubation at pH 9.1 caused approximately a 1000-fold shift (NEEDLEMAN and JOHNSON, 1973). The concentration-dependence for induction of GTN tolerance is shown in Fig. 1. Tolerance induced by various concentrations of GTN and GDN after 2 hrs of incubation at alkaline pH are expressed as a shift in the ED_{25} of challenge doses of GTN; GDN has about 1/100 of the tolerance-inducing potency of GTN. These findings are consistent with the vasodilator potencies of GTN and GDN (BOGAERT et al., 1968; NEEDLEMAN et al., 1968).

Table 2. *Cross-tolerance induced by various organic nitrates.* Strips were incubated for 2 hrs (37° C) at pH 9.3 in the presence of 50 μg of organic nitrate per ml. Curves were run after 1 hr and five to six washes. (NEEDLEMAN and JOHNSON, 1973)

Treatment	ED_{25} (% Relaxation)		
	GTN	Isoproterenol	$NaNO_2$
	ng/ml	ng/ml	ng/ml
Control	2	2	20
Isosorbide dinitrate	25	2	
Butanetriol trinitrate	350	2	
Erythrityl tetranitrate	3100	2	
Mannitol hexanitrate	1500	—	
GTN	350	2	20
Pentaerythrityl trinitrate	350	2	

2. Cross-Tolerance

Organic nitrates administered *in vivo* result in cross-tolerance to other organic nitrates (CRANDALL et al., 1931; SCHELLING and LASAGNA, 1967). The ability of other organic nitrates to induce cross-tolerance to GTN and non-nitrate vasodilators was studied by incubation of aortic strips with several nitrates at a concentration of 50 μg/ml for 2 hrs at pH 9.3 (NEEDLEMAN and JOHNSON, 1973). The data (Table 2) show that all organic nitrates studied induce tolerance under these conditions. The most potent inducers are erythrityl tetranitrate and mannitol hexanitrate. Isosorbide dinitrate induced the least tolerance. Despite the large shift in GTN-sensitivity, no change in responsiveness to either sodium nitrite or isoproterenol was observed, therefore, inorganic nitrite cannot represent the active core of organic nitrate esters.

The *in vitro*-model of organic nitrate tolerance has many characteristics in common with *in vivo*-induced tolerance; these include: specificity for vascular smooth muscle; cross-tolerance to other organic nitrates; lack of cross-tolerance to isoproterenol, inorganic nitrite and papaverine; time- and dose-dependency of the induction; and similar rates of reversal in both models (NEEDLEMAN, 1970).

3. Effect of pH on the Interaction between Glyceryl Trinitrate and Tissue Sulfhydryl Groups

The reaction of organic nitrates with sulfhydryl-containing molecules proceeds according to the following reaction:

$$RONO_2 + 2R'SH \rightarrow R'SSR' + ROH + NO_2^- .$$

This reaction proceeds much more rapidly at alkaline pH. Incubation of GTN (100 μg/ml) with glutathione (1 mM) yielded eight times more nitrite at pH 9.4 than at pH 7.4. The pH-dependence of the tolerance-induction suggested that the mechanism of tolerance may involve oxidation of a sulfhydryl in the GTN-receptor. At pH 9.4, the concentration of titratable aortic SH groups is increased in untreated aortic

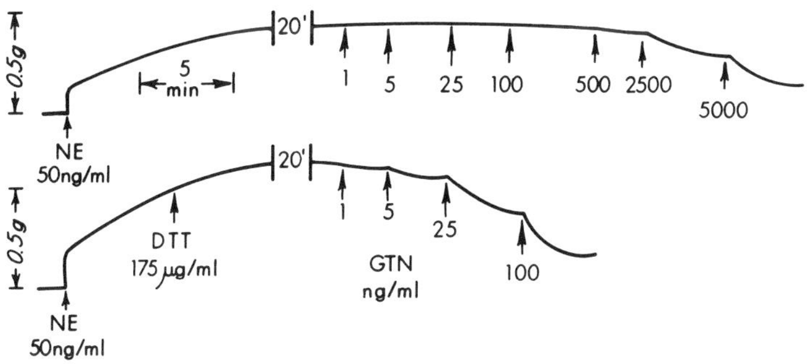

Fig. 2. *In vitro*-reversal of *in vivo*-induced tolerance to GTN. (NEEDLEMAN and JOHNSON, 1973 with permission from Williams and Wilkins)

strips. Upon incubation of GTN with aortic strips at pH 9.4, more NO_2^- is formed and the tissue shows a net loss of titratable SH groups not observed at pH 7.4 (NEEDLEMAN and JOHNSON, 1973)

4. Reversal of Tolerance to Glyceryl Trinitrate

If the tolerance induced by incubation at alkaline pH is due to oxidation of a sulfhydryl group in the nitrate receptor, then disulfide reducing agents should be able to convert GTN-tolerant strips into GTN-responsive strips. The exposure of GTN-tolerant (induced *in vitro*) rabbit aortic strips to the disulfide reducing agent dithiothreitol made the strips just as responsive as control strips (NEEDLEMAN and JOHNSON, 1973).

The critical experiment in the verification of the hypothesis was to demonstrate that tolerance induced *in vivo* by chronic administration of GTN can be reversed by dithiothreitol. Thoracic aortas removed from GTN-tolerant (100 mg of GTN per kg, s.c. three times daily for 3 days) rats showed an approximately 500-fold shift in their sensitivity to GTN *in vitro*. Aortic strips were removed from the GTN-tolerant rats and initial dose-response curves did not show clear relaxation until a dose of 2500 ng of GTN per ml. In the second dose-response curve (shown in Fig. 2), the upper aortic strip from a tolerant rat was untreated and remained unresponsive to GTN, whereas the lower tolerant strip, which was treated with dithiothreitol, showed almost normal responsiveness to GTN. Dithiothreitol did not have any effect on the sensitivity of control strips to GTN (NEEDLEMAN and JOHNSON, 1973).

5. Working Hypothesis

A unifying hypothesis developed to explain this observation is illustrated in Fig. 3. Organic nitrates react with reduced SH groups (reaction enhanced *in vitro* at alkaline pH) in the vascular smooth muscle receptor leading to the formation of a disulfide linkage (produced and maintained by chronic exposure to GTN) and the release of inorganic nitrite. This reaction thus converts the nitrate receptor to the disulfide form, which presumably has a lower affinity for GTN. A confirming test of this hypothesis is the ability to convert the inactive disulfide form of the nitrate receptor

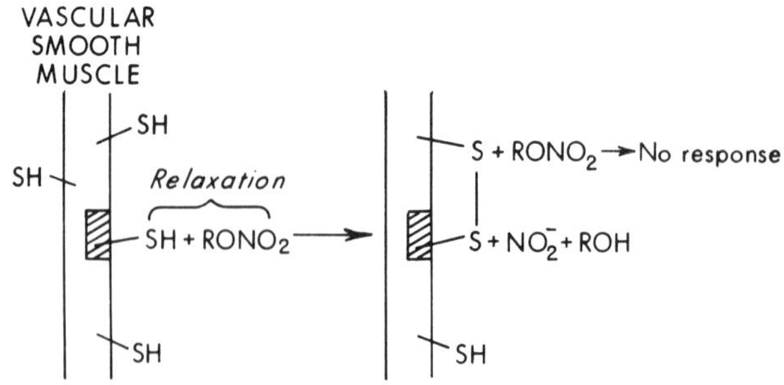

Fig. 3. Schematic diagram of the reaction of GTN with SH groups in its vascular receptor. Abbreviations: $RONO_2$, organic nitrate; ROH, denitrated metabolite. (NEEDLEMAN and JOHNSON, 1973, with permission from Williams and Wilkins)

(induced *in vitro*) to the "active" (i.e., GTN-responsive) reduced form with dithiothreitol. The validity of the model and the hypothesis are further strengthened by the dramatic reversal by dithiothreitol of tolerance in aortic strips taken from animals made tolerant *in vivo* by chronic administration of GTN. Thus, tolerance to GTN seems to be the result of a chemical alteration of the receptor induced by the drug. Such GTN-tolerant aorta strips are still fully responsive to other vasodilator compounds (papaverine, sodium nitrite, sodium nitroprusside, isoproterenol, and 3′5′-cyclic adenosine monophosphate (cAMP), thereby indicating that the organic nitrates react at a specific receptor site distinct from receptor sites for other relaxants.

III. Sulfhydryl Requirement for Relaxation of Vascular Smooth Muscle

Studies into the mechanism of induction of organic nitrate tolerance seem to indicate that tissue thiol groups were either an intimate part of specific vasodilator receptor sites or played a regulatory role in vasodilator-receptor interactions. GTN-tolerant strips are still responsive to other vasodilator compounds (papaverine, sodium nitrite, sodium nitroprusside, isoproterenol and cAMP), thereby indicating that the organic nitrates react at a specific receptor site distinct from receptor sites for other relaxants.

A. The Effect of Ethacrynic Acid on Vascular Effects of GTN and Other Vasodilators

Rabbit thoracic aortic strips were standaridized at pH 7.4 by means of GTN dose-response curves and then incubated in Krebs-bicarbonate solution (at pH 7.4) for 1 hr (37° C) with no addition (controls), or with added ethacrynic acid, furosemide or GTN. These strips were then extensively washed for 1 hr and GTN dose-response curves were retested. Under these conditions, ethacrynic acid produced a profound refractoriness to GTN (1000-fold nonparallel shift in the GTN dose-response curve) presumably due to alkylation of tissue thiol groups. Furosemide, also a potent diuretic, presumably has the same effect as ethacrynic acid on renal ion transport, but furosemide does not react with SH groups and was without effect on GTN responsiveness. As GTN induces tolerance *in vitro* at pH 9.4 there is a simultaneous decrease in tissue SH and an increase in NO_2^- formation. At pH 7.4 GTN produced minimal tolerance and has a lesser effect on the SH-groups of the aorta, while ethacrynic acid induces refractoriness to GTN, inhibits NO_2^- formation and lowers aorta-SH (NEEDLEMAN et al., 1973).

The reaction of ethacrynic acid with rabbit thoracic aortic strips was not specific for GTN and comparably reduced the response of the blood vessel to isoproterenol and inorganic nitrite, as well as to sodium nitroprusside, cAMP, papaverine, acetaldehyde and diamide (NEEDLEMAN et al., 1973). On the other hand, ethacrynic acid at the concentration used did not substantially decrease sensitivity to either norepinephrine or KCl, but it did somewhat alter the shape of the contractile curve.

B. Vasodilator Potency and Sulfhydryl Reactivity

The vasodilator potency of a number of compounds was evaluated on norepinephrine-contracted rabbit aortic strips. Some of these compounds are known vasodilators and others were tested because they are known to oxidize or alkylate SH groups. GTN, isoproterenol and sodium nitroprusside relaxed the norepinephrine-contracted blood vessels at such very low concentrations that they could not be acting by nonspecific sulfhydryl reactivity. Similarly, sodium nitrite and cAMP produce vasodilation that does not appear to rely on direct oxidation of SH. On the other hand, diamide, hydrogen peroxide and acetaldehyde produce vascular relaxation at about the same concentrations required to oxidize reduced glutathione *in vitro* (NEEDLEMAN et al., 1973). Thus, there appeared to be two distinct vasodilation responses: one activated by direct interaction with a specific receptor site and not necessarily requiring SH-oxidation as a primary event and a second group of nonspecific vasodilators in which vasodilation is correlated with ability to react with SH-groups.

C. Working Hypothesis

These data lead to the development of the working hypothesis and model of drug-induced vasodilation shown in Fig. 4 (NEEDLEMAN et al., 1973). Some drugs interact with specific receptor sites in vascular smooth muscle. Isoproterenol relaxes smooth muscle by activation of beta-receptors, possibly by activation of adenyl cyclase, and this effect is blocked both by the specific beta-antagonist, propranolol, or by desensitization after high doses of isoproterenol (FLEISH and TITUS, 1972).

The observation that cAMP-induced vasodilation is blocked by ethacrynic acid indicates that the SH-sensitive intermediate, which is being alkylated by ethacrynic acid is not adenyl cyclase and that in a vasodilation sequence involving cAMP (isoproterenol, papaverine) the blockade by ethacrynic acid is at a step subsequent to adenyl cyclase activation. Organic nitrates also appear to have specific receptors in that chronic exposure of blood vessels *in vivo* or *in vitro* induces a specific tolerance to nitrate, showing no cross-tolerance to other vasodilators (histamine, isoproterenol, papaverine, NO_2^-, diamine, cAMP, etc.) (NEEDLEMAN and JOHNSON, 1973). Toler-

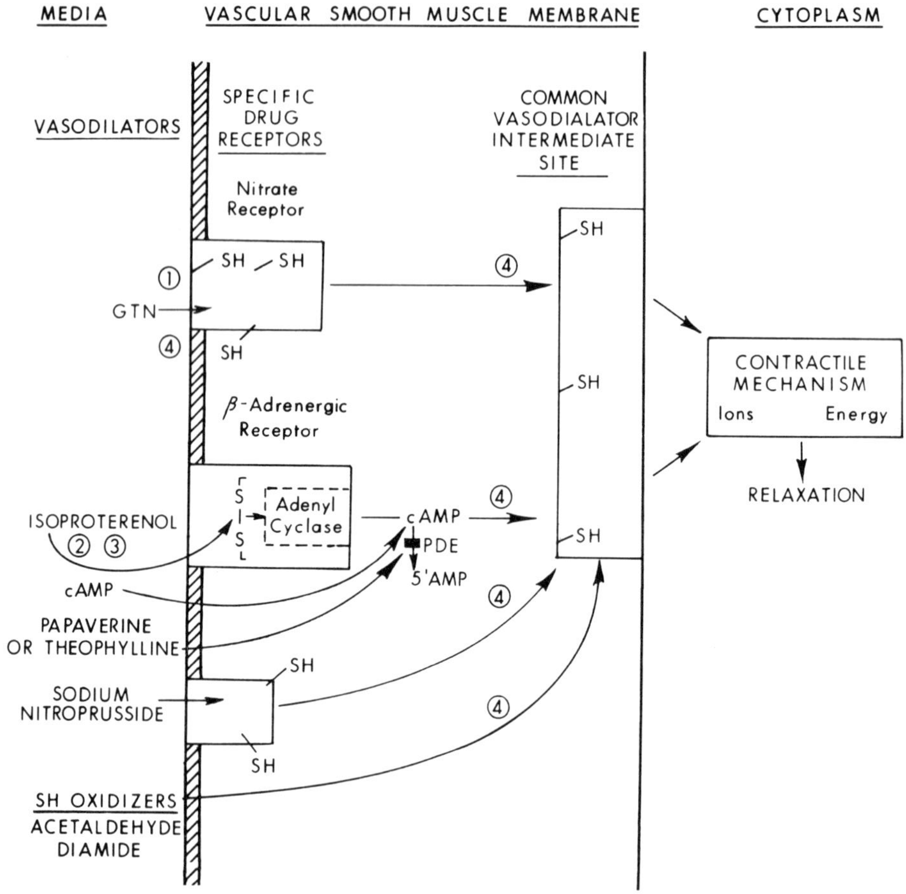

Fig. 4. Schematic diagram of the interrelationship between vasodilators and tissue components. The following abbreviations have been used: GTN, glyceryl trinitrate; cAMP, cyclic 3′5′-adenosine monophosphate; and PDE, phosphodiesterase (being inhibited by papaverine or theophylline). The numbers of the scheme indicate the following: *1* blocked by GTN tolerance; *2* blocked in isoproterenol tachyphylaxis; *3* blocked by propranolol; and *4* blocked by ethacrynic acid. (NEEDLEMAN et al., 1973 with permission from Williams and Wilkins)

ance or tachyphylaxis (without cross-tolerance to other vasodilators) to a particular drug serves as a useful tool in delineating specific drug receptor sites, especially because there is a lack of specific antagonists for many vasodilators.

Besides "specific receptors," vasodilators may hypothetically act through a common intermediate reaction involving critical SH groups within the tissue. Ethacrynic acid probably blocks SH groups throughout the tissue, but must be acting at a common intermediate to block both "specific" and "non-specific" vasodilators. The SH intermediate site may only be a regulatory site and could anatomically actually be a part of specific drug receptors and/or part of the contractile apparatus.

IV. Biochemical Actions of Organic Nitrates

A. Effect of Organic Nitrates on Electron Transport and Phosphorylation in Mitochondria (Sulfhydryl-Rich Organelle)

The effects of various nitrates on cellular respiration in vascular smooth muscle have been reported. The ATPase activity of rabbit aorta was inhibited by glyceryl trinitrate (GTN) and amyl nitrite but not by sodium nitrite (KRANTZ et al., 1951). GTN did not inhibit the dephosphorylating enzymes from dog coronary arteries (CARR et al., 1953). Amyl nitrite and sodium nitrite depressed oxygen uptake by beef coronary arteries, whereas the pharmacologically inactive sodium nitrate did not alter the respiration rate (BRAHEN and KRANTZ, 1955).

HUNTER et al. (1953) demonstrated that mannitol hexanitrate (MHN) inhibited oxidative phosphorylation in isolated rat liver mitochondria. GTN and erythrityl tetranitrate (ETN) were less effective. The uncoupling potency of organic nitrates was not related to the rate of degradation of the organic nitrates, because denitration with glutathione was most rapid for MHN and slowest for GTN (HUNTER and FORD, 1955).

Low concentrations of organic nitrates that are potent vasodilators (MHN, ETN, PETN, GTN) caused loss of respiratory control of tightly coupled rat liver mitochondria (NEEDLEMAN and HUNTER, 1966). With organic nitrates of moderate to low pharmacologic activity (isosorbide dinitrate, 1,2-glyceryl dinitrate, pentaerythritol trinitrate, and sodium nitrite), high concentrations were required to produce loss of respiratory control. The nitrates that are inactive as coronary dilators (glyceryl mononitrate, and potassium nitrate) did not affect oxidative phosphorylation even at very high concentrations (NEEDLEMAN and HUNTER, 1966). A comparison of organic nitrate effects is shown in Table 3. There was a correlation between (a) the ability of nitrates to produce loss of respiratory control in liver or heart mitochondria, (b) the rate of reaction with GSH in the presence of liver organic nitrate reductase (NEEDLEMAN and HUNTER, 1965), and (c) their oil-water partition coefficient. In these studies, the water-soluble $NaNO_2$, GMN, and KNO_3 showed very low or no activity. The organic nitrate esters with higher oil-water coefficients exhibited greater potency in affecting liver or heart mitochondrial respiration and a more rapid enzymatic denitration.

BOIME and HUNTER (1971) studied the selective action of organic nitrates at different sites in electron transport and oxidative phosphorylation in isolated rat liver mitochondria. The primary effect of GTN was to inhibit electron transport by liver mitochondria in the presence of ADP. GTN had little or no effect on succinate oxidation rates or the ADP:O ratio. Thus, GTN inhibited the response to ADP only with an NAD-dependent substrate (such as 3-hydroxybutyrate) and the action of GTN appears to be selective for the NADH dehydrogenase region of the electron transport chain. MHN, on the other hand, possessed generalized uncoupling activity and it accelerated the oxygen consumption rate with succinate just as it did with the NAD-linked substrate (3-hydroxybutyrate, but without ADP). ETN appeared to be intermediate between MHN and GTN in the liver mitochondrial effects produced (BOIME and HUNTER, 1971). LEVY (1970) also observed differences between various organic nitrates and their effects on the myocardial uptake of oxygen *in vitro*. MHN, iditol hexanitrate, and sorbitan tetranitrate stimulated oxygen consumption in isolated

Table 3. Correlation between various organic nitrate effects. The following abbreviations are used: reduced glutathione (GSH), glyceryl trinitrate (GTN), glyceryl dinitrate (GDN), glyceryl mononitrate (GMN), mannitol hexanitrate (MHN), erythrityl tetranitrate (ETN), pentaerythritol tetranitrate (PETN), pentaerythritol trinitrate (PETRIN), and isosorbide dinitrate (ISD). The liver mitochondria data was obtained from NEEDLEMAN and HUNTER (1966), the V_{max} values with liver GSH-organic nitrate reductase were obtained from NEEDLEMAN and HUNTER (1965). The oil-water partition coefficient represents the ratio of nitrate concentrations after equilibration between equal volumes of cottonseed oil and distilled water. PETN was insoluble in both phases, whereas $NaNO_2$ and KNO_3 were insoluble in the oil phase

Nitrate	Conc. for loss of respiratory control, liver		V_{max} liver GSH-organic nitrate reductase		Oil-water partition coefficient
	μM	Relative potency	mmole/kg/min	Relative potency	
MHN	27	19.6	830	6.9	486
ETN	270	2.5	358	3.0	326
PETN	500	1.1	1.4	—	Insoluble
GTN	530	1.0	120	1.0	115
ISD	1500	0.35	21.5	0.18	41
1,2-GDN	4000	0.13	5.0	0.04	—
PETRIN	4200	0.12	9.1	0.08	24
$NaNO_2$	6700	0.08	—	—	0
GMN	No effect at 16.7 mM	—	0.7	<0.01	2.8
KNO_3	No effect at 33.4 mM	—	—	—	0

rabbit atria, whereas GTN decreased oxygen uptake, while ISD and ETN had no effect consistent with the mitochondrial data obtained by BOIME and HUNTER (1971).

BLUM et al. (1971) compared the potency of a large number of organic nitrate esters as vasodilators and for their effects on terminal electron transport with rat heart Keilin-Hartree preparations. GTN was the most potent specific vasodilator. GTN also inhibited the NADH-oxidase activity of the Keilin-Hartree preparations, but ISD, ETN, MHN were less potent. Galactiol and mannitol pentanitrates were several times more potent than GTN as NADH oxidase inhibitors, but the pentanitrates were inactive vasodilators, suggesting no correlation between this biochemical effect and pharmacologic activity.

B. Monoamine Oxidase (MAO) Inhibition by Organic Nitrates

GTN administered *in vivo* inhibited MAO activity of rat heart mitochondria. GTN also inhibited the MAO activity in isolated mitochondria prepared from either heart, liver, or brain tissues of the rat (OGAWA et al., 1967). Organic nitrates were analyzed kinetically and found to be competitive antagonists of MAO and their inhibitor constants (Ki) were: GTN — 0.64 mM, ETN — 1.83 mM, MHN — 3.85, and ISD — 61.6 (OGAWA and GUDBJARNASON, 1968). A relationship between Ki values of organic nitrates and the dose of these drugs as anti-anginal agents was observed. GTN, propylene glycol dinitrate and ethylene glycol dinitrate were competitive inhibitors of MAO in rabbit liver mitochondria, while their metabolites had no such effect (KALIN and KYLIN, 1969). BLUM et al. (1971) reported that the concentrations required for 50% inhibition of rat heart mitochondria *in vitro* were: 2 mM for GTN; 5 mM for MHN; above 20 mM for ISD; 2 mM for pentaerythritol trinitrate; and 0.5 mM for mannitol pentanitrate. EGASHIRA et al. (1971) observed that high concentrations of $NaNO_2$ inhibited MAO activity in rat liver and brain mitochondria.

A comparison of the metabolic effects of GTN with those of the monoamine oxidase inhibitor, tranylcypromine, was performed in the unanesthetized rabbit (KYPSON and HAIT, 1971). Administration of either GTN or tranylcypromine caused simultaneously elevation of plasma free fatty acids, glycerol, lactate, and pyruvate, but the fatty acid and glycerol elevation were blocked by reserpine and propanolol. Thus, the metabolic effects of GTN and the monoamine oxidase inhibitor *in vivo* were comparable (KYPSON and HAIT, 1971). On the other hand, WALDECK (1970) compared GTN to the MAO inhibitor nialamide in rats or mice receiving ^{14}C-tyramine. Nialamide but not GTN increased the labeled octopamine formed in the heart. GTN did not affect the uptake or retention of catecholamines in the heart. KABIN et al. (1969) were also unable to demonstrate that nitrates *in vivo* caused MAO inhibition, nor did nitrates effect uptake, storage, release, and synthesis of catecholamines. It appears, therefore, that relatively high concentrations of organic nitrate can inhibit mitochondrial MAO *in vitro*, but that adequate concentrations cannot be reached *in vivo* to cause an inhibition of MAO.

JAKSCHIK and NEEDLEMAN (1973) incubated GTN with rat liver mitochondria and observed a concentration-dependent inhibition of monoamine oxidase activity. In comparable experiments, other nitrates (ETN, ISD, and MHN) inhibited the enzyme. The apparent mechanism by which organic nitrates inhibit MAO is by means of the redox reaction between the esters and the enzyme SH groups. The disulfide-reducing agent, dithiothreitol, was effective in partially protecting against the MAO inhibition produced by the organic nitrates. The concentrations of GTN required to produce detectable effects on rat liver mitochondrial respiration were the same as those required to inhibit MAO (JAKSCHIK and NEEDLEMAN, 1973), but these concentrations were greater than those required to affect the smooth muscle of blood vessels.

C. Glyceraldehyde-3-Phosphate Dehydrogenase

JAKSCHIK and NEEDLEMAN (1973) studied the reaction between the SH-rich enzyme glyceraldehyde-3-phosphate dehydrogenase (GAPDH) and GTN. Fig. 5a shows that GTN caused a dose-dependent inhibition of GAPDH. Ethacrynic acid, which alkylates SH groups, in equimolar concentrations caused approximately the same inhibition as GTN. The disulfide-reducing agent, dithiothreitol, protected the enzyme fully from inhibition by GTN (Fig. 5b). When dithiothreitol was added to a reaction inhibited by GTN, an immediate reversal occurred (Fig. 5c). At pH 7.4, the direct interaction between GTN and dithiothreitol proceeds very slowly and there is minimal loss due to this non-enzymatic redox reaction. At a more alkaline pH (greater than pH 8) the non-enzymatic reaction between organic nitrates and SH compounds is greatly accelerated; thus, the primary mechanism by which GTN inhibits GAPDH is by a concentration-dependent sulfhydryl oxidation.

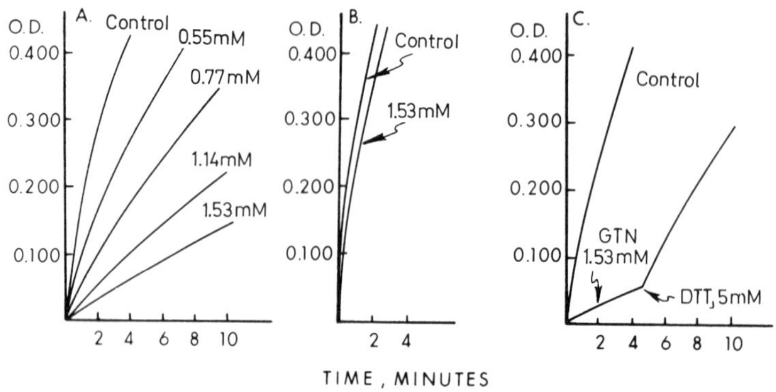

Fig. 5. (A) Glyceraldehyde-3-phosphate dehydrogenase (GAPDH) inhibition by GTN. GAPDH was incubated alone and with GTN (concentrations are shown on the Fig.) for 30 min at 37° C. The reactions were started by adding glyceraldehyde-3-P and recorded continuously. (B) Dithiothreitol (DTT) protection of GAPDH inhibition by GTN. GAPDH was incubated with 0.2 mM DTT without and with 1.53 mM GTN for 30 min at 37° C. (C) DTT reversal of GAPDH inhibition. GAPDH was incubated without and with 1.53 mM GTN. At the time indicated DTT, 5 mM, was added to the reaction mixture containing 1.53 mM GTN. (JAKSCHIK and NEEDLEMAN, 1973, with the permission of Academic Press)

D. Plasma Sulfhydryl Denitration of Organic Nitrates

Organic nitrates have been demonstrated to undergo a sulfhydryl-dependent denitration reaction when incubated with plasma; this reaction appears to be independent of GSH. DI CARLO et al. (1970) demonstrated a rat plasma enzyme that slowly degraded GTN and was inhibited by p-chloromercuribenzoate, iodoacetamide, and silver nitrate. POSADAS DEL RIO and HUNTER (1973) also described a GSH-independent enzyme in blood serum that degrades organic nitrates and was not inhibited by p-chloromercuribenzoate or iodoacetamide.

JAKSCHIK and NEEDLEMAN have shown (unpublished) that MHN markedly decreased plasma SH-levels, while generating inorganic nitrite. Ethacrynic acid (a sulfhydryl-alkylating agent, markedly reduced NO_2-formation (useful measure of the redox reaction of organic nitrates with SH), indicating that ethacrynic acid had access to (and formed a covalent linkage with) the plasma SH groups that react with organic nitrates.

E. Hemoglobin and GSH Oxidation by Nitrite

A prominent feature of organic nitrate or inorganic nitrite toxicity is the oxidation of the iron in hemoglobin to methemoglobin (ferrihemoglobin). The formation of methemoglobin by organic nitrates has been studied for over a century (HAY, 1883; HALDANE et al., 1897). WILHELMI (1942) suggested that organic nitrates must be degraded to inorganic nitrite in order to produce methemoglobin, whereas MARSHALL (1945) suggested that the intact nitrate ester formed methemoglobin directly. CLARK and LITCHFIELD (1973) observed that the methemoglobin formed after injection of GTN or ethylene glycol dinitrate was equivalent to that produced from inorganic nitrite infusions simulating the blood concentration anticipated by the denitration of the intact esters. They concluded that the hemoglobin oxidation, which occurs after administration of organic nitrates, reflects primarily the metabolic formation of inorganic nitrite.

The exposure of intact erythrocytes to inorganic nitrite ion has been found to cause the oxidation of oxyhemoglobin to methemoglobin (KEILIN and HARTREE, 1946) and of reduced glutathione (GSH) to oxidized glutathione (KEILIN and HARTREE, 1946; VELLA, 1959). HARLEY and ROBIN (1962) showed that GSH-depletion does not occur when nitrite and erythrocytes are incubated in the presence of an active pentose phosphate pathway. They observed that high concentrations of nitrite caused increased rates of oxidative destruction of hemoglobin, with formation of Heinz bodies, as well as loss of osmotic integrity. They suggested that nitrate acts by oxidation of the sulfhydryl groups of globin.

Pretreatment with methylene blue protects animals against death produced by nitrite and attenuates the methemoglobinemia (SMITH and LAYNE, 1969). Endogenous ascorbate levels partially determines susceptibility to nitrite toxicosis (KOCIBA and SLEIGHT, 1970), as evidenced by the higher incidence of methemoglobinemia, death and spontaneous abortions that occurred in ascorbate-deficient guinea pigs treated with inorganic nitrite.

BAUMEL et al. (1974) reported that sodium nitrite potentiated the action of barbiturates by decelerating hepatic biotransformation and by altering central nervous system sensitivity. These effects of $NaNO_2$ appeared to be the result of a tissue hypoxia caused by the formation of methemoglobin.

F. Effect of Organic Nitrates on Adenyl Cyclase

The action of a number of vasodilators has been attributed either to the activation of adenyl cyclase or the inhibition of phosphodiesterase. Glyceryl trinitrate (GTN) and sodium nitroprusside caused only a slight increase in 3′5′-cyclic adenosine monophosphate when aortic strips were exposed to very high concentrations of these dilator compounds (TRINER et al., 1971, 1972). BRODY and DIAMOND (1967) observed that GTN inhibited rat uterine motility without affecting either phosphorylase *a* activity or adenyl cyclase. Isoproterenol and erythrityl tetranitrate were reported to inhibit the activation of arterial glycogen phosphorylase (NAMM, 1971). On the other hand, LEVY and WILKENFELD (1968) found that theophylline, which inhibits phosphodiesterase, potentiated the inhibitory response of the uterus to GTN. ANDERSON (1973) observed that relaxation of rabbit colon smooth muscle by GTN or papaverine was preceded by an increase in cAMP content of the muscle. He found that papaverine but not GTN reduced the phosphodiesterase activity. Similarly, sodium nitrite did not effect phosphodiesterase activity in coronary vessels (KUKOVETZ et al., 1969). Thus, there is no little or no compelling evidence to indicate that the vasodilation caused by GTN is mediated by alterations in the levels of cyclic AMP.

Acknowledgement: The research performed by the authors was supported by U.S.P.H.S. grant HE-11771.

References

ANDERSSON, R.: Cyclic AMP as a mediator of the relaxing action of papaverine, nitroglycerine, diazoxide, and hydralazine in intestinal and vascular smooth muscle. Acta Pharmacol. Toxicol. **32**, 321—336 (1973).

BAUMEL, I. P., PITTERMAN, A., PATEL, G., DEFEO, J. J., HARBANS, L.: Mechanisms underlying potentiation of barbiturate action by sodium nitrite in the mouse: The role of methemoglobin-induced hypoxia. J. Pharmacol. Exp. Ther. **188**, 481—489 (1974).

BLUM, S. W., QUINN, J. B., HOWE, B. B., HEFNER, M. A., WINBURY, M. M.: Pharmacologic and biochemical evaluation of organic nitrates: Attempted correlation of activities. J. Pharmacol. Exp. Ther. **176**, 684—691 (1971).

BOGAERT, M. G.: Tolerance towards glyceryl trinitrate (Trinitrin) in rabbits. Arch. Int. Pharmacodyn. Ther. **172**, 228—230 (1968).

BOGAERT, M. G., DESCHAEPDRYVER, A. F.: Tolerance towards glyceryl trinitrate (Trinitrin) in dogs. Arch. Int. Pharmacodyn. Ther. **171**, 221—224 (1968).

BOIME, I., HUNTER, F. E., JR.: Effects of glycerol trinitrate, mannitol hexanitrate and erythritol tetranitrate on electron transport and phosphorylation in liver mitochondria. Biochem. Pharmacol. **20**, 533—545 (1971).

BRAHEN, S., KRANTZ, J. C., JR.: Respiration of coronary arteries and nitrites. Arch. Int. pharmacodyn. **104**, 29—32 (1955).

BRODY, T. M., DIAMOND, J.: Blockade of biochemical correlates of contraction and relaxation in uterine and intestinal smooth muscle. Ann. N. Y. Acad. Sci. **139**, 772—780 (1967).

CARR, C. J., BELL, F. K., BRADYHOUSE, M. F., KRANTZ, J. C., JR.: The effect of vasodilators upon the dephosphorylating enzymes of dogs coronary arteries. J. Pharmacol. exp. Ther. **108**, 385—392 (1953).

CLARK, D. G.: The supersensitivity of the rat cardiovascular system to epinephrine after repeated injections of ethylene glycol dinitrate. Toxicol. appl. Pharmacol. **17**, 433—442 (1970).

CLARK, D. G.: Effects of ethylene glycol dinitrate on pituitary-adrenocortical function in the rat. Toxicol. appl. Pharmacol. **21**, 355—360 (1972).

CLARK, D. G., LITCHFIELD, M. H.: Metabolism of ethylene glycol dinitrate (ethylene dinitrate) in the rat following repeated administration. Brit. J. Industr. Med. **26**, 150—155 (1969).

CLARK, D. G., LITCHFIELD, M. H.: Role of inorganic nitrite in methemoglobin formation after nitrate ester administration to the rat. Brit. J. Pharmacol. **48**, 162—168 (1973).

CRANDALL, L. A., JR., LEAKE, C. D., LOWENHART, A. S., MUEHLBERGER, C. W.: Acquired tolerance to and cross tolerance between the nitrous and nitric acid esters and sodium nitrite in man. J. Pharmacol. exp. Ther. **41**, 103—120 (1931).

DIAMOND, J., BRODY, T. M.: Effect of catecholamines on smooth muscle motility and phosphorylase activity. J. Pharmacol. exp. Ther. **159**, 202—211 (1966).

DICARLO, F. J., MELGER, M. D.: Nitroglycerin biotransformation by rat blood serum. Biochem. Pharmacol. **19**, 1371—1379 (1970).

EGASHIRA, T., TAKANO, K., SHIMIZU, K., KUROSAWA, Y., KAMIJO, K.: Effect of sodium nitrite on monoamine oxidase activity in rat liver and brain. Jap. J. Pharmacol. **21**, 274—276 (1971).

ELBRIGHT, G. E.: The effects of nitroglycerin on those engaged in its manufacture. J. Amer. med. Ass. **62**, 201—202 (1914).

EPSTEIN, S. E.: Angina pectoris: Pathophysiology, evaluation, and treatment. Ann. intern. Med. **75**, 263—296 (1971).

FLEISCH, J. H., TITUS, E.: The prevention of isoproterenol desensitization and isoproterenol reversal. J. Pharmacol. exp. Ther. **181**, 425—433 (1972).

FORSSMAN, S., MASRELIEZ, N., JOHANNSON, G., SUNDELL, G., WILANDER, O., BOSTROM, G.: Untersuchungen des Gesundheitszustandes von Nitroarbeitern bei drei schwedischen Sprengstoffabriken. Arch. Gewerbepath. Gewerbehyg. **16**, 157—177 (1958).

GROSS, E., BOCK, M., HELBRUNG, F.: Zur Toxikologie des Nitroglykols im Vergleich zu der des Nitroglycerins. Arch. exp. Path. Pharmak. **200**, 271—304 (1942).

HALDANE, J., MAKGILL, R. H., MAVROGORDATO, A. E.: The action as poisons of nitrites and other physiologically related substances. J. Physiol. (Lond.) **21**, 160—189 (1897).

HARLEY, J. D., ROBIN, H.: The effect of the nitrite ion on intact human erythrocytes. Blood **20**, 710—721 (1962).

HASEGAWA, H., SATO, M.: Experimental study on nitroglycol poisoning in rabbits. J. Biochem. (Tokyo) **54**, 58—64 (1963).

HAY, M.: The chemical nature and physiological action of nitroglycerin. Practitioner **30**, 422—433 (1883).

HEPPEL, L. A., HILMOE, R. J.: Metabolism of inorganic nitrite and nitrate esters. II. The enzymatic reduction of nitroglycerin and erythritol tetranitrate by glutathione. J. biol. Chem. **183**, 129—138 (1950).

HERMAN, A. G., BOGAERT, M. G.: Organic nitrates: Tolerance at the level of the vascular smooth muscle. Arch. Int. Pharmacodyn. **192**, 200—202 (1971).

HUNTER, F. E., JR., FORD, L.: Nitrite formation by enzymatic reaction of mannitol hexanitrate with glutathione. J. Pharmacol. exp. Ther. **113**, 186—191 (1955).

HUNTER, F. E., JR., KAHANA, S., FORD. L.: Effect of inorganic and organic nitrites and nitrates on aerobic phosphorylation in liver mitochondria. Fed. Proc. **12**, 221 (1953).

JAKSCHIK, B. A., NEEDLEMAN, P.: Sulfhydryl reactivity of organic nitrates: Biochemical basis for inhibition of glyceraldehyde-P-dehydrogenase and monoamine oxidase. Biochem. Biophys. Res. Commun. **53**, 539—544 (1973).

KALIN, M., KYLIN, B.: Organic nitrate explosives as monoamine-oxidase inhibitors. Arch. Environ. Hlth **18**, 311—318 (1969).

KALIN, M., KYLIN, B., MALMFORS, T.: The effect of nitrate explosives on adrenergic nerves. Arch. Environ. Hlth **19**, 32—35 (1969).

KEILIN, D., HARTREE, E. F.: Spectroscopic study of the permeability and lysis of red blood corpuscles. Nature (Lond.) **157**, 210—214 (1946).

KOCIBA, R. J., SLEIGHT, S. D.: Nitrite toxicosis in the ascorbic acid-deficient guinea pig. Toxicol. appl. Pharmacol. **16**, 424—429 (1970).

KRANTZ, J. C., JR., CARR, C. J., BRYANT, H. H.: Alkyl nitrites XIV. The effect of nitrites and nitrates on arterial adenosine triphosphatase. J. Pharmacol. exp. Ther. **102**, 16—21 (1951).

KUKOVITZ, W. R., POCH, G., JUAN, H.: The role of phosphodiesterase inhibition and the mechanism of coronary dilation by drugs. Fourth Int. Congr. Pharmacol., pp. 170. Basel: Schwabe and Co. 1969.

KYPSON, J., HAIT, G.: Metabolic effects of nitroglycerin and tranylcypromine in unanesthetized rabbits. Proc. Soc. exp. Biol. (N.Y.) **136**, 285—289 (1971).

LANG, S., JOHNSON, E. M., JR., NEEDLEMAN, P.: Metabolism and vascular response of glyceryl trinitrate in the eviscerated rat. Biochem. Pharmacol. **21**, 422—424 (1972).

LEVY, J. V.: Effect of organic nitrates on myocardial oxygen consumption *in vitro*. Brit. J. Pharmacol. **38**, 743—748 (1970).

LEVY, B., WILKENFELD, B. E.: The potentiation of rat uterine inhibitory response to noradrenaline by theophylline and nitroglycerine. Brit. J. Pharmacol. **34**, 604—612 (1968).

MARSHALL, C. R.: The mode of action of nitric esters. J. Pharmacol. exp. Ther. **83**, 106—119 (1945).

MCGUINNESS, B. W., HARRIS, L.: "Monday head": An interesting occupational disorder. Brit. med. J. 1961 II., **2**, 245—247.

MYERS, H. B., AUSTIN, V. T.: Nitrite toleration. J. Pharmacol. exp. Ther. **36**, 227—230 (1929).

NAMM, D. H.: The activation of glycogen phosphorylase in arterial smooth muscle. J. Pharmacol. exp. Ther. **178**, 299—310 (1971).

NEEDLEMAN, P.: Tolerance to the vascular effects of glyceryl trinitrate. J. Pharmacol. exp. Ther. **171**, 93—102 (1970).

NEEDLEMAN, P., BLEHM, D. J., HARKEY, A. B., JOHNSON, E. M., JR., LANG, S.: The metabolic pathway in the degradation of glyceryl trinitrate. J. Pharmacol. exp. Ther. **179**, 347—353 (1971).

NEEDLEMAN, P., BLEHM, D. J., ROTSKOFF, K. S.: Relationship between glutathione-dependent denitration and the vasodilator effectiveness of organic nitrates. J. Pharmacol. exp. Ther. **165**, 286—288 (1969).

NEEDLEMAN, P., HARKEY, A. B.: Role of endogenous glutathione in the metabolism of glyceryl trinitrate by isolated perfused rat liver. Biochem. Pharmacol. **20**, 1867—1876 (1971).

NEEDLEMAN, P., HUNTER, F. E., JR.: The transformation of glyceryl trinitrate and other nitrates by glutathione organic nitrate reductease. Molec. Pharmacol. **1**, 77—86 (1965).

NEEDLEMAN, P., HUNTER, F. E., JR.: Effects of organic nitrates on mitochondrial respiration and swelling: Possible correlations with the mechanism of pharmacologic action. Molec. Pharmacol. **2**, 134—143 (1966).

NEEDLEMAN, P., JAKSCHIK, B. A., JOHNSON, E. M., JR.: Sulfhydryl requirement for relaxation of vascular smooth muscle. J. Pharmacol. exp. Ther. **187**, 324—331 (1973).

NEEDLEMAN, P., JOHNSON, E. M., JR.: Mechanism of tolerance development to organic nitrates. J. Pharmacol. exp. Ther. **184**, 709—715 (1973).

NEEDLEMAN, P., KRANTZ, J. C., JR.: The biotransformation of nitroglycerin. Biochem. Pharmacol. **14**, 1225—1230 (1965).

OGAWA, K., GUDBJARNASON, S.: A correlation between the inhibition of monoamine oxidase activity and the relief of angina pain by organic nitrates. Arch. Int. pharmacodyn. **172**, 172—182 (1968).

OGAWA, K., GUDBJARNASON, S., BING, R. J.: Nitroglycerin (glyceryl trinitrate) as a monoamine oxidase inhibitor. J. Pharmacol. exp. Ther. **155**, 449—455 (1967).

POSADAS DEL RIO, F., HUNTER, F. E., JR.: GSH-organic nitrate ester reductase-purification and properties. Fed. Proc. **32**, 733 (1973).

RUSH, M. L., LANG, W. J., RAND, M. J.: Studies on compensatory reflexes and tolerance to glyceryl trinitrate (GTN). Europ. J. Pharmacol. **16**, 148—155 (1971).

SMITH, R. P., LAYNE, W. R.: A. comparison of the lethal effects of nitrite and hydroxylamine in the mouse. J. Pharmacol. exp. Ther. **165**, 30—35 (1969).

STEWART, D. D.: Tolerance to nitroglycerine. J. Amer. med. Ass. **44**, 1678—1681 (1905).

TRINER, L., NAHAS, G. G., VULLIEMOZ, Y., OVERWEG, N. I. A., VEROSKY, M., HABIF, D. V., NGAL, S. H.: Cyclic AMP and smooth muscle function. Ann. N. Y. Acad. Sci. **185**, 458—476 (1971).

TRINER, L., VULLIEMOZ, Y., VEROSKY, M., HABIF, D. V., NAHAS, G. G.: Adenyl cyclase-phosphodiesterase system in arterial smooth muscle. Life Sci. **11**, 817—824 (1972).

VELLA, F.: Observations on spontaneous hemolysis in shed blood. Experientia (Basel) **15**, 433—435 (1959).

VIGLIANI, E. C., CAVAGNA, G., LOCATI, G., FOA, V.: Biological effects of nitroglycol on the metabolism of catecholamines. Arch. Environ. Hlth **16**, 477—483 (1968).

WALDECK, B.: Failure to demonstrate monoamine oxidase inhibition by glyceryl trinitrate *in vivo*. Acta Pharmacol. Toxicol. **28**, 406—412 (1970).

WILHELMI, H.: Studien über Methaemoglobinbildring. XXIII. Mitteilung, Blutwirkung aliphatischer Salpetersäureester. Arch. exp. Pathol. Pharmakol. **200**, 305—323 (1942).

ZELIS, R., MASON, D. T.: Demonstration of nitrite tolerance: attenuation of the venodilator response to nitroglycerin by the chronic administration of isosorbide dinitrate. Circulation **40**, Suppl. III, 221 (1969).

CHAPTER 7

Physiology and Pathophysiology of the Coronary Circulation and the Role of Nitroglycerin

BERTRAM PITT

With 11 Figures

I. Normal Physiology

A. Myocardial Oxygen Supply and Demand

Under normal circumstances there is a balance between myocardial oxygen supply and demand. A schematic illustration of current concepts of this relationship is shown in Fig. 1. In the presence of a normal coronary circulation any increase in oxygen demands is met by a concomitant increase in oxygen delivery. If, however, oxygen demands should exceed delivery ischemia results. The factors controlling oxygen demand have been recently reviewed [1] and will not be discussed further. Oxygen delivery is dependent upon the extraction of oxygen across the myocardium and coronary blood flow. Since oxygen extraction is near maximal in the myocardium, any major increase in oxygen demands must be met by an increase in coronary blood flow.

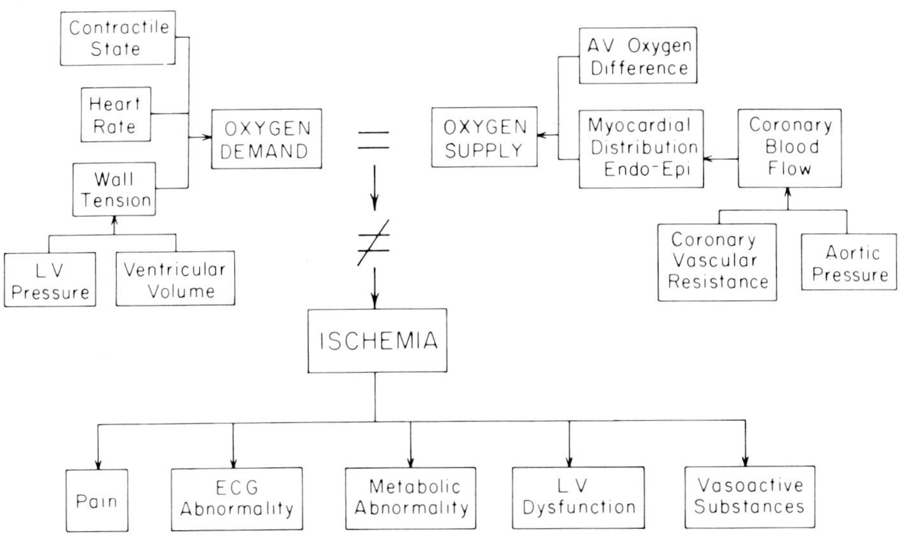

Fig. 1. Schematic diagram of the relation between myocardial oxygen supply and demand

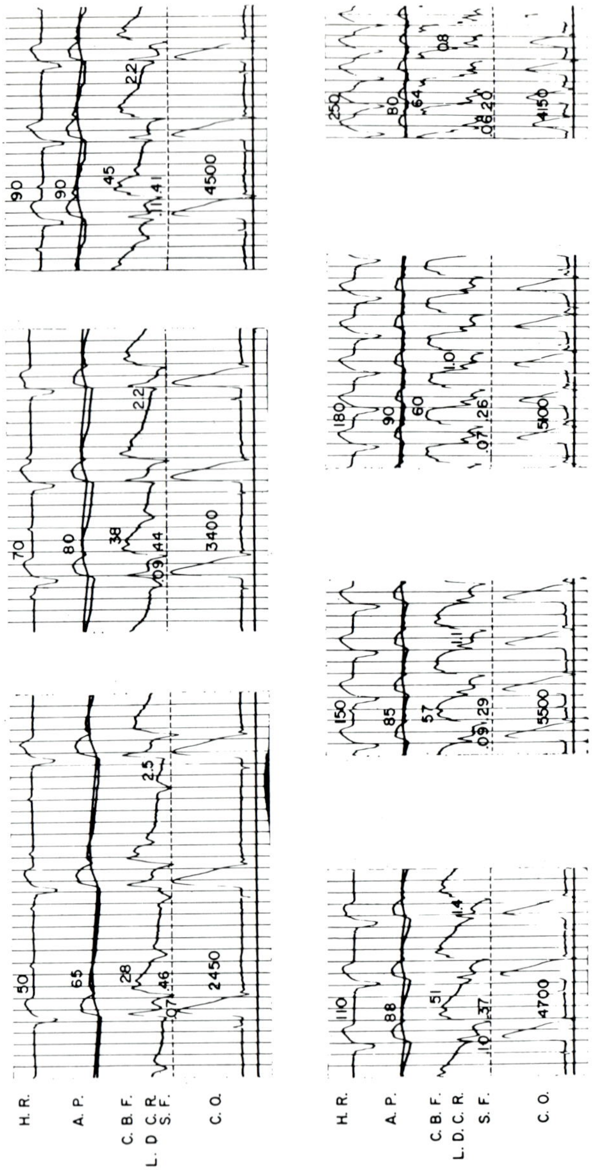

Fig. 2. Effect of increasing heart rate on coronary blood flow in a conscious dog. *HR* heart rate (beats/min), *AP* aortic pressure (mm Hg), *CBF* left circumflex coronary blood (ml/min) obtained by an electromagnetic flow transducer. *LDCR* late diastolic coronary resistance (units), *SF* stroke coronary flow (ml), *CO* cardiac output (ml/min). (From PITT et al., Ref. [2])

An example of the coronary flow response to an increase in heart rate in a normal conscious dog is shown in Fig. 2. When heart rate is increased from 50 to 150 beats/min both coronary flow and cardiac output tend to increase. At heart rates above 150 beats/min cardiac output begins to fall because of inadequate venous return, but coronary blood flow continues to rise up to 300 beats/min [2]. Not only does flow continue to rise up to this rate but it can be shown that there is still a reserve capacity

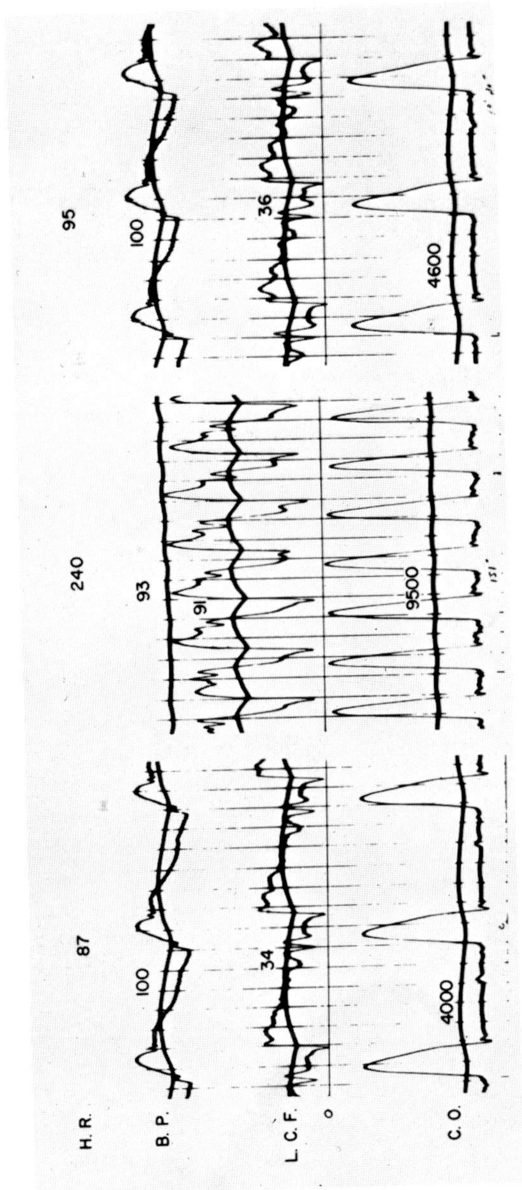

Fig. 3. Effect of exercise on coronary blood flow in the conscious dog. The left hand panel shows the resting values, the middle panel during treadmill exercise, and the right hand panel during recovery from exercise. *HR* heart rate (beats/min), *BP* aortic blood pressure (mm Hg), *LCF* left circumflex coronary blood flow (ml/min), *CO* cardiac output (ml/min). (From PITT and GREGG, unpublished observations)

for the coronary bed to dilate at a heart rate of 300 beats/min [2]. Increases in oxygen demands by exercise (Fig. 3) or excitement (Fig. 4) also lead to an increase in coronary flow [3—5]. In this instance the increased demands are due to a combination of factors that tend to increase all of the three major determinants of oxygen demand.

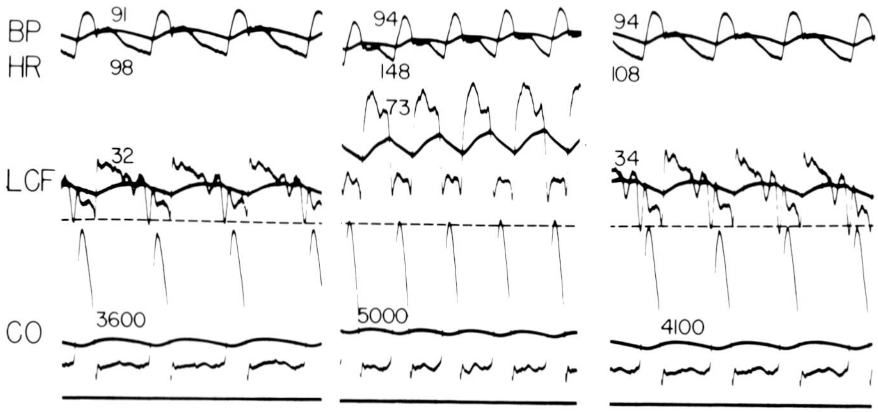

Fig. 4. Effects of excitement on coronary blood flow in the conscious dog. The left had panel shows the values at rest, the middle panel during excitement caused by auditory stimulation, and the right hand panel during recovery. Abbreviations are the same as Fig. 3 (From PITT and GREGG, unpublished observations)

B. Adrenergic Innervation of the Coronary Arteries

Another illustration of the effects of increased oxygen demand on coronary flow can be seen after sympathetic nerve stimulation [6]. The effects of stimulation of the stellate ganglion on the coronary circulation (Fig. 5) are of interest in that they demonstrate the presence of both alpha- and beta-adrenergic receptor activity in the coronary circulation. Within 2 to 3 seconds of stimulation there is a decrease in coronary flow that is immediately followed by an increase in flow, which persists as long as the stimulation is continued. The initial decrease in flow is thought to be due to direct stimulation of the alpha-adrenergic receptors in the coronary artery by norepinephrine. The increase in flow accompanying the increase in heart rate and contractility is due to "secondary metabolic vasodilatation," i.e., the increased oxygen demands result in release of metabolites, such as adenosine or prostaglandins, which overcome the tendency for direct vasoconstriction and cause vasodilatation. The distribution of alpha- and beta-receptor activity in the coronary circulation has been investigated by Zuberbuhler and Bohr in isolated vascular strips [7]. They have shown that there is a decrease in alpha-receptor density as one moves from the ostia of the major epicardial coronary arteries peripherally toward the intramuscular arterioles. While beta-receptor activity can also be demonstrated in the major epicardial coronary arteries, there is no alpha-receptor activity in the arterioles. As will be described below, the presence of alpha-adrenergic receptors in the major epicardial arteries provides a mechanism whereby "coronary spasm" could be produced.

C. Reactive Hyperemia

A study of the effects of transient coronary artery occlusion is of value in our understanding of the pathophysiology of ischemic heart disease. When a coronary

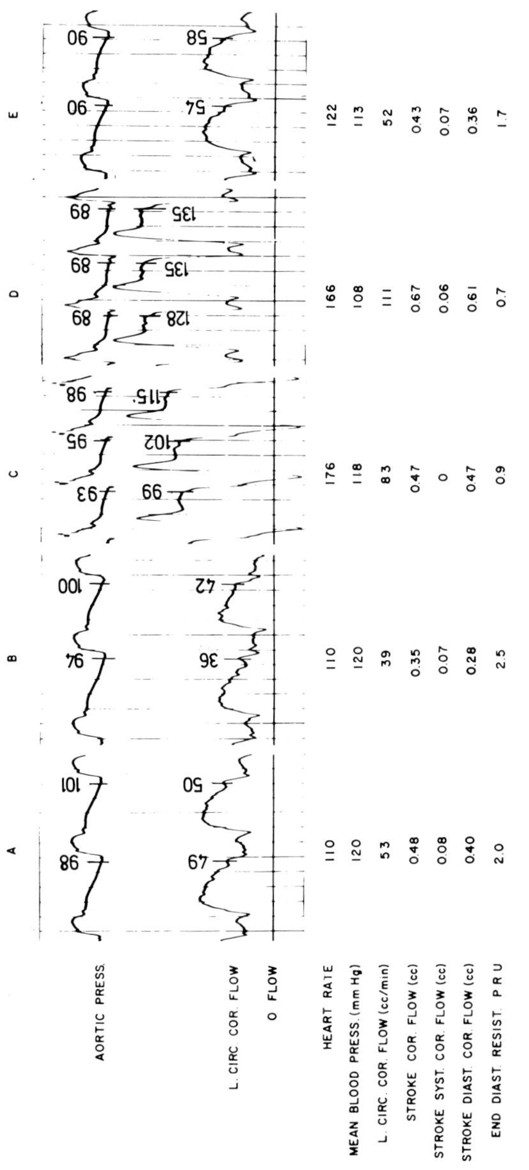

Fig. 5A–E. Effect of stellate ganglion stimulation on coronary blood flow in the conscious dog. Panel (A) shows the resting values, panel (B) during the initial period of increased coronary vasoconstriction. Panels (C) and (D) during the period of secondary metabolic vasodilatation and panel (E) during recovery. (From GRANATA et al., Ref. [6])

artery is occluded for a period of 10 seconds or more and then the occlusion is abruptly released, a characteristic response, "reactive hyperemia," can be seen, as illustrated in Fig. 6. The increase in flow after release of the occlusion is more than that lost during the period of occlusion [8]. The overpayment of flow and oxygen may be greater than twice that lost. If a coronary artery is occluded for progressively longer periods of time, the total period of increased flow and the total flow repaid is increased. The magnitude of the early increase in peak flow — peak

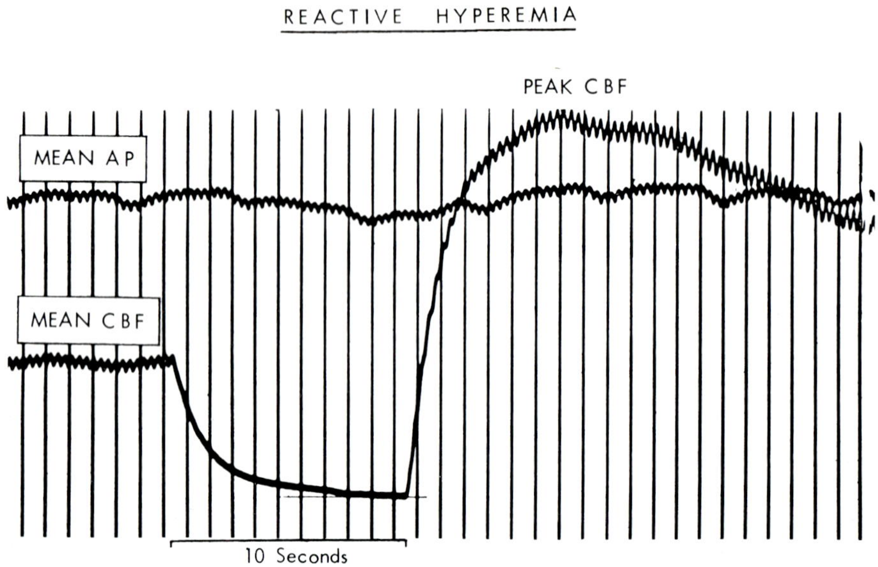

Fig. 6. Effect of transient coronary artery occlusion on coronary blood flow. The upper tracing is the mean aortic pressure (AP) and the lower tracing, mean coronary blood flow obtained with an electromagnetic flow transducer. Note the rise in flow following release of the ten second interruption in coronary flow. The peak coronary blood flow following relief of the occlusion is the point of maximal coronary vasodilatation

reactive hyperemia — does not, however, increase with increasing periods of coronary occlusion. The peak flow during reactive hyperemia is the maximal coronary vasodilatation possible at a given perfusion pressure. Peak reactive hyperemic flow may be three to five times resting flow and represents the reserve capacity of the coronary circulation to dilate above resting conditions. The metabolic factor thought to be responsible for reactive hyperemic flow is adenosine [9]. Proof of this hypothesis, however, has been difficult to accumulate because of the presence of adenosindeaminase which rapidly destroys adenosine as it enters the circulation. Inhibition of this enzyme by agents such as dipyridamole leads to marked coronary vasodilatation almost equivalent to reactive hyperemia. Prostaglandins and the kinins [10, 11] have also been implicated in the metabolic mediation of this response; however it is now too early to determine their role in the regulation of the coronary circulation vis-à-vis adenosine.

II. Pathophysiology of Ischemic Heart Disease

Coronary Occlusion

The principles described above are essential to an understanding of the effects of coronary artery narrowing and occlusion. The effect of coronary artery narrowing on resting coronary flow and the reserve capacity of the coronary bed to dilate are shown in Fig. 7. As described above, the reserve capacity of the coronary bed to

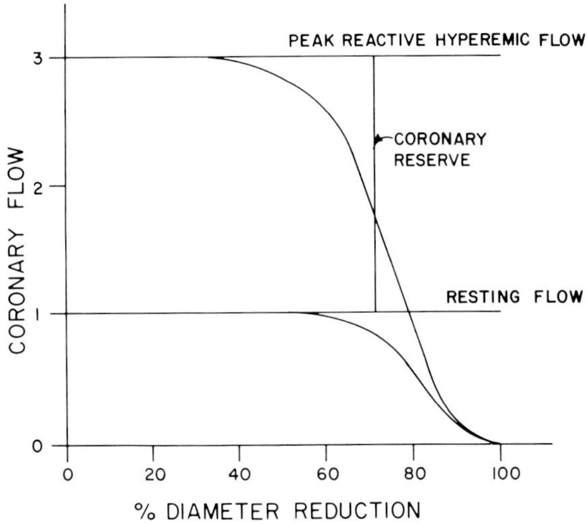

Fig. 7. Schematic illustration of the effects of coronary artery narrowing on resting coronary flow and peak reactive hyperemic flow. At a point approximately 70% narrowing, resting flow is relatively unchanged while peak reactive hyperemic flow and therefore the reserve capacity of the coronary bed to dilate is severely reduced. (From KLOPP et al., unpublished observations)

dilate, as reflected by peak reactive hyperemic flow, is three to five times resting flow. As a major coronary artery is progressively narrowed, resting flow tends to remain at control levels, while peak reactive hyperemic flow diminishes [12]. At a point of 60%-narrowing of a coronary artery (depending on the extent of the segment narrowed) resting flow may be unchanged, while peak reactive hyperemic flow is reduced to less than one-half of its original value. If a patient with a narrowing of a major coronary artery, such as the left anterior descending coronary artery, has a 60%-narrowing on arteriography, we would expect that under resting conditions his flow would be normal. If oxygen demands tripled as a result of exercise, coronary flow would tend to increase, but it could not increase to a degree sufficient to supply the oxygen demands, because the reserve vasodilator capacity would have been partially exhausted in attempting to maintain resting flow. At approximately 70%-narrowing of the coronary lumen the point of "critical stenosis" is reached, i.e., degree of occlusion at which resting coronary flow is essentially unchanged but reactive hyperemic flow is almost completely eliminated. At this point the reserve capacity has been completely expended in attempting to maintain resting flow. If there is a further reduction in coronary artery lumen to 80 or 90%, resting flow falls. At this point there is an imbalance between oxygen supply and demand. This would result in either prolonged chest pain at rest, indicating the presence of myocardial ischemia, or a decrease in local demands for oxygen. A local reduction in oxygen-demands can be accomplished by reducing regional myocardial wall motion. At angiography, a patient with such a lesion can be seen to have reduced myocardial wall motion. A further reduction in coronary artery lumen could result in myocardial infarction. Figure 7 also illustrates the futility of attempting to increase flow to an ischemic area by a coronary vasodilator. The patient with a 60%-reduction in arterial lumen may still be able to increase flow to some degree in response to a vasodilator. The patient with a 70- to 90%-obstruction may not respond at all, since the reserve vasodilator capacity has been expended in maintaining resting flow.

Once ischemia occurs as a result of a discrepancy between oxygen supply and demands, a number of pathophysiologic events occur which in themselves can further affect the coronary circulation. During angina pectoris, there is an almost invariable increase in left ventricular end-diastolic pressure [13]. End-diastolic pressure may rise to 20 to 40 mm Hg during spontaneous angina. In part, this is due to decreased regional myocardial function resulting in an increased left ventricular end diastolic volume, to a decrease in myocardial compliance [14] and to delayed relaxation [15]. The increase in end-diastolic pressure during ischemia may affect the distribution of flow within the ischemic area. Under normal conditions flow is relatively evenly distributed across the myocardium between the subendo- and epi-cardium. At rest, approximately 15% of coronary flow occurs during systole and 85% during diastole. The systolic portion of coronary flow is distributed mainly to the epicardial region, while the diastolic portion supplies both the epi- and subendocardial areas. During systole, when intramyocardial pressure is high, there is an insufficient pressure differential to force blood into the deeper layers of the myocardium. During diastole there is a pressure gradient that is sufficient to cause flow to the deeper layers of the myocardium. In the presence of a significant coronary artery obstruction a pressure drop occurs across the obstruction, which is related to both the severity and extent of the obstruction. Coronary perfusion pressure in the presence of an obstructing lesion is not aortic pressure, but the pressure distal to the lesion. This pressure may be in the range of 40 to 60 mm Hg in the presence of an approximataly 70%-narrowing of a coronary artery. At rest this pressure may be adequate to perfuse the myocardium evenly. During stress there may be a further drop in perfusion pressure and an increase in the left ventricular and diastolic pressure. The effective coronary perfusion pressure under these circumstances may be inadequate to perfuse the subendocardium. In calculating the effective coronary perfusion pressure, it should be noted that the down-stream pressure in the coronary bed, under normal conditions, is not right atrial or coronary sinus pressure, but rather intramyocardial tissue pressure. Coronary sinus pressure can be increased up to the level of myocardial tissue pressure without altering the distribution of coronary flow [16]. When coronary sinus pressure is increased above tissue pressure it becomes the down-stream pressure, and any further increases in coronary sinus pressure may cause an alteration in flow distribution. The myocardial tissue pressure is greatest in the inner and middle third of the myocardium and diminishes toward the epicardial surface. During myocardial ischemia, when left ventricular end-diastolic pressure reaches levels of 20 to 40 mm Hg, the inner layers of the ventricular wall, supplied by a vessel with a low perfusion pressure, may not be adequately perfused. We have termed this mechanism the "diastolic crunch" [17]. This relationship between coronary artery perfusion pressure and tissue pressure, as reflected by end-diastolic pressure, may also be of importance in circumstances in which an area of myocardium is perfused by a collateral vessel. The pressure from a collateral vessel beyond a complete coronary artery obstruction, "peripheral coronary pressure," has

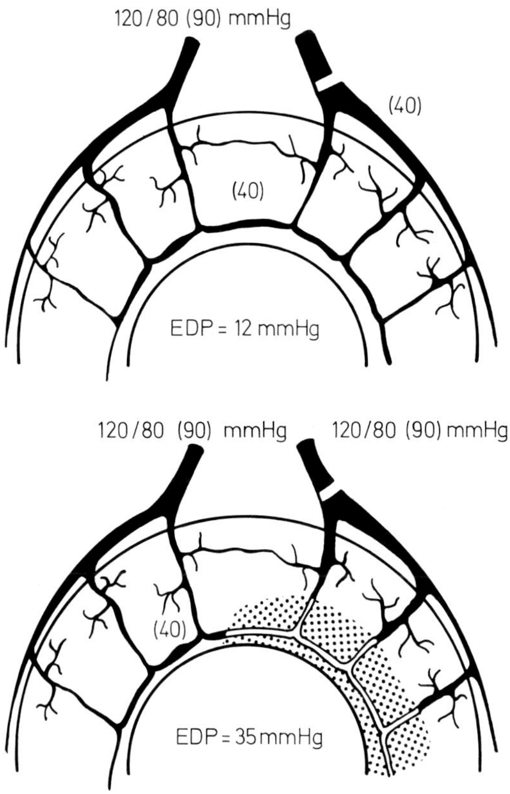

Fig. 8. Schematic illustration of the effects of ischemia on collateral flow. In the upper panel mean pressure in the vascular area supplied by the occluded vessel is 40 mm Hg, as is flow in the subendocardial collateral vessels. In the lower panel during ischemia left ventricular end diastolic pressure (EDP) hat risen to 35 mm Hg. Under these circumstances the flow through the collateral channels may be inadequate since the 40 mm Hg pressure in the collaterals may be insufficient to perfuse the vascular bed in the area of the occluded vessel

been found to be in the range of 40 to 60 mm Hg. Under resting conditions, this pressure may be adequate to perfuse the myocardium. During stress, the presence of collateral flow may prevent or delay the onset of ischemia. As the level of stress increases with an accompanying increase in heart rate, or under conditions prone to cause hypotension, such as anesthesia, the subendocardium may be inadequately perfused, with resultant ischemia. Once ischemia is manifest, left ventricular end-diastolic pressure increases and can cause mechanical compression of the collateral vessels in the subendocardium, which would further aggravate the imbalance between oxygen supply and demand (Fig. 8). Studies of regional myocardial blood flow in man using xenon-133 and a scintillation camera [18] have shown that once ischemia develops during pacing-induced angina, the flow to the ischemic region decreases below control values. This decrease in flow to the ischemic area below control may in part be explained by mechanical compression of the subendocardial

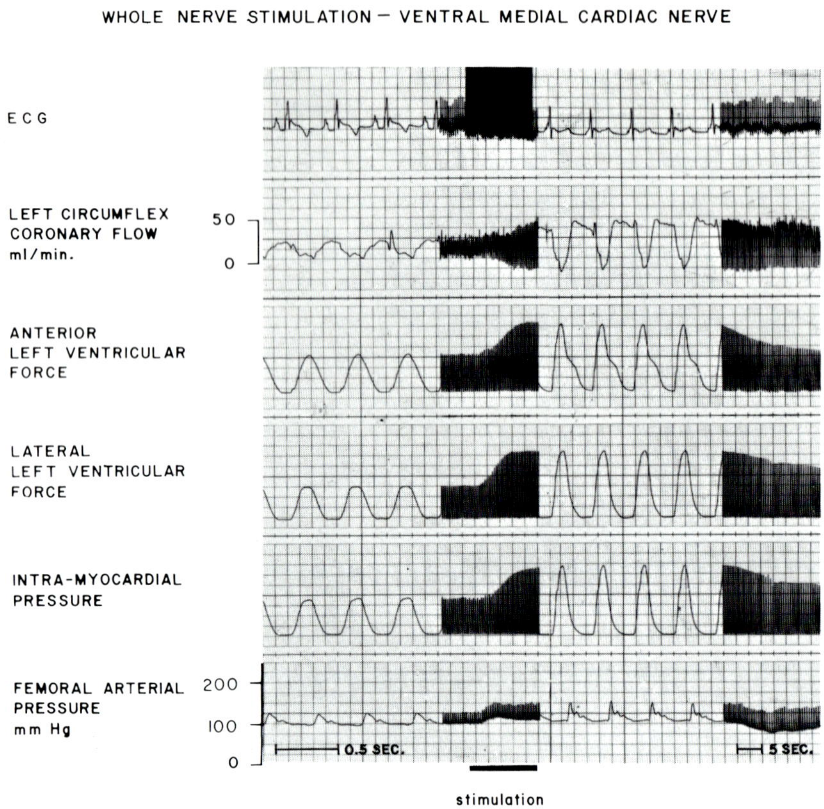

Fig. 9. Effect of stimulation of the ventral medial cardiac nerve on coronary blood flow in the anesthetized dog. Nerve stimulation results in an increase in myocardial force, systemic pressure, and coronary, blood flow. The increase in coronary blood flow is thought to be due to secondary metabolic vasodilatation. (From SHAW, ARMOUR, RANDALL, and PITT, unpublished observations)

vessels by myocardial tissue pressure, which acutely increases during ischemia. Reduction of left ventricular end-diastolic pressure by agents such as nitroglycerin, could result in relief of the mechanical compression and an increase in flow to the subendocardium.

Other manifestations of myocardial ischemia must also be considered. The typical electrocardiographic manifestations of angina pectoris, i.e., ST-segment depression have been shown to be due to subendocardial ischemia [19]. ST-segment elevation occurring during an anginal episode, such as in Prinzmetal variant angina, suggests transmural ischemia. The transmural ischemia that occurs in patients with Prinzmetal angina often occurs in the absence of demonstrable coronary artery lesions and is thought to be due to coronary artery spasm. While the exact neural pathways involved in spasm have not been elucidated, reflex pathways have been found that could lead to ischemia in the absence of obstructive coronary artery

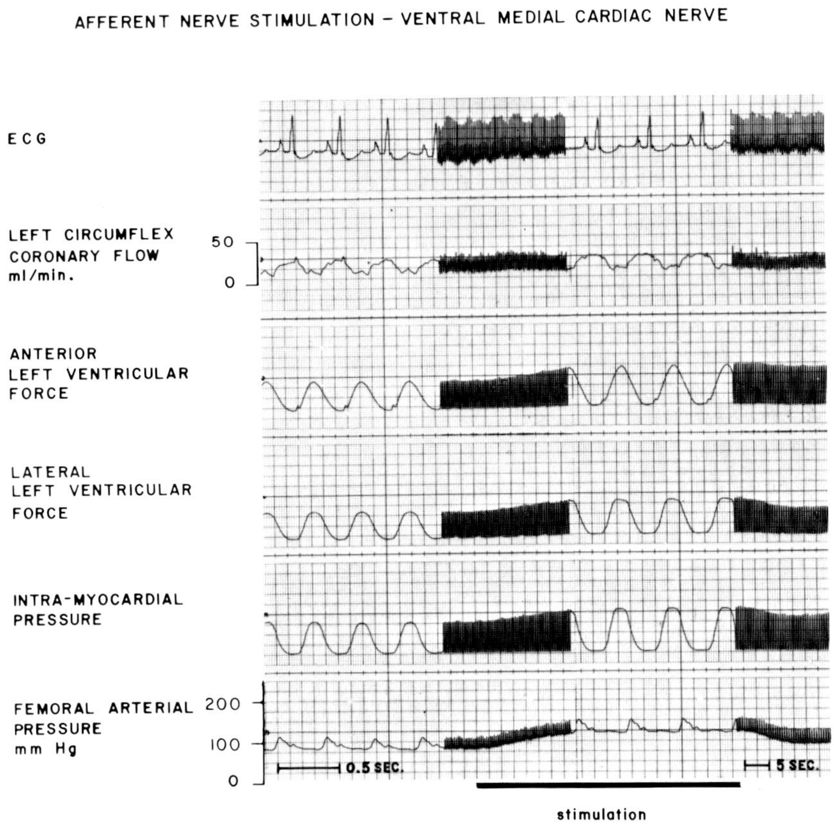

Fig. 10. Effect of stimulation of the afferent end of the cut ventral medial cardiac nerve in an anesthetized dog. In contrast to the experiment in Fig. 9, note the failure of coronary blood flow to increase despite an increase in myocardial force and systemic pressure. This suggests a discrepancy between myocardial oxygen demands and supply. (From SHAW, ARMOUR, RANDALL, and PITT, unpublished observations)

lesions [20, 21]. As mentioned above, stimulation of the stellate ganglion results in an initial decrease in flow followed by secondary metabolic vasodilatation [6]. If, however, one of the local sympathetic nerves is stimulated other effects can be seen. When the intact ventromedial sympathetic nerve is stimulated (Fig. 9), myocardial contractility and systemic pressure increase with an accompanying increase in coronary blood flow. If, however (Fig. 10), the nerve is cut and the afferent end stimulated, the increase in contractility and systemic pressure is not accompanied by the expected increase in flow [22]. Thus, there is a discrepancy between oxygen demand and supply and the expected "secondary metabolic vasodilatation" does not occur. These studies hold promise for future investigation into the occurence of myocardial ischemia without obstructive coronary artery disease.

During ischemia there are also metabolic and humoral factors that are of importance. Measurements of intramyocardial gas tension by the mass spectrometer have shown that pCO_2 increases markedly in ischemic regions of myocardium [23]. This increase in pCO_2 is directly correlated with the intramyocardial ST-segment changes [21]. Recent studies have shown that the accumulation of pCO_2 may cause a decrease in myocardial function independent of pH [22]. Thus, the mechanism for the local decrease in myocardial wall motion during ischemia, referred to earlier, may in part be related to the increase in pCO_2.

III. Action of Nitroglycerin in Relieving Myocardial Ischemia

The pathophysiological mechanisms discussed above are of importance in understanding how anti-anginal agents such as nitroglycerin work. Nitroglycerin has three major vascular sites of action: (1) coronary arteries, (2) peripheral arteries, and (3) peripheral veins. Although nitroglycerin causes coronary vasodilatation, it is unlikely that in view of the relationship described in Fig. 7 that its major action in relieving ischemia is due to coronary vasodilatation. First, in the presence of a critical or subcritical coronary artery lesion the reserve vasodilator capacity of the coronary bed is already almost completely exhausted in maintaining resting flow. Nitroglycerin may cause some increase in flow, but this increase is limited by the remaining vascular reserve present with the given degree of stenosis. Secondly, when given directly into the coronary arteries in a concentration sufficient to cause an increase in flow nitroglycerin does not relieve angina pectoris [25]. Nitroglycerin causes a reduction in myocardial oxygen demands by reducing wall stress. Both systolic pressure and ventricular volume are reduced by nitroglycerin. It is likely that the reduction in ventricular volume due to venous dilatation is more important than the reduction in arterial pressure due to arterial dilatation. The reduction in arterial pressure after sublingual nitroglycerin is transient lasting 10 to 15 min, the reduction in ventricular volume may last up to 30 min [26]. Also, it should be pointed out that a reduction in aortic pressure by other agents, which are arterial dilators, has not been shown to be effective in relieving angina. Although arterial vasodilators may reduce oxygen demands by a reduction in wall stress, this appears to be balanced in part by a reduction in coronary perfusion pressure and, hence, in oxygen supply. A precipitous reduction in arterial pressure, occasionally caused by nitroglycerin, but more frequently by amyl nitrite, may actually cause angina pectoris. The reduction in ventricular volume and therefore wall stress by nitroglycerin can be significantly increased by placing the patient in the upright position. In the supine position, sublingual nitroglycerin results in a 4- to 5%-reduction in volume compared to approximately a 20%-reduction in the sitting position [26]. This suggests that patients with severe ischemia, such as those with unstable angina, should be kept in the sitting position if maximal nitrate effect is desired. The reduction in oxygen demands after the administration of organic nitrates, can be further enhanced by the concomitant administration of an agent such as propranolol. The reduction in arterial pressure after nitroglycerin is often accompanied by a reflex tachycardia, which would tend to increase oxygen demands. If nitroglycerin is given after beta-adrenergic receptor blockade, the reflex tachycardia is prevented, and oxygen demands are reduced to a greater degree than would occur if either was given alone. Although the over-all reduction in myocardial oxygen demands by nitroglycerin is of

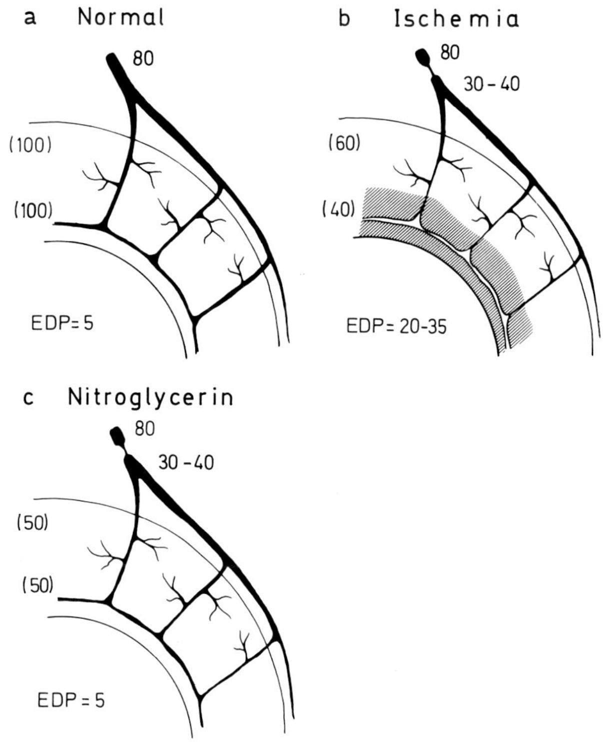

Fig. 11a—c. Schematic illustration of the effects of ischemia and nitroglycerin on the distribution of myocardial blood flow. In panel (a), under normal conditions, there is a mean pressure of 80 mm Hg in the coronary artery and flow is evenly distributed to the outer and inner layers of the myocardium. The numbers in parenthesis are the flow values. The left ventricular end diastolic pressure (EDP) is 5 mm Hg. In panel (b) the perfusion pressure beyond the coronary artery narrowing is 30 to 40 mm Hg and may in part contribute to a relatively greater decrease in blood flow to the deeper layers of the myocardium. Panel (c) shows the effect of nitroglycerin. After the initial arterial hypotension venous dilatation persists with a resultant reduction in EDP. Under these circumstances, there may be a redistribution of flow to the subendocardium without a total increase in flow. (From Becker and Pitt, Ref. [17])

importance, its effects on regional flow must also be considered [27] (Fig. 11). As described above, myocardial ischemia is often most severe in the subendocardium. Nitroglycerin causes a reduction in left ventricular end-diastolic pressure as a result of venous dilatation. The reduction in end-diastolic pressure reduces myocardial tissue pressure and increases effective coronary perfusion pressure. This, in turn, could account for the relative increase in subendocardial flow seen after nitroglycerin. The relative increase in subendocardial flow may occur with only a minimal, or no increase in total coronary blood flow [27]. Nitroglycerin may also have important direct effects on collateral vessels [28]. Aside from its direct effect in dilating large collateral vessels, nitroglycerin could increase collateral flow to an ischemic region by reducing end-diastolic pressure and, therefore, the mechanical compression of collaterals in the subendocardium. This mechanism may be of greater importance in man than in the dog with experimental ischemia. In man there is an extensive subendocardial collateral plexus that would be subject to compression, while in the dog the collateral vessels are to a greater extent located in the subepicardial region.

IV. Use of Nitroglycerin in Myocardial Infarction

Although nitroglycerin has been widely used as an anti-anginal agent, it has not been recommended for use in patients with myocardial infarction. Recent studies have shown, however, that nitroglycerin [29, 30] and other vasodilators [31] may improve ventricular performance in patients with myocardial infarction complicated by congestive heart failure. Nitroglycerin results in a reduction in left ventricular end-diastolic pressure from values of 20 to 30 mm Hg to the normal range of 10 to 15 mm Hg with only a small drop in arterial pressure and maintenance or improvement in cardiac output [30]. A reduction in left ventricular end-diastolic pressure, with the maintenance or improvement in stroke work, results in relief of pulmonary congestion and suggests an improvement in ventricular performance. In patients with a normal heart or those with myocardial infarction not complicated by manifest left ventricular failure, a reduction in left ventricular afterload by an arterial vasodilator does not lead to an improvement in ventricular performance. In these patients, ventricular performance is adequate and can easily overcome normal peripheral resistance or impedance. If, however, peripheral resistance is increased, the normal heart's performance may decrease. Conversely, if peripheral resistance is decreased in a patient with severely depressed cardiac function, ventricular performance will improve since a relatively large percentage of cardiac work must be expended in overcoming the normal peripheral resistance. Reduction in ventricular afterload may also be of value in patients with papillary muscle dysfunction or rupture [32]. Afterload reduction may also be of value in patients with shock secondary to left ventricular infarction. In this situation, the vasodilator should be given in conjunction with diastolic augmentation so as to maintain diastolic coronary perfusion pressure while reducing systolic pressure.

Although nitroglycerin does not improve ventricular performance in patients with myocardial infarction not complicated by manifest left ventricular failure, there may be reasons to administer it even to these patients. Experimental studies have shown that nitroglycerin can minimize the size of an infarct and can increase the threshold for ventricular fibrillation [33]. These effects are even more pronounced if the hypotension resulting from nitroglycerin administration is prevented by the concomitant administration of a peripheral vasoconstrictor, such as methoxamine or phenylephrine [33]. The beneficial effects of nitroglycerin under these circumstances are not due to a reduction in ventricular afterload but possibly to a direct effect on the coronary collateral vessels [28].

If nitroglycerin is to be used in patients with acute myocardial infarction, it should be given intravenously [30] rather than sublingually. When administered by the sublingual route, its effects upon arterial pressure are unpredictable. Severe hypotension may occur after sublingual administration, which may cause a reduction in coronary perfusion pressure and cause further ischemia. Secondly, the duration of action by the sublingual route is relatively short. When given by the intravenous route, a more prolonged reduction in left ventricular end diastolic pressure and improvement in ventricular performance can achieved without the occurrence of the reflex tachycardia seen after sublingual administration [30].

References

1. SONNENBLICK, E. H., SKELTON, C. L.: Oxygen consumption of the heart: Physiologic principles and clinical implications. Mod. Conc. cardiovasc. Dis. **40**, 9 (1971).
2. PITT, B., GREGG, D. E.: Coronary hemodynamics effects of increasing ventricular rate in the unanesthetized dog. Circulation Res. **22**, 753 (1968).
3. PITT, B., GREGG, D. E.: Effect of exercise at fixed ventricular rate on the coronary hemodynamics in the unanesthetized dog. Circulation **34**, 188 (1966) (Abstract).
4. PITT, B., GREGG, D. E.: Effect of excitement at fived ventricular rate on the coronary hemodynamics in the unanesthetized dog. Physiologist **9**, 267 (1966) (Abstract).
5. PITT, B.: Effect of beta adrenergic receptor blockade on the coronary circulation of the unanesthetized dog. Cardiovascular Beta Adrenergic Responses, edited by KATTUS, ROSS, and HALL. Los Angeles: UCLA Press 1970.
6. GRANATA, L., OLSSON, R. A., HUVOS, A., GREGG, D. E.: Coronary in flow and oxygen useage following sympathetic nerve stimulation in the unanesthetized dog. Circulation Res. **16**, 114 (1965).
7. ZUBERBUHLER, R. C., BOHR, D. F.: Responses of coronary smooth muscle to catecholamines. Circulation Res. **16**, 431 (1965).
8. OLSSON, R. A., GREGG, D. E.: Myocardial reactive hyperemia in the unanesthetized dog. Amer. J. Physiol. **208**, 224 (1965).
9. RUBIO, R., BERNE, R. M., KATORI, M.: Release of adenosine in reactive hyperemia of the dog heart. Amer. J. Physiol. **216**, 56 (1969).
10. TALESNIK, J., SUNAHARA, F. A.: Enhancement of metabolic dilatation by aspirin-like substances by suppression of prostaglandin feedback control. Nature (Lond.) New. Biol. **244**, 351 (1973).
11. PITT, B., MASON, J., CONTI, C. R., COLMAN, R. W.: Observations on the plasma kallikrein system during myocardial ischemia. Trans. Amer. Ass. Physns **82**, 98 (1969).
12. KHOURI, E. M., et al.: Flow in the major branches of the left cronary artery during experimental coronary insufficiency in the unanesthetized dog. Ciculation Res. **23**, 99 (1968).
13. FRIESINGER, G. C., CONTI, C. R., PITT, B.: Ventricular hemodynamics during spontaneous angina pectoris. Circulation **36, II**, 93 (1967).
14. DWYER, E. M.: Left ventricular pressure volume alterations and regional disorders of contraction during myocardial ischemia induced by atrial pacing. Circulation **42**, 111 (1970).
15. MCLAWRIN, L. P., ROLETT, E. L., GROSSMAN, W.: Impaired left ventricular relaxation during pacing-induced ischemia. Amer. J. Cardiol. **32**, 751 (1973).
16. SCHARF, S., BROMBERGER-BARNEA, B., PERMUTT, S.: Distribution of coronary venous flow. J. appl. Physiol. **30**, 657 (1971).
17. BECKER, L., PITT, B.: Regional myocardial blood flow, ischemia, and anti-anginal drugs. Ann. Clin. Res. **3**, 353 (1971).
18. MASSERI, A., PESCOLA, A., CONTINI, C., L'ABBATA, A.: Regional alterations of myocardial perfusion in angina pectoris. Circulation **38, IV**, 65 (1973 (Abstract).
19. SCHEUER, J. L.: Coronary insufficiency and relations between hemodynamic electrical and biochemical parameters. Circulation Res. **18**, 178 (1966).
20. ARMOUR, J. A., RANDALL, W. C.: A cardio-cardiac reflex in dog. Fed. Proc. **32**, 331 (1973).
21. SHAW, J., PITT, B.: Peripheral mechanisms involved in a cardiocardiac reflex. Fed. Proc. **32**, 331 (1973).
22. Unpublished observations: SHAW, J., ARMOUR, J. A., RANDALL, W. C., and PITT, B.
23. FLAHERTY, J. T., KHURI, S. F., O'RIORDAN, J. B., PITT, B., GOTT, V. L.: Quantitation of myocardial ischemia by intramyocardial carbon dioxide oxygen electrograms. Fed. Proc. **33**, 335 (1974).

24. BISHOP, E. L., WEISFELDT, M. L., ROSS, R. S.: Effects of pH and PCO_2 on performance of hypoperfused myocardium. Fed. Proc. **33**, 890 (1974).
25. GANZ, W., MARCUS, H. S.: Fairlure of intra coronary nitroglycerin to alleviate pacing induced angina. Circulation **48**, 880 (1972).
26. FORTUIN, N. J., CHATHAM, F., PITT, B.: Noninvasive evaluation of effects of nitroglycerin on determinants of myocardial oxygen consumption. Clin. Res.
27. BECKER, L., FORTUIN, N. J., PITT, B.: Effect of ischemia and anti-anginal drugs on the distribution of microspheres in the canine left ventricle. Circulation Res. **28**, 263 (1971).
28. GOLDSTEIN, R. E., STINSON, E. B., SCHERER, J. L., SENINGEN, R. P., GREHL, T. M., EPSTEIN, S. E.: Intraoperative coronary collateral function in patients with coronary occlusive disease. Circulation **49**, 298 (1974).
29. GOLD, H. K., LEINBACH, E. C., SANDERS, G. A.: Use of sublingual nitroglycerin in congestive heart failure following myocardial infarction. Circulation **46**, 839 (1972).
30. FLAHERTY, ., REID, P., KELLY, D. T., TAYLOR, D., WEISFELDT, M., PITT, B.: Intravenous nitroglycerin in acute myocardial infarction. Circulation **48**, 4.104 (1973) (Abstract).
31. FRANCIOSA, J. A., GUIHA, N. H., LIMAS, C. J., RODRIGUERA, E., COHN, J. N.: Improved left ventricular function during nitroprusside infusion in acute myocardial infarction. Lancet **1972 I**, 650.
32. CHATTERJEE, K., PARMLEY, W. W., SWAN, H. J. C., BERMAN, G., FORESTER, J., MARCUS, H. S.: Beneficial effects of vasodilator agents in severe mitral regurgitation due to dysfunction of subvalvular apparatus. Circulation **48**, 684 (1973).
33. EPSTEIN, S. E., GOLDSTEIN, R. E., REDWOOD, D. R., KENT, K. M., SMITH, E. R.: The early phase of acute myocardial infarction: Pharmacologic aspects of therapy. Ann. intern. Med. **78**, 918 (1973).

CHAPTER 8

Mechanism of Action of Nitroglycerin: Coronary, Cardiac, and Systemic Effects

STEPHEN F. VATNER and GUY R. HEYNDRICKX

With 14 Figures

I. Introduction

The salutary action of nitrates in the treatment of angina pectoris has been recognized for over a century since the classic reports of BRUNTON (1867) and MURRELL (1879). The historical background of nitrates is reviewed in detail in another chapter of this book. Despite the frequent, daily administration to patients with coronary disease and many investigations of these drugs in patients and experimental animals, their mechanism of action is still incompletely understood. This is in part because nitrates affect systemic vessels and the heart as well as coronary vessels. Mindful of the manifold effects of nitroglycerin which include peripheral vascular and myocardial factors, all interacting simultaneously with the direct coronary vascular effects of the drug in the control of the coronary circulation, it is perhaps understandable that a unified concept regarding the mechanism of action of nitrates has not evolved.

BRUNTON (1867) initially attributed the beneficial effects of amyl nitrite in the relief of angina pectoris to its hypotensive action and recommended it as a substitute for phlebotomy in this situation. Subsequently, attention focused on its direct coronary vasodilating action. Accordingly, when coronary vasospasm was a popular concept in the pathogenesis of angina pectoris, nitroglycerin was thought to be effective by inducing coronary dilation and relief from vasospasm. More recently the bulk of opinion has shifted back to the early views of Brunton, i.e., that the beneficial effects of nitrates are derived primarily from their peripheral actions and not necessarily due to their direct effects on the coronary circulation. However, in light of recent data demonstrating that nitrates affect the regional distribution of coronary flow, the coronary bed has again been advocated as an important site for the action of nitroglycerin.

It is clear that knowledge of the mechanism of action of nitrates must be derived from an understanding of the manner in which these drugs act on the heart and systemic circulation as well as on the coronary vascular bed. In addition, since nitroglycerin reduces arterial pressure, it elicits a variety of reflex effects which also affect the heart and coronary vessels. Finally, the evidence that the drug may act differently in the presence and absence of diseased coronary vessels must be considered. With this in mind the discussion of nitroglycerin's various mechanisms of action will focus first on a) its overall effects on the coronary circulation in the normal heart and b) in the presence of coronary artery disease, and then will be followed by a discussion of its effects on c) collateral vessels and on the distribution of myocardial blood flow. The next part of this review will discuss nitroglycerin's action on d) the heart and systemic circulation. Finally, the effects of nitroglycerin on e) cardiac function in the presence of severe myocardial ischemia and myocardial infarction will be summarized. Two important points must be kept in mind throughout. First, although for the purpose of clarity this review is divided into several sections, the coronary vascular effect of nitrates cannot be dissociated from simultaneous effects on the major determinants of myocardial oxygen consumption, i.e., cardiac rate, contractility and left ventricular wall tension, since these latter variables along with coronary perfusion pressure are intimately involved in the regulation of coronary blood flow and vascular resistance (BRAUNWALD, 1969, 1971). Secondly, the effects of nitrates vary considerably with the dose and route of administration. This latter point may resolve some of the discrepancies observed from different investigations.

II. Action on the Coronary Circulation

A. Normal Circulation

As long as 60 years ago it was observed by VOEGTLIN and MACHT (1913—1914) that nitroglycerin relaxed the isolated coronary artery as well as other vessels. These observations were extended to the intact anesthetized dog by BOYER and GREEN (1941) using an optically recording flowmeter and to the conscious dog by ESSEX et al. (1940). In both of these studies substantial coronary vasodilatation was observed after administration of nitrates. While these, as well as a number of subsequent studies have demonstrated that coronary vasodilation occurs following nitroglycerin in intact animals, the magnitude of nitroglycerin's coronary vasodilating action has been underestimated for several reasons.

1. Time Course of Action

First of all, when the drug is administered intravenously in a bolus, the peak rise in coronary flow occurs rapidly (Fig. 1). Accordingly, techniques that possess a limited response time, such as many of the indirect methods used to measure coronary blood flow in man, e.g., nitrous oxide or Rubidium^{86}, might miss the striking, transient rise in coronary blood flow that occurs. This short-lived, but impressive, coronary vasodilator effect is accompanied by an increase in coronary venous oxygen saturation and a reduction in the coronary arterio-venous oxygen difference (Fig. 2), indicating that nitroglycerin acts to dilate coronary vessels directly and not secondarily in response to increased myocardial metabolic demands. This point is best demonstrated by Fig. 3 and 4. Figure 3 shows typical simultaneous responses of left ventricular dimensions and velocity, pressures and *dP/dt*, coronary flow and heart rate in response to an intravenous bolus dose of nitroglycerin, 40 μg/kg, in a conscious dog. Figure 4 summarizes these results in a series of conscious animals. In both figures it is evident at point "A" that coronary flow has increased substantially prior to any systemic or left ventricular effects of the drug, which might affect the coronary vascular bed secondarily.

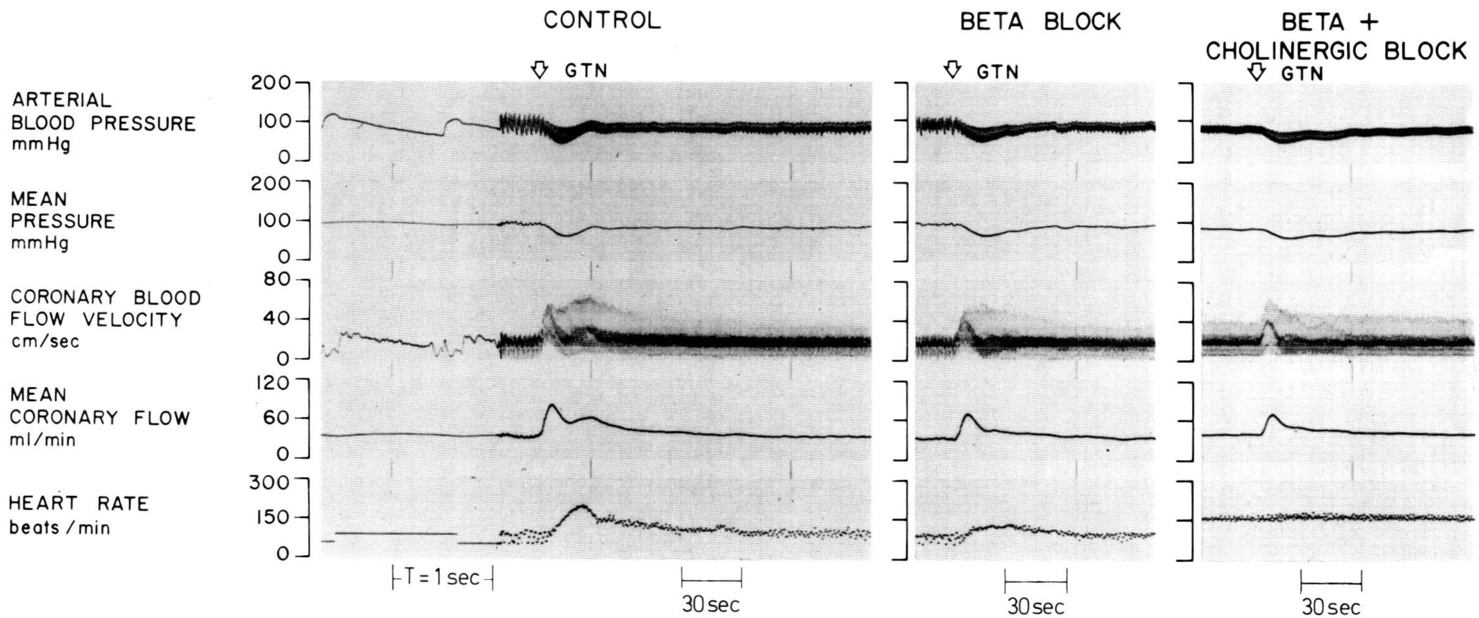

Fig. 1. The effects of nitroglycerin, 20 μg/kg, intravenously in a healthy, conscious dog instrumented for phasic and mean measurements of arterial pressure and coronary blood flow. The responses to the same dose of nitroglycerin are compared in the control state (left panel), after beta adrenergic blockade with propranolol, 1 mg/kg, (middle panel) and after combined blockade with propranolol and atropine (right panel). Note that nitroglycerin in the conscious animal produces a sustained increase in coronary flow. In the control state a secondary peak for coronary flow is evident, which is due to the reflex chronotropic and inotropic effects and is abolished by autonomic blockades

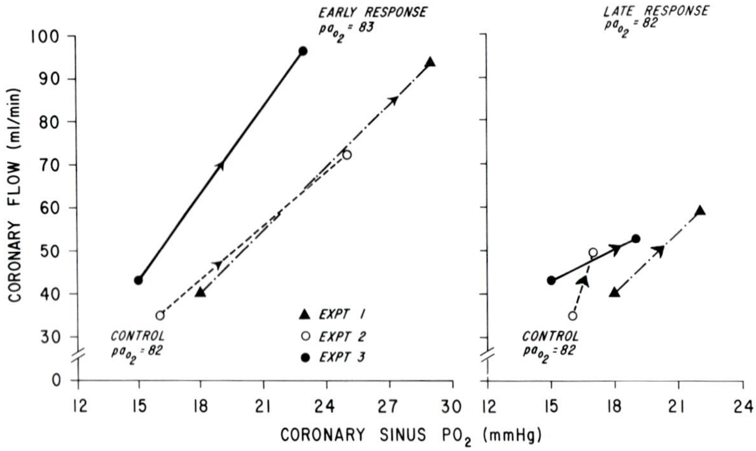

Fig. 2. The average of three determinations of coronary sinus oxygen values for each of three dogs are plotted against their coronary flow responses. The early response to intravenous nitroglycerin (left panel) can be compared with the later effects (right panel). The simultaneous average values for arterial pO_2 are noted. The early response to intravenous nitroglycerin involves a direct dilator effect on coronary vessels and a narrowing of arterio-venous oxygen difference, whereas the later phase of coronary dilatation is secondary to increase in myocardial metabolic demands, i.e. increased heart rate and contractility and is not associated with substantial narrowing of coronary arterio-venous oxygen difference. (Reprinted with permission from the Journal of Clinical Investigation, VATNER et al., 1972)

2. Effects of Anesthesia

Secondly, the experimental preparation used is important to consider. Most studies in animals have been conducted in anesthetized preparations, in which the effects of the general anesthetic and surgical manipulation may have acted to dilate the coronary bed prior to nitroglycerin. Moreover, the hypotensive effects of nitroglycerin (as well as any hypotensive stimulus)are accentuated in the open chest anesthetized animal, in which reflex control of the circulation is attenuated. The effect of anesthesia on circulatory control has recently been reviewed (VATNER and BRAUNWALD). For instance, when arterial pressure is lowered reflexly by electrical stimulation of the carotid sinus nerves, the recovery period for arterial pressure is considerably longer in anesthetized as compared to conscious animals (VATNER et al., 1971). Similarly, with nitroglycerin the depression of arterial pressure is augmented in anesthetized open chest preparations. One of the primary determinants of coronary blood flow is the coronary perfusion pressure, i.e., the diastolic arterial pressure. Since arterial pressure is depressed to a greater extent and for a longer period than in the conscious state, less of an elevation in coronary flow would be expected in the anesthetized state if an equal reduction in coronary resistance occurred.

3. Reflex Effects

Furthermore, it must be considered that a substantial portion of the increase in coronary flow and reduction in coronary resistance after nitroglycerin adminis-

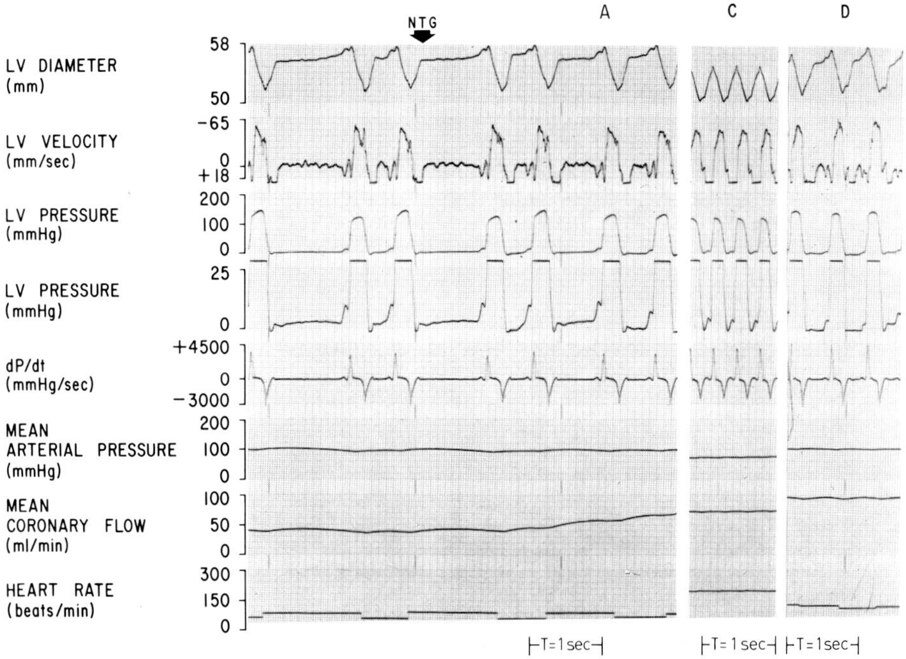

Fig. 3. A typical response to intravenous nitroglycerin (NTG), 40 μg/kg, in a conscious dog. The phasic wave forms for left ventricular diameter, velocity, systolic and diastolic pressures, *dP/dt*, are shown simultaneously with mean arterial pressure, mean coronary flow, and heart rate. Waveforms in the control period prior to nitroglycerin are shown in the left panel. The early rise in coronary flow that occurs prior to systemic or left ventricular function changes is also shown in the left panel (A). The response of the left ventricle and coronary bed during the peak hypotensive action of the drug is shown in the middle panel (C), and the second phase of coronary dilation that occurs with the peak inotropic response is shown at the right (D). (Reprinted with permission from the Journal of Clinical Investigation, VATNER et al., 1972)

tered to the unanesthetized dog is due to reflex effects, i.e., the reflex increases in heart rate and myocardial contractility that occur after the fall in arterial pressure (VATNER et al., 1972). The positive inotropic and chronotropic actions increase myocardial oxygen consumption and increase coronary blood flow on this basis (Figs. 1, 5 and 6). This secondary rise in coronary blood flow after intravenous nitroglycerin has been rarely observed in studies in anesthetized animals (CHARLIER, 1971). Thus, the attenuation of the reflex response and the prolongation of the depression of arterial pressure tend to mask the coronary vasodilator effects of nitroglycerin in the anesthetized animal more than in the conscious animal. In fact, a biphasic coronary response to nitroglycerin is often observed in the anesthetized preparation, after a brief initial increase in coronary flow, flow generally falls below control values as shown in Fig. 3 in CHARLIER'S review (1971). This biphasic effect has never been observed in our experience when the drug is administered to conscious animals (Figs. 1, 5 and 6), in which coronary blood flow remains above control during the entire response.

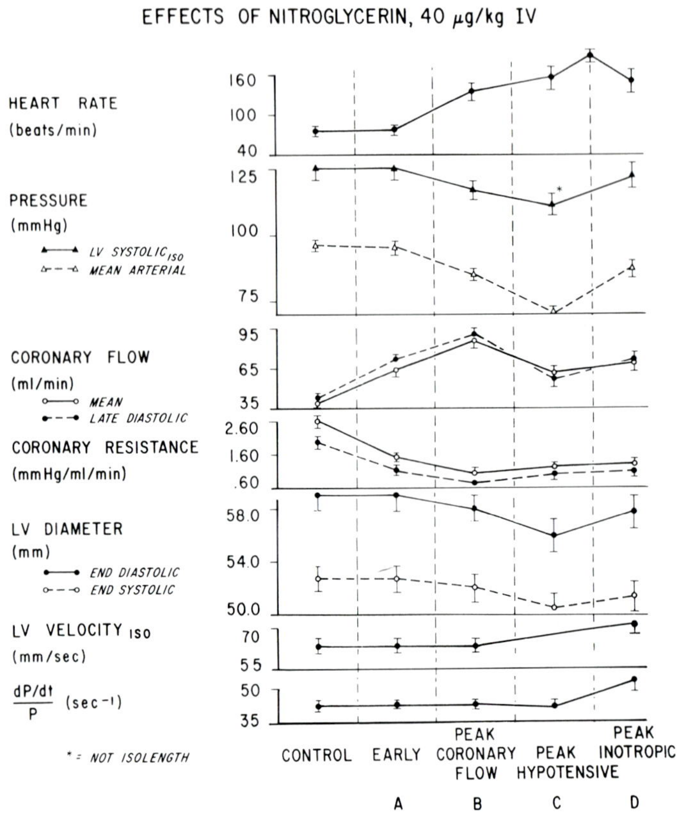

Fig.4. The normal response to intravenous nitroglycerin, 40 μg/kg, is shown for heart rate, isolength left ventricular systolic pressure and mean arterial pressure, mean and late diastolic coronary flow and resistance, end-diastolic and end-systolic diameters, isolength velocity and $(dP/dt)/P$. The average control values are shown in the first panel. The early increase in coronary flow and decrease in coronary resistance that occurred prior to systemic or left ventricular changes are shown next (A). The simultaneous effects on the left ventricle and systemic circulation are compared during the peak coronary vasodilatation response (B). Effects during the peak hypotensive action of intravenous nitroglycerin are shown next (C). The second phase of coronary vasodilatation that occurred with the peak inotropic response are shown at the right (D). (Reprinted with permission from the Journal of Clinical Investigation, VATNER et al., 1972)

4. Dose Response and Route of Administration

There is an additional reason for which the coronary vasodilator effects of nitroglycerin have been underestimated in the past, which relates to the dose delivered to the coronary circulation and to the route of administration. While intracoronary nitroglycerin easily elicits a striking coronary vasodilator response in most experimental preparations, the same response is not as easily demonstrated when the drug is administered intravenously for the reasons outlined above. However, coronary vasodilation is even less obvious when the drug is administered sublingually, as it is almost always used in patients (BING et al., 1964; COHEN et al., 1965; LUEBS et al.,

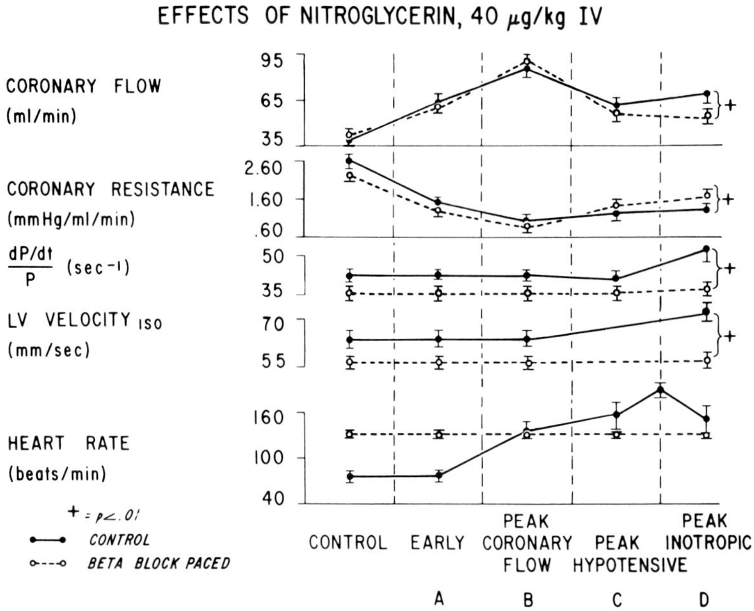

Fig. 5. The normal responses (solid lines) and those after beta blockade and heart rate held constant with atrial pacing (broken lines) are compared after intravenous nitroglycerin, 40 μg/kg, on mean coronary flow and resistance, $(dP/dt)/P$, isolength velocity, and heart rate. Note that preventing reflex effects does not substantially affect the early or peak coronary effects, but modifies the later coronary response. (Reprinted with permission from the Journal of Clinical Investigation, VATNER et al., 1972)

1966; LICHTLEN et al., 1966; KNOEBEL et al., 1968; CARSON et al., 1969). There are several reports of studies conducted in anesthetized preparations by ECKENHOFF and HAFKENSCHIEL (1947); VYDEN et al. (1970); GILLIS and MELVILLE (1971) or in man using indirect methods for measuring coronary blood flow, such as the study by KNOEBEL et al. (1968) in which no changes in coronary flow or resistance were noted after sublingual nitroglycerin. This is understandable when it is considered that the relative increase in coronary blood flow and decrease in coronary vascular resistance is much less after sublingual than intravenous nitroglycerin (Fig. 7). In the absence of reflex positive inotropic and chronotropic effects, the direct coronary dilation effect of sublingual nitroglycerin is minor (VATNER et al., 1972). Thus, since only a 25% rise in coronary blood flow is observed when nitroglycerin was administered sublingually to normal conscious dogs (Fig. 5), it is reasonable that such a small response might not be observed using techniques that do not measure coronary flow directly and continuously or even with flowmeters in anesthetized open chest preparations, in which reflex responses to nitroglycerin are blunted.

5. Summary of Coronary Effects in the Normal Heart

In summary, when a sufficiently large dose of nitroglycerin is delivered to the normal heart, striking coronary vasodilation is observed. Two distinct mechanisms of coro-

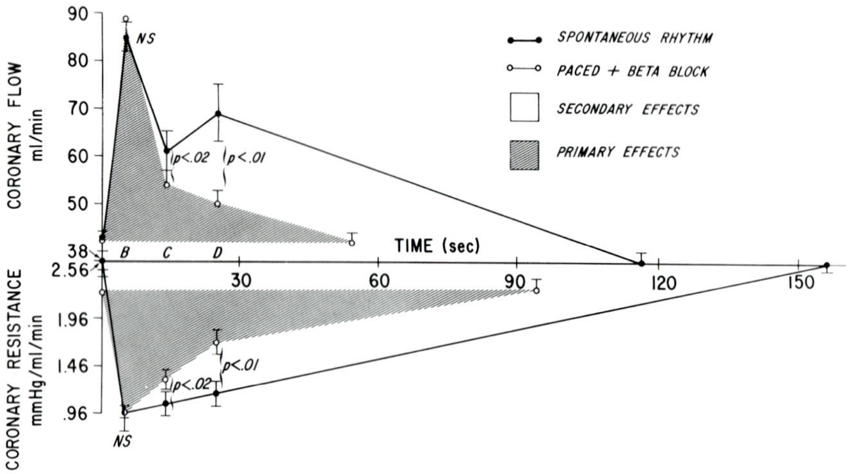

Fig. 6. The relative contributions of the direct and secondary effects of intravenous nitroglycerin, 40 μg/kg, to the responses of coronary flow (top) and coronary resistance (bottom) are shown. The smaller shaded area represents the direct action of the drug on coronary vessels, while the amount due to secondary effects is shown by the clear areas. (Reprinted with permission from the Journal of Clinical Investigation, VATNER et al., 1972)

nary vasodilation can be identified. First, a direct dilating action on coronary vascular smooth muscle results in primary vasodilation, unassociated with changes in cardiac rate or contractility and is accompanied by a reduction in the coronary arteriovenous oxygen difference (Figs. 1 and 2). In addition, a major component of coronary vasodilation secondary to increased myocardial metabolic demands is observed (Fig. 6). This portion of the increase in coronary flow and reduction in coronary resistance can be abolished by preventing the reflex chronotropic and inotropic effects that arise in response to an abrupt reduction in arterial pressure (Fig. 6). These same mechanisms are responsible for coronary vasodilation after sublingual nitroglycerin. However, the magnitude of the coronary vascular effects following sublingual nitroglycerin are considerably less than those following intravenous administration (Fig. 7), due to the smaller quantity of drug delivered to the heart and also to the resultant reduction in the intensity of the reflexes that can be elicited in response to a fall in arterial pressure that is more gradual in onset and smaller in magnitude.

B. Effects on the Ischemic Heart

To fully understand the action of nitrates on the ischemic heart, the pathogenesis of angina pectoris must be reviewed, which has been done elsewhere in this volume. While it is generally agreed that nitroglycerin dilates coronary vessels in the normal heart, there is no general agreement as to its effects on those vessels in the ischemic heart. For many years, as pointed out by WEGRIA et al. (1951); HONIG et al. (1960); CHARLIER (1961), it was held that nitroglycerin, which had been shown to dilate normal coronary vessels, also dilated coronary vessels in the ischemic heart and that

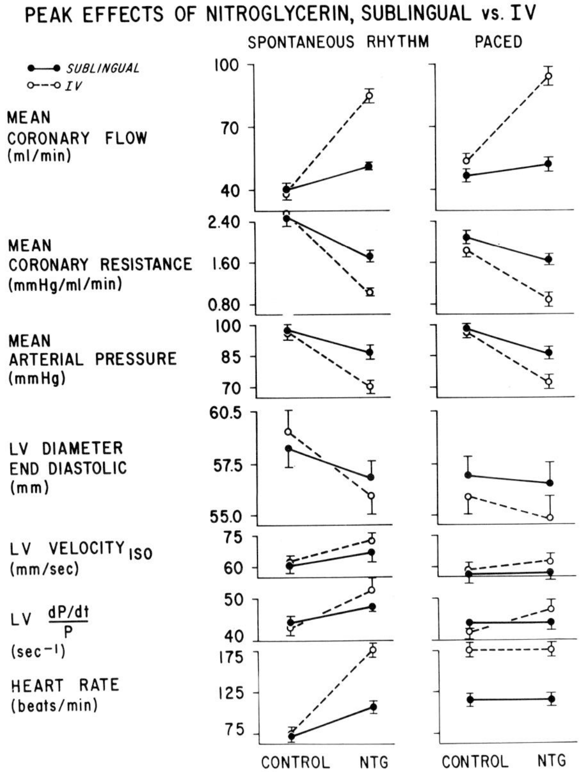

Fig. 7. Peak responses to nitroglycerin (NTG), 40 μg/kg, are compared for the intravenous (broken lines) and sublingual (solid lines) routes of administration in spontaneous rhythm (left panel) and when heart rate was maintained constant (right panel). There was no significant difference between the control values before nitroglycerin when administered sublingually or intravenously, but all the changes after intravenous nitroglycerin were significantly greater ($p < 0.01$). (Reprinted with permission from the Journal of Clinical Investigation, VATNER et al., 1972)

this dilatation allowed flow to increase to the ischemic area. The studies of GORLIN et al. (1959) suggested that nitroglycerin failed to dilate coronary vessels in patients with coronary artery disease. In these patients coronary vascular resistance was found to be essentially fixed; after sublingual nitroglycerin resistance did not change significantly and in several patients coronary flow actually fell. GORLIN and coworkers (1959) then concluded that "nitrites probably relieve pain in some manner other than general coronary dilatation", for instance by reducing myocardial oxygen demands. On the other hand, several investigators have demonstrated that nitroglycerin dilates the coronary bed even in the presence of myocardial ischemic disease (COWAN et al., 1969; LIKOFF et al., 1964). Some studies have observed that nitrates can increase coronary blood flow in patients with coronary artery disease (BERNSTEIN et al., 1966; COWAN et al, 1969), while others have noted in patients (PARKER et al., 1971) and in animals (MALINDZAK et al., 1970) with coronary insufficiency that nitroglycerin failed to change coronary blood flow as arterial pressure fell, indicating that coronary vasodilatation must have occurred. In fact, since it is now generally felt that nitroglycerin reduces myocardial oxygen demands by reducing arterial pressure and preload and pari passu the myocardial demand for coronary blood flow, i.e., a reduction of metabolically induced vasodilation would be expected. Thus, in the face of falling myocardial oxygen demands where demand for coronary flow is less, an observed reduction or no change in coronary resistance reflects coronary dilatation and actually underestimates the extent to which the drug dilates coronary vessels.

Since coronary artery disease is generally patchy in nature, the key question is not whether the coronary bed as a whole dilates with nitroglycerin, but rather whether the dilatation occurs in the vessels supplying the ischemic area, i.e., where more blood is needed, or whether the dilatation is occurring in vessels supplying normal myocardium, i.e., where excess flow may be superfluous or may even deprive the ischemic myocardium of blood flow through a vascular "steal". The latter is essentially what has recently been observed in a study by Ganz and Marcus (1972), who reported that intracoronary nitroglycerin increased coronary blood flow in patients with coronary artery disease but failed to relieve angina pectoris induced by pacing. In contrast, when nitroglycerin was administered intravenously, coronary flow failed to increase but relief from pacing induced anginal pain rapidly occurred associated with the fall in arterial pressure. These investigators, therefore support the earlier conclusion of Gorlin et al. (1959), that nitroglycerin acts through its peripheral rather than its direct coronary vascular effects. The possibility also exists, however, that nitroglycerin exerts its beneficial action by different mechanisms, depending on the etiology of the coronary insufficiency. In the case of angina pectoris induced by coronary vasospasm, nitroglycerin could relieve the constriction and improve myocardial perfusion, thereby ameliorating the anginal episode. It must be pointed out, however, that while it has been speculated that coronary vasospasm may be etiologically responsible for angina, this has not been demonstrated with regularity, except in the special case of patients with Prinzmetal's atypical angina. In some of these patients nitroglycerin dilates the constricted coronary vessels and relieves the pain, as shown in a recent report by Oliva et al. (1973). However, in the more common situation, in which angina is associated with a maximally dilated bed, as occurs in chronic obstructive coronary artery disease, the effects of nitroglycerin on the coronary circulation would be beneficial only if it resulted in a redistribution of coronary flow or an increase in collateral blood flow.

C. Regional and Collateral Coronary Effects

Ischemic heart disease is generally not uniform, but is most commonly patchy and localized to one or several areas; in the involved portions of the myocardium the severity of the disease is frequently variable. The ultimate goal of the use of nitroglycerin in ischemic heart disease is to restore the balance between oxygen demand and supply in the ischemic areas of the heart.

When an area of the myocardium is inadequately perfused, a more appropriate balance between local oxygen delivery and requirements is unlikely to occur through increased oxygen extraction since it is already maximal or nearly so (Gregg and Fischer 1963; Berne 1964), but may be achieved by (1) increased total coronary blood flow with a proportional increase in flow to the ischemic region, (2) constant total coronary blood flow with redistribution of blood flow from a normal area to the ischemic area through the collateral circulation, (3) reduction of oxygen requirements of the whole heart or specifically in the ischemic area or (4) some combination of the three aforementioned mechanisms. An increase in total coronary blood flow does not necessarily result in an increase in perfusion of the ischemic area. Considering that the resistance vessels in the ischemic area may already be maximally dilated due to the potent coronary dilator stimulus provided by local hypoxia, a reduction in total coronary resistance in the remaining normal vessels secondary to a vasodilator may produce a vascular "steal" and thereby reduce perfusion of the ischemic zone, unless an extensive collateral circulation redistributes blood from the normal zone to the ischemic area (Fig. 8). The capability for developing collateral circulation, in order to supply additional blood flow not only depends on the site of the obstruction in the coronary vascular bed, but also upon the time course and the evolution of the disease and varies among different species (SCHAPER, 1971). The remaining mechanism, a reduction of oxygen requirements, can be achieved mainly by the peripheral effects of nitroglycerin that will be discussed below. In light of the observations in patients with coronary disease, showing that nitroglycerin failed to increase total coronary flow (GORLIN et al., 1959; BING et al., 1964; GANZ and MARCUS, 1972) and considering the experiments conducted by KIRK and HONIG (1964a, b) indicating that coronary blood flow is not homogeneously distributed across the wall of the left ventricle, considerable attention has been directed to the effects of nitrates on regional myocardial blood flow distribution.

1. Effects of Nitroglycerin on Large and Small Coronary Vessels

The total coronary resistance consists of the resistance of the large epicardial vessels (denoted as "A" in Fig. 8) on the one hand and of the smaller coronary arteries (denoted as "C" in Fig. 8) and arterioles on the other. WINBURY et al. (1969) indicated that the resistance of the large vessels normally constitutes approximately only 5% of the total resistance. This means that the total coronary resistance is localized almost entirely in the small vessels and that the resistance of the large vessels is not a limiting factor of blood supply, unless the lumen is obstructed by more than 50%. FAM and MCGREGOR (1964, 1968) assessed the amount of blood available to an ischemic area through collateral vessels by measuring the volume of retrograde flow distal to a coronary occlusion. They demonstrated in anesthetized dogs that nitroglycerin increases retrograde blood flow distal to a chronic occlusion of a branch of the left coronary artery and that resistance in the large conductive vessels fell more than in the arteriolar resistance vessels in the normal myocardium. They concluded that nitroglycerin acts primarily by dilating large conductive vessels, which is presumed to promote an increase in blood flow to the ischemic area through collateral channels (denoted as "B" in Fig. 8). LEIGHNINGER et al. (1959) also demonstrated enhanced coronary backflow after nitroglycerin. The study of WINBURY et al. (1969), emphasizes the importance of this observation. These investigators also found that nitroglycerin produced a prolonged dilatation of the large coronary arteries, which persisted up to 12 min, while the small coronary arteries showed only a transient dilatation that had disappeared by 2 min, and which was actually followed by an increase in small vessel resistance at 12 min. This selectivity of action

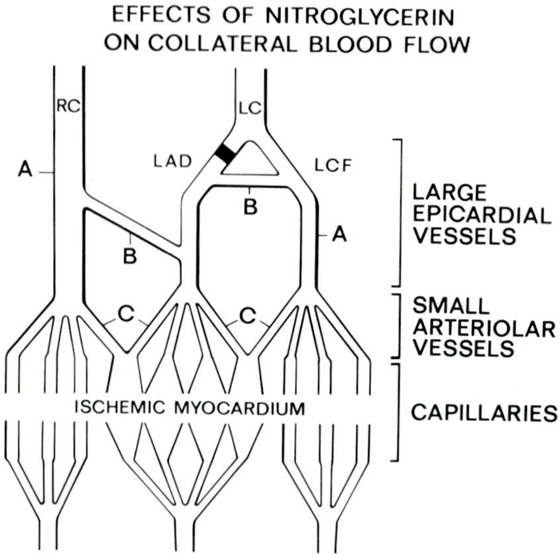

Fig. 8. A schematic representation of the coronary circulation with an obstruction in one of the major vessels, in this case the left anterior descending (LAD). Nitroglycerin is thought to improve the blood supply to the ischemic myocardium by dilating large epicardial vessels (A) and collateral channels (B), while having a lesser transient effect on the resistance vessels of the normal myocardium (C)

upon the large vessels is even more pronounced when expressed as the ratio of large vessel resistance to total vessel resistance (RL/RT). Nitroglycerin, administered intravenously, only increases the ratio during the first 2 min, due to a relatively greater depression of small vessel resistance, but decreased the ratio at 12 min. As a result of these findings the authors suggested that in contrast with the non-nitrate vasodilators such as dipyridamole and chromonar, the nitrates act primarily on the large epicardial conductive vessels, which do not participate to as great an extent in the instantaneous regulation of coronary blood flow as do the smaller resistance vessels. Corroborative evidence for the hypothesis of FAM and MCGREGOR and of WINBURY et al. was provided by experiments of SCHNAAR and SPARKS (1972) using isolated strips of coronary arteries, which showed that nitroglycerin produced a more prolonged relaxation in the strips from the large vessels. COHEN and KIRK (1973a), using a constant flow technique to monitor directly changes in the coronary vascular resistance also found a transient dilatation of the small vessels and a more sustained dilatation of the large vessels, thereby supporting the findings of FAM and MCGREGOR (1964, 1968); WINBURY et al. (1969). With infusion of nitroglycerin the small vessels exhibited tachyphylaxis, while the large vessels did not (COHEN and KIRK, 1973a). From these observations the authors concluded that the vasodilator effect of nitroglycerin on the small vessels is compensated for by their autoregulatory properties. The large epicardial vessels do not appear to participate in this autoregulation, as previously shown by WINBURY et al. (1969); FAM and MCGREGOR (1964, 1968).

Several investigators have demonstrated the important dilator action of nitroglycerin on the large epicardial vessels in the dog as well as in man with and without coronary artery disease by cineangiographic techniques (LEHAN et al., 1966; WEST and GUZMAN, 1959; LIKOFF et al., 1964; GENSINI et al., (1962). Studies by WEST and GUZMAN (1959); LIKOFF (1964); GENSINI (1962); OLIVA (1973) and their respective collaborators have demonstrated dilation of large coronary vessels after nitroglycerin in patients with coronary artery disease. Thus, it is generally held that nitrates can dilate large coronary vessels even in the presence of coronary atherosclerosis.

2. Effects of Nitroglycerin on Collateral Vessels

An important compensatory mechanism in response to coronary atherosclerosis by the human heart is the development of collateral circulation. Since patients utilizing nitroglycerin for the relief of angina pectoris generally have developed collateral channels, considerable attention has been directed to the possibility that nitroglycerin acts on these vessels (denoted as "B" in Fig. 8).

A recent study in a model of chronic myocardial ischemia by COHEN et al. (1973b) has demonstrated that regional contractility increased in an ischemic zone after administration of nitroglycerin. They felt that the augmentation of regional contractility reflected an increase in local myocardial blood flow through collateral channels. However, in the presence of global myocardial ischemia, nitroglycerin did not improve regional contractility, suggesting that nitroglycerin is able to dilate collateral vessels only when the area of the myocardium that supplies these collateral vessels is not in itself ischemic. The dilatation of collaterals is more sustained than the dilatation of the normal resistance vessels in the nonischemic portion of the heart, resulting in an increase in collateral flow and a redistribution of blood towards the ischemic area. However, when the entire myocardium is ischemic, all channels are already maximally dilated and nitroglycerin can no longer exert a vasodilator effect. This finding of increased myocardial perfusion in ischemic zones after nitroglycerin has recently been confirmed in patients with coronary artery disease studied in the course of operation by HORWITZ et al. (1971); GOLDSTEIN et al. (1973). WINBURY et al. (1969); LINDER and SEEMAN (1967) have also demonstrated that nitroglycerin dilates coronary collaterals in the presence of acute myocardial ischemia. WINBURY et al. (1969), felt that collateral blood flow is enhanced passively, since the study by MAUTZ and GREGG (1937) showed that collateral vessels have little smooth muscle and therefore, exhibit only minor vasoactive properties. SCHAPER (1971) has recently pointed out that collateral vessels may exhibit smooth muscle in small quantities and thus could respond directly to a vasodilator.

In contrast to the general opinion that nitroglycerin does dilate collateral vessels are the studies by BECKER et al. (1971), who found no evidence for this phenomenon, but rather observed improved myocardial perfusion of ischemic areas through transmural redistribution of blood flow rather than through collateral channels. While the discrepancy between these two groups of investigators cannot be easily reconciled, it is of interest that in all of these studies nitroglycerin improved the perfusion of the ischemic area.

3. Effects of Nitroglycerin on Regional Myocardial Blood Flow

A great deal of work has recently been done on the transmural distribution of the coronary blood flow in the normal heart as well as in the presence of ischemia. Considerable controversy still exists regarding the normal transmural distribution of myocardial blood flow, which may be due to differences in methodology (MOIR, 1972). Studies using clearance of local injection of diffusible isotopes into the myocardium by BRANDI et al. (1966) and other investigators, based on determinations of local tissue oxygen tension in different layers of the myocardium as indices of regional blood flow by KIRK and HONIG (1964b) and by WEISS and WINBURY (1973) have shown that the subendocardium is normally less well perfused than the subepicardium, supporting a number of clinical and pathological observations emphasizing the vulnerability of the endocardium to ischemic injury (FRIEDBERG, 1966; HORN et al., 1950; JENNINGS et al., 1960). On the other hand, studies using intravascular diffusible isotopes by MATHES and RIVAL (1971); YIPINTSOI et al. (1973) and radioactive microspheres by YIPINTSOI et al. (1973); DOMENECH et al. (1969); BECKER et al. (1971); KJEKSHUS (1973); COBB et al. (1974) have shown that the endocardium is normally at least as well perfused as the epicardium; the ratio between subendocardial flow and the subepicardial flow actually slightly exceeding 1. The discrepancy in these results is apparently due to the use of two different groups of methods, i.e., whether the indicator is injected intravenously, as with microspheres and Rubidium^{86} or whether the indicator is directly injected into the myocardium. Both methods have been criticized and, although much evidence is in favor of at least an even perfusion of the subendocardium and the subepicardium, no definite answer is available. Regardless of the method used, it is generally agreed that there is a differential perfusion of the subendocardium and subepicardium in the ischemic heart. When coronary flow is limited, the subendocardium becomes ischemic first, MOIR (1972). This fits with the clinical and pathological observations of FRIEDBERG (1966); HORN et al. (1950); JENNINGS et al. (1960).

The effects of nitroglycerin on the transmural distribution of myocardial blood flow has been investigated both in the normal and ischemic heart. WEISS and WINBURY (1973) suggest that nitroglycerin increases the subendocardial blood flow in the normal heart. BECKER et al. (1971) also found a redistribution of coronary flow after nitroglycerin, favoring the subendocardium both in the well perfused and ischemic portion of the heart. Ischemia on the other hand has been reported by KJEKSHUS (1973); FORMAN et al. (1973) to alter the transmural blood flow distribution following an experimental coronary artery occlusion, subendocardial flow being reduced more than subepicardial. MATHES and RIVAL (1971) found that only when the subendocardial region was ischemic did administration of nitroglycerin reverse the abnormal flow distribution by increasing the flow in the subendocardium more than in the subepicardium. WINBURY and GOBEL (1967) have also indicated that nitroglycerin is able to improve subendocardial blood flow, presumably by acting on the precapillary sphincters, resulting in an increase in endocardial perfusion. Thus, the bulk of evidence suggests that nitroglycerin improves perfusion of the subendocardium in the presence of ischemia.

This conclusion is based primarily on studies in which there is no epicardial/endocardial flow gradient in the normal myocardium but a selective reduction in subendocardial flow with ischemia. It is of interest to note that this improvement cannot be related to the concomitant fall in arterial perfusion pressure, since it has been shown clearly that a reduction in coronary perfusion pressure reduces subendocardial blood flow while sparing subepicardial flow (BUCKBERG et al., 1972; GRIGGS and CHEN, 1974). FORMAN et al. (1973), who monitored the contractile force of the deep and superficial layers used this as an index of regional blood flow to the subendocardium and subepicardium. After constricting a branch of the left anterior descending coronary artery acutely up to the point that any further constriction reduced contractile force in the deep layers only and not in the superficial layers, the intravenous or intracoronary administration of nitroglycerin caused a significant reduction in the contractile force only in the subendocardium, which the authors felt reflected a reduction in subendocardial blood flow without a change in subepicardial flow. This hypothesis was supported by the myocardial distribution of Rubidium^{86}, which showed a decrease in the ratio of flow in the subendocardium to the flow in the subepicardium after nitroglycerin. This observation suggests that in these circumstances nitroglycerin does not act on the already fully dilated vessels in the subendocardium but only dilated the subepicardial vessels causing a "steal" of blood from the subendocardium to the subepicardium. The conclusions from this investigation do not agree with those of WINBURY et al. (1969); BECKER et al. (1971); MATHES and RIVAL (1971), all of whom found that in the ischemic heart nitroglycerin preferentially increases blood flow to the subendocardium. These latter studies demonstrating enhanced endocardial flow following nitrates are consistent with the clinical effects of nitrates, i.e., they relieve myocardial ischemia, whereas the findings of FORMAN et al. (1973) would indicate that this action of nitroglycerin is deleterious and could actually intensify the myocardial ischemia, which is not consistent with the commonly observed clinical response, but could explain the rare instances in which a paradoxical effect of nitroglycerin has been observed (RUSSEK et al., 1955).

The exact mechanism by which nitroglycerin redistributes blood flow from the subepicardium to the subendocardium in an ischemic region has not been completely elucidated. Under normal conditions intramyocardial pressure during diastole, which is closely related to left ventricular end-diastolic pressure, is considerably lower than the coronary perfusion pressure. An increase of left ventricular end-diastolic pressure, however, as frequently occurs during ischemia, may interfere more with the normal blood flow in the subendocardial than in the subepicardial layers, resulting in an intensification of subendocardial ischemia. Nitroglycerin, by reducing left ventricular size and end-diastolic pressure, as discussed below, reduces the extravascular compression, which would tend to improve subendocardial circulation.

III. Systemic and Cardiac Effects

A. Systemic Effects

Nitroglycerin has a potent vasodilating action on peripheral arterial vessels. In addition the drug has been shown in both experimental animals and man to dilate post capillary vessels (ÅBLAD and JOHNSSON, 1963), including the large veins (WILKINS et al., 1937; MASON and BRAUNWALD, 1965). This is in contrast to amyl nitrite which exhibits similar actions on the arterial circulation, but has an opposite effect on the venous side. In contrast to sublingual nitroglycerin, amyl nitrite induces an increase in venous tone, which can be blocked by guanethidine and reserpine, supporting the concept that this venoconstriction is mediated via adrenergic pathways, which may be provoked by baroreceptor stimulation. MASON and BRAUNWALD (1965) concluded from these observations that the beneficial effect of nitrates in angina pectoris is probably not related to its effect on the venous system, since nitroglycerin and amyl nitrite both alleviate angina, but have opposing effects on venous resistance. It is generally agreed that nitroglycerin reduces pulmonary vascular resistance (PINKERSON et al., 1963; NAJMI et al., 1967; AVIADO et al., 1968). Arterial pressure as well as total systemic resistance fall with either sublingual or intravenous nitroglycerin, while cardiac output may fall slightly after sublingual nitroglycerin (WILLIAMS et al., 1965; BRAUNWALD et al., 1964; BERNSTEIN et al., 1966) or actually increase slightly with intravenous nitroglycerin as shown by O'ROURKE et al. (1971) in the conscious dog. It is clear that one of nitroglycerin's most important actions is to dilate peripheral vessels. The reductions in systemic and pulmonary vascular resistances are responsible for many of nitroglycerin's effects on the heart, in particular the reflex changes in contractility and cardiac rate that occur.

B. Cardiac Effects

Nitroglycerin's effects on cardiac output and cardiac work appear to be related to the dose and route of administration of the drug as well as to the different experimental techniques for measuring cardiac output. In general most investigators find that cardiac output falls slightly (WILLIAMS et al., 1965; BRAUNWALD et al., 1964; BERNSTEIN et al., 1966; PARKER et al., 1971; KNOEBEL et al., 1968; FERRER et al., 1966) or does not change significantly (BRACHFELD et al., 1959; NAJMI et al., 1967; PARKER et al., 1966; COWAN et al., 1969; HOESCHEN et al., 1966; BENCHIMOL et al., 1965) with sublingual nitroglycerin both in the normal and ischemic heart. Since all agree that nitrates reduce arterial pressure, it follows that a reduction in left ventricular work occurs and this has been reported by WILLIAMS et al. (1965); BRAUNWALD et al. (1964); BERNSTEIN et al. (1966); BRACHFELD et al. (1959); NAJMI et al. (1967); PARKER et al. (1966, 1971); COWAN et al. (1969); KNOEBEL et al. (1968); FERRER et al. (1966); HOESCHEN et al. (1966); BENCHIMOL et al. (1965). As was pointed out earlier, the effects on the coronary circulation vary with the dose and route of administration as well as the extent to which reflex effects are elicited. Similarly, cardiac output, which is an important determinant of left ventricular work, shows little change or a slight decrease when nitroglycerin is administered sublingually to patients but increases significantly if the drug is administered intravenously to the conscious dog as shown by O'ROURKE et al. (1971) or when a large dose of amyl nitrite is inhaled in man as indicated by PERLOFF et al. (1963). Considering that nitroglycerin is most frequently administered therapeutically by the sublingual route, the fact that left ventricular work falls in this situation is important and must be considered as a major mechanism by which the drug alleviates myocardial ischemia. On the other hand a recent study in our laboratory (BERGERON et al., 1975) demonstrated that cardiac output never fell with intravenous nitroglycerin in conscious dogs even at sufficiently small doses, which simulate blood levels obtained following sublingual administration.

The critical question, as BRAUNWALD (1969, 1971) and SARNOFF and coworkers (1958) have pointed out, is not what happens to cardiac output and perhaps even external cardiac work, but rather how the drug affects the major determinants of myocardial oxygen consumption. The conclusions regarding the effects of nitroglycerin on myocardial oxygen consumption are conflicting, most likely due to the difficulties inherent in measuring this variable precisely. GORLIN and coworkers (1959) have demonstrated that sublingual nitroglycerin increases myocardial oxygen consumption in normal subjects, but this has not been found by others. Myocardial oxygen consumption has generally been shown to fall slightly after intravenous nitroglycerin to an anesthetized dog (MARCHETTI et al., 1964; GANZ and FRŎNEK, 1961) as well as in normal man (GORLIN et al., 1959) and in patients with coronary artery disease (BERNSTEIN et al., 1966; PARKER et al., 1971; HOESCHEN et al., 1966). In order to understand why nitroglycerin has never been shown to cause a large reduction in myocardial oxygen demands, it would be most helpful in reviewing the opposing effects of nitrates on the major determinants of myocardial oxygen consumption, i.e., (1) cardiac rate, (2) contractility, and (3) left ventricular wall tension, all of which can be measured more accurately than myocardial oxygen consumption itself.

The effects on left ventricular wall tension depend upon nitroglycerin's effects on cardiac pressure and size. Administered either sublingually or intravenously nitrates reduce cardiac size (GORDON and WELLS, 1924; BECK and HOLMAN, 1925; BRANDT et al., 1952; WILLIAMS et al., 1965; FRICK et al., 1962; O'ROURKE et al, 1971; VATNER et al., 1972). This effect has been demonstrated repeatedly in man utilizing radiographic techniques; WILLIAMS et al. (1965) measured cardiac size radiographically in patients after radiopaque markers had been sutured to the heart and demonstrated that sublingual nitroglycerin reduced cardiac size. These findings have been confirmed after intravenous and sublingual nitroglycerin in intact conscious animals (Figs. 3, 4 and 7) using ultrasonic transit-time dimension gauges for measuring left ventricular diameter (O'ROURKE et al., 1971; VATNER et al., 1972).

Three major causes for the reduced cardiac size must be considered; (1) increased inotropic response, (2) increased chronotropic response and (3) decreased cardiac afterload. The first mechanism probably plays a minor role, since cardiac size still decreases after the reflex positive inotropic effects are prevented with propranolol (VATNER et al., 1972). Moreover, cardiac size decreases after sublingual nitroglycerin, where reflex inotropic responses are minor. Through nitroglycerin's hypotensive action, arterial pressure falls and heart rate rises reflexly. Tachycardia limits diastolic filling time and thereby causes cardiac size to diminish (HIGGINS et al., 1973). Thus, since heart rate rises substantially after intravenous nitroglycerin and slightly following sublingual nitroglycerin, tachycardia is a significant mechanism for the reduction in cardiac size that occurs with nitroglycerin. However, it is not the sole mechanism, since it has also been shown that at a constant heart rate nitroglycerin still reduces cardiac size, albeit to a lesser degree (Fig. 7). Furthermore, after a bolus dose of nitroglycerin given intravenously, cardiac size remains depressed for several minutes after heart rate returns to control (VATNER et al., 1972). Thus, the ability of nitroglycerin to decrease cardiac size must be due to a great extent to concomitant reduction in afterload which occurs through nitroglycerin's peripheral vasodilating action. The reduction in afterload as well as the reflex tachycardia that occurs contribute significantly to nitroglycerin's effects on cardiac size. The finding that nitroglycerin decreases cardiac size has been given considerable importance in explaining the beneficial effects of the drug (WILLIAMS et al., 1965; PARKER et al., 1966, 1971), since the decrease in cardiac size and pressure leads to a reduction in left ventricular wall tension, a principal determinant of myocardial oxygen consumption

(BRAUNWALD, 1969, 1971). The favorable effects on subendocardial tension, as alluded to above are of particular importance in restoring balance between myocardial oxygen demand and supply in the subendocardium.

C. Inotropic Effects

While it is generally felt that nitroglycerin has little direct inotropic effect, BERGAMASCHI and GLÄSSER (1963), AVIADO et al. (1968), and DARBY et al. (1958, 1960) have indicated that the drug may decrease contractility slightly due to a direct depressant action while GILLIS and MELVILLE (1970), RAAB and LEPESCHKIN (1950); RAAB and HUMPHREYS (1947) found an adrenergic blocking effect. The evidence indicating that nitroglycerin reduces contractility by an adrenergic blocking effect is based on the finding that beta adrenergic agonists exert less positive inotropic responses after pretreatment with nitroglycerin. Since anginal attacks are frequently associated with an increase in adrenergic activity, the finding that nitroglycerin blocks this action would be important in understanding the mechanism of nitroglycerin in angina pectoris. However, these studies have been conducted in anesthetized preparations in which reflex effects are considerably depressed. When the drug is administered intravenously into conscious animals as shown in Figs. 3 and 4, nitroglycerin elicits a significant increase in myocardial contractility, the increases in dP/dt and velocity of myocardial fiber shortening follow the reductions in cardiac size and arterial pressure suggesting that the afferent path involves baroreceptor stimulation. This reflex positive inotropic response occurs through an efferent path involving beta adrenergic stimulation, since it is abolished after propranolol (Fig. 5).

Besides the reflex sympathetic action that increases contractility, two other mechanisms might be considered in explaining the positive inotropic response to the drug. The first is the BOWDITCH phenomenon, i.e., the positive inotropic effect that occurs with increasing cardiac rate, as demonstrated by BOWDITCH in 1871 and by WOODWORTH in 1902. The second is the positive inotropic effect due to the increase in coronary blood flow that occurs, which has been considered by BACANER et al. (1971) and TEMPLETON et al. (1972) as a stimulus that augments contractility. However, neither of these alternative explanations are attractive, when it is considered that after propranolol pretreatment, heart rate along with coronary blood flow still increase, whereas indices of contractility such as peak dP/dt, $dP/dt/P$ or velocity of myocardial fiber shortening do not increase (Fig. 5). This suggests that the BOWDITCH mechanism and any possible effects of increased myocardial perfusion play little if any role in mediating the positive inotropic response.

The reflex positive inotropic effect, although seemingly important when arterial pressure is reduced rapidly after a bolus of intravenous nitroglycerin, is of much less significance when the drug is administered sublingually (Fig. 7). The gradual fall in arterial pressure produced by sublingual nitroglycerin elicits only a minor augmentation of contractility as shown by VATNER et al. (1972), which cannot counteract the tendency for myocardial oxygen consumption to fall in conjunction with the concomitant reduction in left ventricular wall tension. Thus, this difference in degree of baroreceptor reflex mediated inotropic response with intravenous versus sublingual nitroglycerin is a further example of how the rate of drug delivery to the circulation alters an important aspect of nitroglycerin's effect. Therefore, when nitroglycerin is administered sublingually the predominant effect is to reduce myocardial oxygen demands despite a minor opposing action involving reflex increases in myocardial contractility.

D. Chronotropic Effects

Nitroglycerin is not considered to possess direct positive or negative chronotropic properties. However, like its inotropic effect it can increase heart rate through reflex mechanisms (VATNER et al., 1974a). Unlike the positive inotropic effects of the drug, the reflex tachycardia cannot be abolished by beta adrenergic blockade alone (Fig. 9) (THAMES and KONTOS, 1970; VATNER et al., 1974a). While the reflex inotropic effects are only sympathetically mediated, the positive chronotropic response is mediated by both sympathetic stimulation and parasympathetic withdrawal, since either atropine or propranolol attenuate the tachycardia but neither alone can abolish this reflex response (Fig. 9).

Both the reflex increases in cardiac rate and contractility are generally undesirable effects in patients with ischemic heart disease, since these changes raise myocardial oxygen consumption and unfavorably affect the balance between myocardial oxygen supply and demand. Accordingly, the combination of propranolol and nitroglycerin has been advocated in the treatment of myocardial ischemia by WIENER et al. (1969). However, despite these reflex effects of nitroglycerin, which act to increase myocardial oxygen consumption, as well as its tendency to cause arterial hypotension and reduce coronary perfusion pressure, the drug remains one of the cornerstones of therapy for angina pectoris. This is probably because the positive chronotropic and inotropic actions of the drug, which appear important when the drug is administered intravenously in an experimental situation, play a much less important role when the drug is administered by the normal therapeutic route, sublingually. In addition, it has been shown by ECKBERG et al. (1971) in patients and by HIGGINS et al. (1972) in experimental animals that cardiac disease alters reflex con-

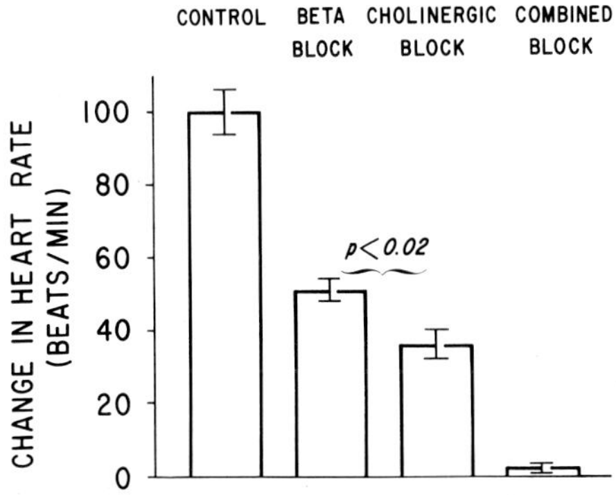

Fig. 9. Comparison of the reflex tachycardia after intravenous nitroglycerin, 20 µg/kg, in a conscious dog before and after autonomic blockades. Without blockade (left) nitroglycerin elicited almost a 100 beat/min rise in heart rate, which was abolished by combined beta and cholinergic blockade (right), but neither by beta nor cholinergic blockades alone (middle)

trol of the circulation. Thus, a similar hypotensive response in a patient with myocardial ischemic disease would be expected to elicit less of a reflex chronotropic and inotropic response than in a normal subject. In conclusion, it would appear that the minor reflex increases in cardiac rate and contractility that occur after sublingual nitroglycerin are not nearly strong enough to counteract the salutary actions of the drug to reduce left ventricular wall tension and left ventricular work, which results in a slight net reduction in myocardial oxygen consumption.

IV. Effects of Nitroglycerin on the Ischemic Myocardium

Clinical studies have demonstrated repeatedly that nitroglycerin improves the ability of the ischemic heart to respond to stress. For instance, nitroglycerin permits increased exercise capacity and can raise the threshold for angina pectoris in response to exercise (Wayne and LaPlace, 1933; Parker et al., 1967, 1971; Detry and Bruce, 1971) or pacing induced tachycardia (Ganz and Marcus, 1972; Linhart et al., 1967; Parker et al., 1969). Detry and Bruce (1971) found that patients with coronary artery disease tolerated a higher pressure-time product, which is an index of myocardial oxygen demand, during exercise before angina appeared and attributed this higher threshold to the reduced cardiac size and left ventricular wall tension that occur with nitroglycerin.

While it is clear that nitroglycerin is extremely useful in the treatment of angina pectoris, its efficacy when administered to patients with acute myocardial infarction is controversial. For many years the use of nitroglycerin has been contraindicated for the alleviation of myocardial infarction pain, since it has been thought that the reduction in arterial pressure and associated tachycardia would be deleterious (Prodger and Ayman, 1932; Sprague and White, 1933; Weiss et al., 1937; Lueth and Hanks, 1938; Dewar and Grimson, 1950; Contro et al., 1952; Russek et al., 1955). While nitroglycerin ameliorates ischemic EKG changes in most patients, Russek et al. (1955) observed that in some patients nitroglycerin causes paradoxical EKG changes, suggesting intensified ischemia. Nitroglycerin, through its action to reduce coronary perfusion pressure, has been implicated in the extension of acute myocardial infarction. In fact, Russek et al. (1955) stated that "the precipitation of acute myocardial infarction should be recognized as a definite risk from overdosage during therapy of the anginal attack".

Recently Epstein and colleagues have forced a reevaluation of the use of nitroglycerin in patients with acute myocardial infarction. Their studies of experimental myocardial infarction in conscious dogs indicate that myocardial ischemic injury as assessed by ST segment elevation, CPK depletion and histological assessment of tissue damage was not augmented by nitroglycerin, but rather that infarct size was contained and actually reduced as long as excessive tachycardia or hypotension did not accompany the nitroglycerin therapy (Smith et al., 1973; Epstein et al., 1973). These investigators then carried these studies further and administered nitroglycerin in combination with a sufficient amount of an alpha adrenergic agonist, e.g. methoxamine, to prevent hypotension and tachycardia. Under these circumstances nitroglycerin always reduced the size of experimentally produced infarcts as evidenced by less ST segment elevation, less CPK-depletion and less histological evidence of tissue

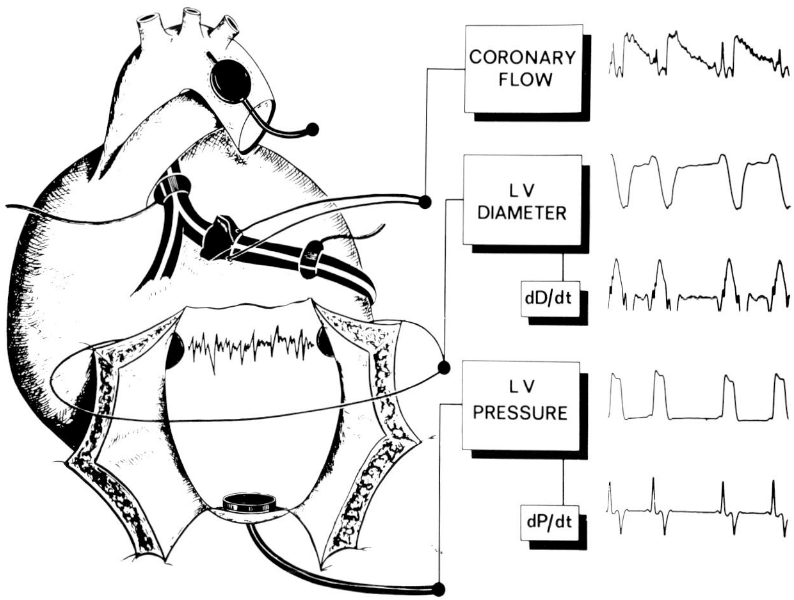

Fig. 10. The instrumentation implanted is shown. A miniature pressure gauge and opposing ultrasonic diameter transducers were implanted in the left ventricle. A Doppler ultrasonic flow probe was implanted on the left circumflex coronary artery along with an occluding cuff. An occluding cuff was also implanted on the main left coronary artery. (Reprinted with permission from Transactions of the Association of American Physicians, VATNER et al., 1973)

necrosis. Studies by WEISSE and coworkers (1972) showed that nitroglycerin could be safely administered to the anesthetized, closed chest dog with myocardial infarction and may even be beneficial as long as cardiogenic shock was not present. KENT et al. (1974) showed that nitroglycerin lowered the ventricular fibrillation threshold in dogs during experimental myocardial infarction. Recently, REID et al. (1971) reported that nitroglycerin reduced the extent of myocardial injury as evidenced by decreased ST-elevation in patients with acute myocardial infarction. Moreover, GOLD and coworkers (1972) showed that nitroglycerin can increase cardiac output in patients with acute myocardial infarction, whose end-diastolic pressures were elevated.

Thus, nitroglycerin can improve function in the heart with regional ischemia and perhaps even with myocardial infarction. It could be that the clinical observations on the deleterious effects of nitroglycerin occurred in patients with diffuse coronary artery disease in which reduction in coronary perfusion pressure can be critical. The possibility that nitroglycerin elicits different effects on cardiac function in the normal and ischemic heart and in particular in the presence of diffuse or global myocardial ischemia, in contrast to regional ischemia was examined in conscious dogs instrumented for the continuous measurement of coronary blood flow and arterial pressure, left ventricular dimensions, pressures and myocardial contractility. In addition, an hydraulic occluder was implanted around the left main coronary artery (Fig. 10), which provided the capability for reducing coronary flow to the

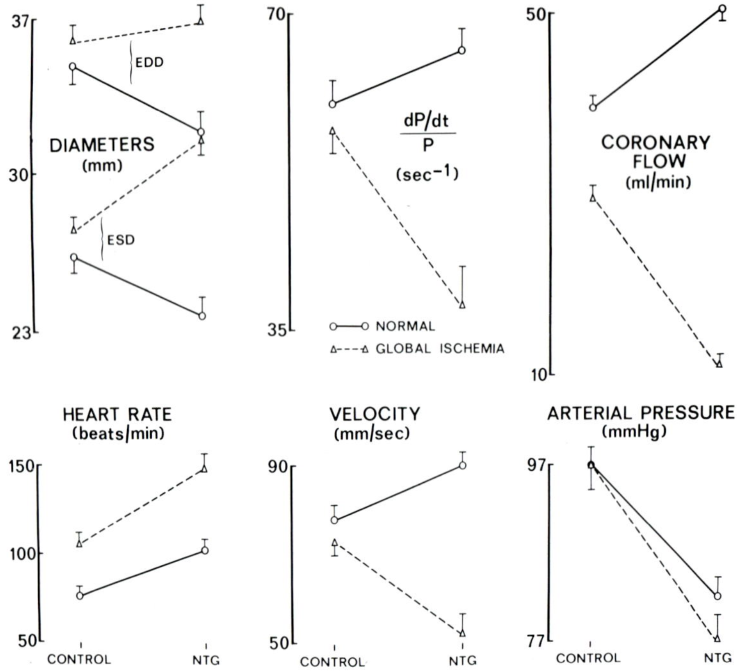

Fig. 11. Comparison of the effects of intravenous nitroglycerin (NTG), 15 μg/kg/min on cardiac function and coronary dynamics in the normal heart (circles and solid lines) and with global myocardial ischemia (triangles and broken lines). Note in the presence of global ischemia the paradoxical effects of nitroglycerin on left ventricular end-diastolic diameter, myocardial contractility and coronary flow. (Reprinted with permission from the Journal of Clinical Investigation, VATNER et al., 1974)

entire left ventricle (the left main coronary artery supplies the left ventricle in the dog), to any desired level. In the normally perfused heart nitroglycerin improved cardiac function along with inducing substantial coronary vasodilation (Figs. 11 and 12). In the presence of marginal global ischemia at rest (approximately a 30% reduction in total coronary inflow) nitroglycerin could no longer dilate the coronary vessels and the reduction in arterial pressure and hence of coronary perfusion caused by the drug was deleterious, and the heart rapidly failed (Figs. 11 and 13) (VATNER et al., 1974b). A reduction in coronary perfusion pressure in the globally ischemic heart is deleterious, since decreasing pressure intensifies ischemia. In fact, the acute cardiac decompensation that was observed was probably due to the associated hypotension, since it was not seen in the same situation when arterial pressure was maintained constant by inflation of an intraaortic balloon. Thus, the paradoxical effects of nitroglycerin noted by RUSSEK et al. (1955) and others in clinical studies where ischemia was intensified by the drug were dramatically demonstrated in a model of global myocardial ischemia (VATNER et al., 1974b).

In contrast to the responses observed in the presence of global myocardial ischemia, nitroglycerin elicited a qualitatively normal response when administered in

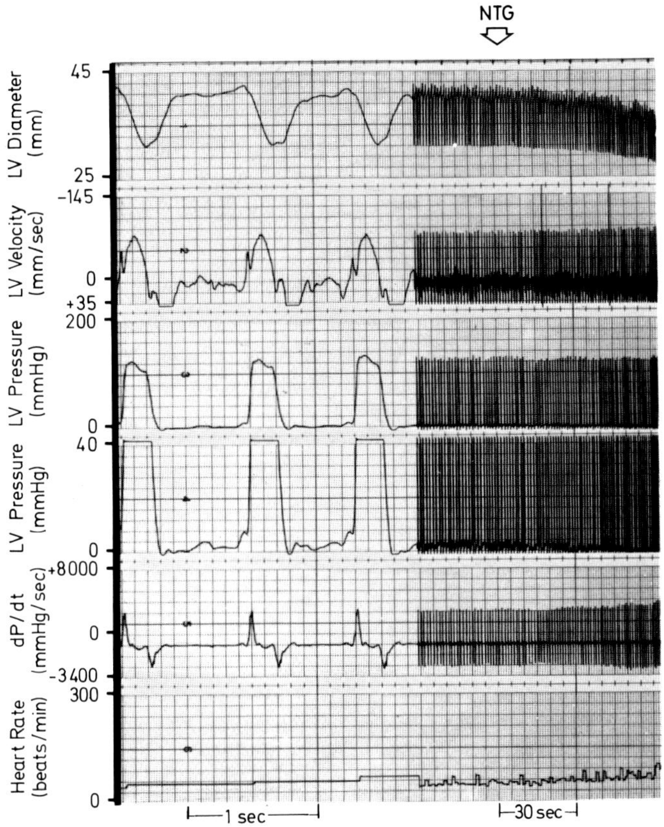

Fig. 12. Typical response to intravenous nitroglycerin, 15 μg/kg/min, in the normal heart. Phasic records of left ventricular diameter, velocity, pressure, end-diastolic pressure *dP/dt* and heart rate are shown. Nitroglycerin decreased cardiac size and increased *dP/dt* and heart rate slightly. (Reprinted with permission from Transactions of the Association of American Physicians, VATNER et al., 1973)

the presence of intense regional ischemia. Regional ischemia was elicited by inflating the hydraulic occluder implanted on the left circumflex coronary artery leaving left anterior descending coronary perfusion intact. In the presence of intense regional ischemia nitroglycerin did not elicit a paradoxical response, but rather local and general myocardial fuction was maintained and overall cardiac size was still able to decrease (Fig. 14). This would fit with the findings of EPSTEIN (1973) and SMITH (1973) and coworkers and WEISSE et al. (1972), who observed a salutary effect of the drug in the presence of myocardial infarction.

V. Summary

Nitroglycerin exerts a number of actions on the circulation. These effects differ depending not only upon the dose and route of administration, i.e., intracoronary, intravenous or sublingual, but also the state of the experimental preparation, i.e.,

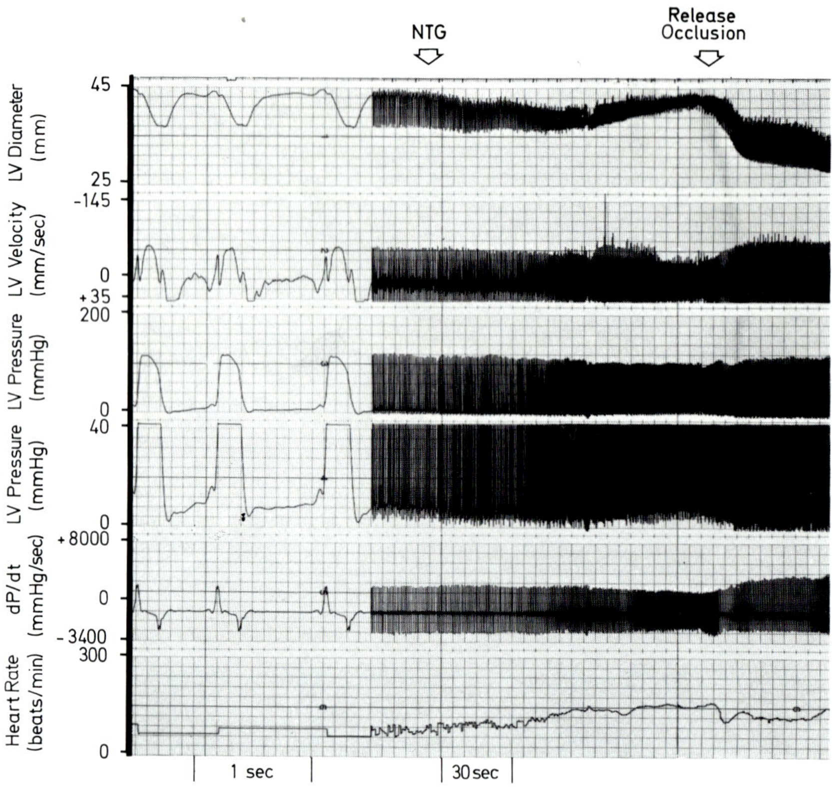

Fig. 13. Response to the same dose of nitroglycerin in the same dog shown in Fig. 12, but in this case with global myocardial ischemia produced by partial occlusion of the main left coronary artery occlusion. Note that after transient initial improvement, function deteriorated, cardiac size rose and *dP/dt* fell. With release of occlusion and return of normal coronary flow cardiac size fell below control and contractility rose above control levels. (Reprinted with permission from Transactions of the Association of American Physicians, VATNER et al., 1973)

conscious or anesthetized and on the presence or absence of coronary artery disease; the drug's action in the presence of coronary insufficiency differ depending upon whether ischemia is local or global.

In the normal conscious dog, an intravenous bolus dose of nitroglycerin elicits striking coronary vasodilatation, consisting of two phases. The first is due to a direct dilating effect on the coronary vessels, since it is not associated with significant increases in the determinants of myocardial oxygen consumption and is accompanied by a substantial augmentation of coronary venous oxygen and reduction in the coronary arterio-venous oxygen difference. The second phase of coronary vasodilatation results from reflex increases in cardiac rate and contractility that occur due to the hypotension and baroreceptor stimulation. Accordingly, this later phase can be prevented by beta adrenergic blockade and maintaining heart rate constant.

While nitroglycerin decreases arterial pressure, total systemic and pulmonary vascular resistance, it also diminishes cardiac size. Nitroglycerin has little if any

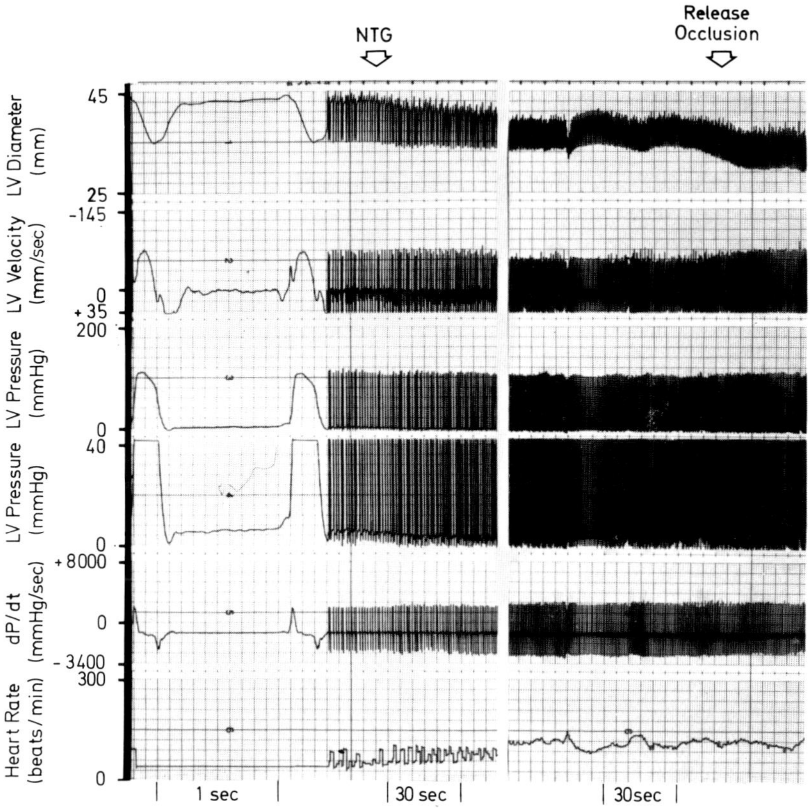

Fig. 14. Response to the same dose of nitroglycerin in the same dog shown in Fig. 12 and 13, but in this case with severe regional ischemia produced by left circumflex coronary artery occlusion. In contrast to the condition of global ischemia, cardiac function improved. When the occlusion was released further improvement in cardiac function occurred. (Reprinted with permission from Transactions of the Association of American Physicians, VATNER et al., 1973)

action on cardiac muscle, but elicits striking reflex tachycardia mediated both by the sympathetic and parasympathetic systems and modest increases in myocardial contractility induced by beta adrenergic receptor stimulation when the drug is administered intravenously as a bolus. These reflex actions of the drug as well as its coronary vasodilator effects are of little if any consequence when a smaller dose of the drug is delivered to the circulation as occurs after sublingual administration. Sublingual nitroglycerin dilates normal coronary vessels by these same mechanisms, but the magnitude of the dilatation is less and the duration of action is more prolonged, while the reflex chronotropic and inotropic responses are attenuated considerably.

There is no unified concept as to nitroglycerin's mechanism of action in alleviating angina pectoris. While it is attractive to attribute the beneficial effects of the drug to its powerful coronary vasodilating action, this has been shown to be an unlikely explanation in the presence of severe myocardial ischemia due to coronary vascular obstruction where vessels may be already maximally dilated in response to the local hypoxic stress. Accordingly, it is generally held that the peripheral vascular effects of the drug, which decrease arterial pressure and left ventricular pressure and size (thereby reducing left ventricular wall tension) are responsible for the beneficial effects. The reduction in left ventricular wall tension would then act to produce a more favorable balance between myocardial oxygen supply and demand in the ischemic heart. Although this appears to be nitroglycerin's most important therapeutic action, its coronary dilating effects cannot be dismissed.

If the coronary effects of nitrates were inconsequential, angina pectoris could be treated equally well with any agent that simply reduces left ventricular wall tension. In fact, phlebotomy which reduces left ventricular work and oxygen demands, primarily by reducing cardiac size and pressure was employed prior to the time of Brunton. However, the weight of recent evidence suggests that nitroglycerin exerts additional beneficial action on the coronary vasculature even if it does not augment total coronary blood flow. Nitroglycerin's ability to improve collateral coronary blood flow and cause a redistribution of coronary flow favoring the ischemic zones of the heart could contribute to the improvement of local oxygen delivery and be in part responsible for the salutary effects of the drug in the treatment of acute myocardial ischemia.

Acknowledgement: We appreciate greatly the help in preparation of the manuscript by V. FOWLER and the advice of Dr. E. BRAUNWALD.

Supported in part by U.S. Public Health Service Grants HL 15416 and HL 1043609 and the National Aeronautics and Space Administration-Ames Research Grant No. 22-036-001.

S. F. VATNER is an Established Investigator of the American Heart Association.

References

ÅBLAD, B., JOHNSSON, G.: Comparative effects of intra-arterially administered hydralazine and sodium nitrite on blood flow and volume of forearm. Acta Pharmacol. (Kbh.) **20**, 1—15 (1963).

AVIADO, D. M., FOLLE, L. E., BELLET, S.: Cardiopulmonary effects of glyceryl trinitrate and isosorbide dinitrate. Cardiologia (Basel) **52**, 287—303 (1968).

BACANER, M. B., LIOY, F., VISSCHER, M. B.: Coronary blood flow, oxygen delivery rate and cardiac performance. J. Physiol. (Lond.) **216**, 111—127 (1971).

BECK, C. S., HOLMAN, E.: The physiological response of the circulatory system to experimental alterations. II. The effect of variations in total blood volume. J. exp. Med. **42**, 681—692 (1925).

BECKER, L. C., FORTUIN, N. J., PITT, B.: Effect of ischemia and antianginal drugs on the distribution of radioactive michrospheres in the canine left ventricle. Circulation Res. **28**, 263—269 (1971).

BENCHIMOL, A., LIGGETT, M. S., DUENAS, A., DIMOND, E. G.: Effect of nitroglycerin on cardiovascular function at fixed and at variable heart rate. Brit. Heart J. **27**, 902—910 (1965).

BERGAMASCHI, M., GLÄSSER, A. H.: Effect of the endecapeptide eledoisin on the coronary blood flow: Comparison with nitroglycerin, bradykinin, and epinephrine in the dog. Circulation Res. **13**, 329—335 (1963).

BERGERON, G., MILLARD, R., HEYNDRICKX, G., VATNER, S. F.: Effects of nitroglycerin on cardiac output and regional flow distribution in conscious dogs. (Abst) Fed. Proc., 1975.

BERNE, R. M.: Regulation of coronary blood flow. Physiol. Rev. **44**, 1—29 (1964).

BERNSTEIN, L., FRIESINGER, G. C., LICHTLEN, P. R., ROSS, R. S.: The effect of nitroglycerin on the systemic and coronary circulation in man and dogs. Myocardial blood flow measured with Xenon 133. Circulation **33**, 107—116 (1966).

BING, R. J., BENNISH, A., BLUEMCHEN, G., COHEN, A., GALLAGHER, J. P., ZALESKI, E. J.: The determination of coronary flow equivalent with coincidence counting technic. Circulation **29**, 833—846 (1964).

BOWDITCH, H. P.: Über die Eigenthümlichkeiten der Reizbarkeit, welche die Muskelfasern des Herzens zeigen. Arb. Physiol. Anstalt Leipzig **6**, 139—176 (1871).

BOYER, N. H., GREEN, H. D.: The effects of nitrites and xanthines on coronary inflow and blood pressure in anesthetized dogs. Amer. Heart J. **21**, 199—214 (1941).

BRACHFELD, N., BOZER, J., GORLIN, R.: Action of nitroglycerin on the coronary circulation in normal and in mild cardiac subjects. Circulation **19**, 697—704 (1959).

BRANDI, G., FAM, W. M., MCGREGOR, M.: Measurement of coronary flow in local areas of myocardium using Xenon 133. J. appl. Physiol. **24**, 446—450 (1968).

BRANDT, J. L., CACCESE, A., DOCK, W.: Slit-kymographic evidence that nitroglycerin decreases heart volume and stroke volume. While increasing the amplitude of ballistocardiographic waves. Amer. J. Med. **12**, 650—658 (1952).

BRAUNWALD, E.: Thirteenth Bowditch lecture. The determinants of myocardial oxygen consumption. Physiologist **12**, 65—93 (1969).

BRAUNWALD, E.: Control of myocardial oxygen consumption. Physiological and clinical considerations. Amer. J. Cardiol. **27**, 416—432 (1971).

BRAUNWALD, E., OLDHAM, H. N., JR., ROSS, J., JR., LINHART, J. W., MASON, D. T., FORT, L., III.: The circulatory response of patients with idiopathic hypertrophic subaortic stenosis to nitroglycerin and to the Valsalva maneuver. Circulation **29**, 422—431 (1964).

BRUNTON, T. L.: Use of nitrite of amyl in angina pectoris. Lancet **2**, 97—98 (1867).

BUCKBERG, G. D., FIXLER, D. E., ARCHIE, J. P., HOFFMAN, J. I. E.: Experimental subendocardial ischemia in dogs with normal coronary arteries. Circulation Res. **30**, 67—81 (1972).

CARSON, R. P., WILSON, W. S., NEMIROFF, M. J., WEBER, W. J.: The effects of sublingual nitroglycerin on myocardial blood flow in patients with coronary artery disease or myocardial hypertrophy. Amer. Heart J. **77**, 579—584 (1969).

CHARLIER, R.: Coronary vasodilators, lst Ed. Oxford-London-New York-Paris: Pergamon Press Ltd. 1961.

CHARLIER, R.: Antianginal drugs. In: Handbook of Experimental Pharmacology. Berlin-Heidelberg-New York: Springer 1971.

COBB, F. R., BACHE, R. J., GREENFIELD, J. C., JR.: Regional myocardial blood flow in awake dogs. J. clin. Invest. **53**, 1618—1625 (1974).

COHEN, A., GALLAGHER, J. P., LUEBS, E.-D., VARGA, Z., YAMANAKA, J., ZALESKI, E. J., BLUEMCHEN, G., BING, R. J.: The quantitative determination of coronary flow with a positron emitter (Rubidium-84). Circulation **32**, 636—649 (1965).

COHEN, M. V., DOWNEY, J. M., SONNENBLICK, E. H., KIRK, E. S.: The effects of nitroglycerin on coronary collaterals and myocardial contractility. J. clin. Invest. **52**, 2836—2847 (1973b).

COHEN, M. V., KIRK, E. S.: Differential response of large and small coronary arteries to nitroglycerin and angiotensin. Circulation Res. **33**, 445—453 (1973a).

CONTRO, S., HARING, O. M., GOLDSTEIN, W.: Paradoxic action of amyl nitrite in coronary patients. Circulation **6**, 250—256 (1952).

COWAN, C., DURAN, P. V. M., CORSINI, G., GOLDSCHLAGER, N., BING, R. J.: The effects of nitroglycerin on myocardial blood flow in man. Measured by coincidence counting and bolus injections of ^{84}Rubidium. Amer. J. Cardiol. **24**, 154—160 (1969).

DARBY, T. D., ALDINGER, E. E.: Further studies of the effects on myocardial energy utilization elicited by nitroglycerin. Circulation Res. **8**, 100—108 (1960).

DARBY, T. D., SPROUSE, J. H., WALTON, R. P.: Evaluation of sympathetic reflex effects on the inotropic action of nitroglycerin, quinidine, papaverine, aminophylline, and isoproterenol. J. Pharmacol. exp. Ther. **122**, 386—395 (1958).

DETRY, J.-M. R., BRUCE, R. A.: Effects of nitroglycerin on "maximal" oxygen intake and exercise electrocardiogram in coronary heart disease. Circulation **43**, 155—163 (1971).

DEWAR, H. A., GRIMSON, T. A.: Khellin in the treatment of angina of effort. Brit. Heart J. **12**, 54—60 (1950).

DOMENECH, R. J., HOFFMAN, J. I. E., NOBLE, M. I. M., SAUNDERS, K. B., HENSON, J. R., SUBIJANTO, S.: Total and regional coronary blood flow measured by radioactive microspheres in conscious and anesthetized dogs. Circulation Res. **25**, 581—596 (1969).

Eckberg, D. L., Drabinsky, M., Braunwald, E.: Defective cardiac parasympathetic control in patients with heart disease. New Engl. J. Med. **285**, 877—883 (1971).

Eckenhoff, J. E., Hafkenschiel, J. H.: The effect of nikethamide on coronary blood flow and cardiac oxygen metabolism. J. Pharmacol. exp. Ther. **91**, 362—369 (1947).

Epstein, S. E., Goldstein, R. E., Redwood, D. R., Kent, K. M., Smith, E. R.: The early phase of acute myocardial infarction: Pharmacologic aspects of therapy. Ann. intern. Med. **78**, 918—936 (1973).

Essex, H. E., Wegria, R. G. E., Herrick, J. F., Mann, F. C.: The effect of certain drugs on the coronary blood flow of the trained dog. Amer. Heart J. **19**, 554—565 (1940).

Fam, W. M., McGregor, M.: Effect of coronary vasodilator drugs on retrograde flow in areas of chronic myocardial ischemia. Circulation Res. **15**, 355—365 (1964).

Fam, W. M., McGregor, M.: Effect of nitroglycerin and dipyridamole on regional coronary resistance. Circulation Res. **22**, 649—659 (1968).

Ferrer, M. I., Bradley, S. E., Wheeler, H. O., Enson, Y., Preisig, R., Brickner, P. W., Conroy, R. J., Harvey, R. M.: Some effects of nitroglycerin upon the splanchnic, pulmonary, and systemic circulations. Circulation **33**, 357—373 (1966).

Forman, R., Kirk, E. S., Downey, J. M., Sonnenblick, E. H.: Nitroglycerin and heterogeneity of myocardial blood flow. Reduced subendocardial blood flow and ventricular contractile force. J. clin. Invest. **52**, 905—911 (1973).

Frick, M. H., Balcon, R., Cross, D., Sowton, E.: Hemodynamic effects of nitroglycerin in patients with angina pectoris studied by an atrial pacing method. Circulation **37**, 160—168 (1968).

Friedberg, C. K.: Diseases of the heart, 3rd ed. Philadelphia: W. B. Saunders Co. 1966.

Ganz, W., Fröněk, A.: The action of nitroglycerin on coronary and systemic haemodynamics and on the oxygen metabolism of the myocardium. Cor et Vasa (Praha) **3**, 107—119 (1961).

Ganz, W., Marcus, H. S.: Failure of intracoronary nitroglycerin to alleviate pacing-induced angina. Circulation **46**, 880—889 (1972).

Gensini, G. G., Di Giorgi, S., Murad-Netto, S., Black, A.: Arteriographic demonstration of coronary artery spasm and its release after the use of a vasodilator in a case of angina pectoris and in the experimental animal. Angiology **13**, 550—553 (1962).

Gillis, R. A., Melville, K. I.: Coronary flow changes and cardiac adrenergic blockade during nitroglycerin infusions. Europ. J. Pharmacol. **13**, 15—22 (1970).

Gillis, R. A., Melville, K. I.: Effects of sublingually and intravenously administered nitroglycerin on the cardiovascular system of the dog. Amer. J. Cardiol. **28**, 38—42 (1971).

Gold, H. K., Leinbach, R. C., Sanders, C. A.: Use of sublingual nitroglycerin in congestive failure following acute myocardial infarction. Circulation **46**, 839—845 (1972).

Goldstein, R. E., Stinson, E. B., Epstein, S. E.: Effects of nitroglycerin on coronary collateral function in patients with coronary occlusive disease. Amer. J. Cardiol. **31**, 135 (1973).

Gordon, B., Wells, G.: The effect of amyl nitrite, bleeding and epinephrin on the blood pressure and the size of the cat's heart. Arch. intern. Med. **33**, 738—741 (1924).

Gorlin, R., Brachfeld, N., MacLeod, C., Bopp, P.: Effect of nitroglycerin on the coronary circulation in patients with coronary artery disease or increased left ventricular work. Circulation **19**, 705—718 (1959).

Gregg, D. E., Fischer, L. C.: Blood supply to the heart. In: Handbook of Physiology. Section 2, volume II. Washington, D. C.: Amer. Physiol. Soc. 1963.

Griggs, D. M., Chen, C. C.: Coronary hemodynamics and regional myocardial metabolism in experimental aortic insufficiency. J. clin. Invest. **53**, 1599—1606 (1974).

Higgins, C. B., Vatner, S. F., Eckberg, D. L., Braunwald, E.: Alterations in the baroreceptor reflex in conscious dogs with heart failure. J. clin. Invest. **51**, 715—724 (1972).

Higgins, C. B., Vatner, S. F., Franklin, D., Braunwald, E.: Extent of regulation of the heart's contractile state in the conscious dog by alteration in the frequency of contraction. J. clin. Invest. **52**, 1187—1194 (1973).

Hoeschen, R. J., Bousvaros, G. A., Klassen, G. A., Fam, W. M., McGregor, M.: Haemodynamic effects of angina pectoris, and of nitroglycerin in normal and anginal subjects. Brit. Heart J. **28**, 221—230 (1966).

Honig, C. R., Tenney, S. M., Gabel, P. V.: The mechanism of cardiovascular action of nitroglycerine. An example of integrated response during the unsteady state. Amer. J. Med. **29**, 910—923 (1960).

HORN, H., FIELD, L. E., DOCK, S., MASTER, A. M.: Acute coronary insufficiency: pathological and physiological aspects. An analysis of twenty-five cases of subendocardial necrosis. Amer. Heart J. **40**, 63—80 (1950).
HORWITZ, L. D., GORLIN, R., TAYLOR, W. J., KEMP, H. G.: Effects of nitroglycerin on regional myocardial blood flow in coronary artery disease. J. clin. Invest. **50**, 1578—1584 (1971).
JENNINGS, R. B., SOMMERS, H. M., SMYTH, G. A., FLACK, H. A., LINN, H.: Myocardial necrosis induced by temporary occlusion of a coronary artery in the dog. Arch. Path. **70**, 82—92 (1960).
KENT, K. M., SMITH, E. R., REDWOOD, D. R., EPSTEIN, S. E.: Beneficial electro-physiologic effects of nitroglycerin during acute myocardial infarction. Amer. J. Cardiol. **13**, 513–516 (1974).
KIRK, E. S., HONIG, C. R.: An experimental and theoretical analysis of myocardial tissue pressure. Amer. J. Physiol. **207**, 361—367 (1964a).
KIRK, E. S., HONIG, C. R.: Nonuniform distribution of blood flow and gradients of oxygen tension within the heart. Amer. J. Physiol. **207**, 661—668 (1964b).
KJEKSHUS, J. K.: Mechanism for flow distribution in normal and ischemic myocardium during increased ventricular preload in the dog. Circulation Res. **33**, 489—499 (1973).
KNOEBEL, S. B., MCHENRY, P. L., ROBERTS, D., STEIN, L.: Myocardial blood flow in man measured by a coincidence counting system and a single bolus of ^{84}Rubidium chloride. Effect of nitroglycerin. Circulation **37**, 932—938 (1968).
LEHAN, P. H., OLDEWURTEL, H. A., WEISSE, A. B., ELLIOTT, M. S., REGAN, T. J.: Relationship of angiographic coronary artery diameter to blood flow. Circulation **33** (Suppl III), 154—155 (1966).
LEIGHNINGER, D. S., RUEGER, R., BECK, C. S.: Effect of glyceryl trinitrate (Nitroglycerin) on arterial blood supply to ischemic myocardium. Amer. J. Cardiol. **3**, 638—646 (1959).
LICHTLEN, P., ROSS, R. S., FRIESINGER, G. C., BERNSTEIN, L.: Die Wirkung von Nitroglyzerin auf die Koronardurchblutung am Menschen, unter Berücksichtigung der Selektiven Koronarangiographie und Messung der Koronardurchblutung mit Xenon 133. Cardiologia (Basel) **48**, 371—373 (1966).
LIKOFF, W., KASPARIAN, H., LEHMAN, J. S., SEGAL, B. L.: Evaluation of "coronary vasodilators" by coronary arteriography. Amer. J. Cardiol. **13**, 7—9 (1964).
LINDER, E., SEEMAN, T.: Effects of persantin and nitroglycerin on myocardial blood flow during temporary coronary occlusions in dogs. Angiologica **4**, 225—255 (1967).
LINHART, J. W., HILDNER, F. J., BAROLD, S. S., LISTER, J. W., SAMET, P.: Left heart hemodynamics during angina pectoris induced by atrial pacing. Circulation **40**, 483—492 (1969).
LUEBS, E.-D., COHEN, A., ZALESKI, E. J., BING, R. J.: Effect of nitroglycerin, intensain, isoptin and papaverine on coronary blood flow in man. Measured by the coincidence counting technic and Rubidium^{84}. Amer. J. Cardiol. **17**, 535—541 (1966).
LUETH, H. C., HANKS, T. G.: Unusual reactions of patients with hypertension to glyceryl trinitrate. Arch. intern. Med. **62**, 97—108 (1938).
MALINDZAK, G. S., GREEN, H. D., STAGG, P. L.: Effects of nitroglycerin on flow after partial constriction of the coronary artery. J. appl. Physiol. **29**, 17—22 (1970).
MARCHETTI, G. V., MERLO, L., ANTOGNETTI, R. M.: The effects of nitroglycerin on the coronary blood flow and oxygen consumption of the myocardium in anesthetized dogs. Amer. J. Cardiol. **13**, 51—57 (1964).
MASON, D. T., BRAUNWALD, E.: The effects of nitroglycerin and amyl nitrite on arteriolar and venous tone in the human forearm. Circulation **32**, 755—766 (1965).
MATHES, P., RIVAL, J.: Effect of nitroglycerin on total and regional coronary blood flow in the normal and ischaemic canine myocardium. Cardiovasc. Res. **5** 54—61 (1971).
MAUTZ, F. R., GREGG, D. E.: Dynamics of collateral circulation following chronic occlusion of coronary arteries. Proc. Soc. exp. Biol. (N. Y.) **36**, 797—801 (1937).
MOIR, T. W.: Subendocardial distribution of coronary blood flow and the effect of antianginal drugs. Circulation Res. **30**, 621—627 (1972).
MURRELL, W.: Nitro-glycerine as a remedy for angina pectoris. Lancet **1879 I**, 80—81.
NAJMI, M., GRIGGS, D. M., JR., KASPARIAN, H., NOVACK, P.: Effects of nitroglycerin on hemodynamics during rest an exercise in patients with coronary insufficiency. Circulation **35**, 46—54 (1967).
OLIVA, P. B., POTTS, D. E., PLUSS, R. G.: Coronary arterial spasm in Prinzmetal angina. New Engl. J. Med. **288**, 745—751 (1973).

O'ROURKE, R. A., BISHOP, V. S., KOT, P. A., FERNANDEZ, J. P.: Hemodynamic effects of nitroglycerin and amyl nitrite in the conscious dog. J. Pharmacol. exp. Ther. **177**, 426—432 (1971).

PARKER, J. O., DI GIORGI, S., WEST, R. O.: A hemodynamic study of acute coronary insufficiency precipitated by exercise. With observations on the effects of nitroglycerin. Amer. J. Cardiol. **17**, 470—483 (1966).

PARKER, J. O., LEDWICH, J. R., WEST, R. O., CASE, R. B.: Reversible cardiac failure during angina pectoris. Hemodynamic effects of atrial pacing in coronary artery disease. Circulation **39**, 745—757 (1969).

PARKER, J. O., WEST, R. O., DI GIORGI, S.: The hemodynamic response to exercise in patients with healed myocardial infarction without angina. With observations on the effects of nitroglycerin. Circulation **36**, 734—751 (1967).

PARKER, J. O., WEST, R. O., DI GIORGI, S.: The effect of nitroglycerin on coronary blood flow and the hemodynamic response to exercise in coronary artery disease. Amer. J. Cardiol. **27**, 59—65 (1971).

PERLOFF, J. K., CALVIN, J., DE LEON, A. C., BOWEN, P.: Systemic hemodynamic effects of amyl nitrite in normal man. Amer. Heart J. **66**, 460—469 (1963).

PINKERSON, A. L., KOT, P. A., KNOWLAN, D. M.: Effect of glyceryl trinitrate on pulmonary vasculature of anesthetized dogs. Proc. Soc. exp. Biol. **113**, 18—20 (1963).

PRODGER, S. H., AYMAN, D.: Harmful effects of nitroglycerin. With special reference to coronary thrombosis. Amer. J. med. Sci. **184**, 480—491 (1932).

RAAB, W., HUMPHREYS, R. J.: Drug action upon myocardial epinephrine-sympathin concentration and heart rate (nitroglycerine, papaverine, priscol, dibenamine, hydrochloride). J. Pharmacol. exp. Ther. **89**, 64—76 (1947).

RAAB, W., LEPESCHKIN, E.: Anti-adrenergic effects of nitroglycerin on the heart. Circulation **1**, 733—740 (1950).

REID, P., FLAHERTY, J., TAYLOR, D., KELLY, D., WEISFELDT, M., PITT, B.: Effect of nitroglycerin on ST segments in acute myocardial infarction. Circulation **48** (Suppl IV), 207 (1973).

RUSSEK, H. I., URBACH, K. F., ZOHMAN, B. L.: Paradoxical action of glyceryl trinitrate (nitroglycerin) in coronary patients. J. Amer. med. Ass. **158**, 1017—1021 (1955).

SARNOFF, S. J., BRAUNWALD, E., WELCH, G. H., CASE, R. B., STAINSBY, W. N., MACRUZ, R.: Hemodynamic determinants of oxygen consumption of the heart. With special reference to the Tension-Time Index. Amer. J. Physiol. **192**, 148—156 (1958).

SCHAPER, W.: The collateral circulation of the heart. Amsterdam-London: North-Holland Publishing Company; New York: American Elsevier Publishing Co., Inc. 1971.

SCHNAAR, R. L., SPARKS, H. V.: Response of large and small coronary arteries to nitroglycerin $NaNo_2$, and adenosine. Amer. J. Physiol. **223**, 223—228 (1972).

SMITH, E. R., REDWOOD, D. R., MCCARRON, W. E., EPSTEIN, S. E.: Coronary artery occlusion in the conscious dog. Effects of alterations in arterial pressure produced by nitroglycerin, hemorrhage and alpha-adrenergic agonists on the degree of myocardial ischemia. Circulation **47**, 51—57 (1973).

SPRAGUE, H. B., WHITE, P. D.: Nitroglycerin collapse-a potential danger in therapy. Report of three cases. Med. Clin. N. Amer. **16**, 895—898 (1933).

TEMPLETON, G. H., WILDENTHAL, K., MITCHELL, J. H.: Influence of coronary blood flow on left ventricular contractility and stiffness. Amer. J. Physiol. **223**, 1216—1220 (1972).

THAMES, M. D., KONTOS, H. A.: Mechanisms of baroreceptor-induced changes in heart rate. Amer. J. Physiol. **218**, 251—256 (1970).

VATNER, S. F., BRAUNWALD, E.: Effect of anesthesia on cardiovascular control. (In preparation.)

VATNER, S. F., FRANKLIN, D., BRAUNWALD, E.: Effects of anesthesia and sleep on circulatory response to carotid sinus nerve stimulation. Amer. J. Physiol. **220**, 1249—1255 (1971).

VATNER, S. F., HIGGINS, C. B., BRAUNWALD, E.: Sympathetic and parasympathetic components of reflex tachycardia induced by hypotension in conscious dogs with and without heart failure. Cardiovasc. Res. **8**, 153—161 (1974a).

VATNER, S. F., HIGGINS, C. B., MILLARD, R. W., FRANKLIN, D.: Direct and reflex effects of nitroglycerin on coronary and left ventricular dynamics in conscious dogs. J. clin. Invest. **51**, 2872—2882 (1972).

VATNER, S. F., MCRITCHIE, R. J., MAROKO, P. R., PATRICK, T. A., BRAUNWALD, E.: Paradoxical effects of isoproterenol, nitroglycerin and exercise in conscious dogs with myocardial ischemia. Trans Ass. Amer. Phycns **86**, 201—213 (1973).

VATNER, S. F., MCRITCHIE, R. J., MAROKO, P. R., PATRICK, T. A., BRAUNWALD, E.: Effects of catecholamines, exercise and nitroglycerin on the normal and ischemic myocardium in conscious dogs. J. clin. Invest. **54**, 563—575 (1974).

VOEGTLIN, C., MACHT, D. I.: The action of nitrites and drugs of the digitalis group on the isolated coronary artery. J. Pharmacol. exp. Ther. **5**, 77—86 (1913—1914).

VYDEN, J. K., CARVALHO, M., BOSZORMENYI, E., LANG, T. W., BERNSTEIN, H., CORDAY, E.: Effect of glyceryl trinitrate (nitroglycerin) on the systemic and coronary circulation of the dog. Amer. J. Cardiol. **25**, 53—58 (1970).

WAYNE, E. J., LAPLACE, L. B.: Observations on angina of effort. Clin. Sci. **1**, 103—129 (1933).

WEGRIA, R., NICKERSON, J. L., CASE, R. B., HOLLAND, J. F.: Effect of nitroglycerine on the cardiovascular system of normal persons. Amer. J. Med. **10**, 414—418 (1951).

WEISS, H. R., WINBURY, M. M: Intracoronary nitroglycerin, pentaerythritol trinitrate and dipyridamole on intramyocardial oxygen tension. Microvasc. Res. **4**, 273—284 (1973).

WEISS, S., WILKINS, R. W., HAYNES, F. W.: The nature of circulatory collapse induced by sodium nitrite. J. clin. Invest. **16**, 73—84 (1937).

WEISSE, A. B., SENFT, A., KHAN, M. I., REGAN, T. J: Effect of nitrate infusions on the systemic and coronary circulations following acute experimental myocardial infarction in the intact dog. Amer. J. Cardiol. **30**, 362—370 (1972).

WEST, J. W., GUZMAN, S. V.: Coronary dilatation and constriction visualized by selective arteriography. Circulation Res. **7**, 527—536 (1959).

WIENER, L., DWYER, E. M., JR., COX, J. W.: Hemodynamic effects of nitroglycerin, propranolol, and their combination in coronary heart disease. Circulation **39**, 623—632 (1969).

WILKINS, R. W., HAYNES, F. W., WEISS, S.: The role of the venous system in circulatory collapse induced by sodium nitrite. J. clin. Invest. **16**, 85—91 (1937).

WILLIAMS, J. F., JR., GLICK, G., BRAUNWALD, E.: Studies on cardiac dimensions in intact unanesthetized man. Circulation **32**, 767—771 (1965).

WINBURY, M M., GOBEL, L. P.: Effect of nitrates on nutritional circulation of heart and hindlimb. Amer. J. Physiol. **212**, 1062—1066 (1967).

WINBURY, M. M., HOWE, B. B., HEFNER, M. A.: Effect of nitrates and other coronary dilators on large and small coronary vessels: An hypothesis for the mechanism of action of nitrates. J. Pharmacol. exp. Ther. **168**, 70—95 (1969).

WOODWORTH, R. S.: Maximal contraction, "staircase" contraction, refractory period, and compensatory pause, of the heart. Amer. J. Physiol. **8**, 213—249 (1902—1903).

YIPINTSOI, T., DOBBS, W. A., JR., SCANLON, P. D., KNOPP, T. J. BASSINGTHWAIGHTE, J. B.: Regional distribution of diffusible tracers and carbonized microspheres in the left ventricle of isolated dog hearts. Circulation Res. **33**, 573—587 (1973).

CHAPTER 9

Use of Nitrates as Antianginal Agents

WILBERT S. ARONOW

Angina pectoris due to coronary artery disease is generally considered to be chest pain due to myocardial ischemia which occurs because the myocardial oxygen demand exceeds the myocardial oxygen supply. An effective antianginal agent should relieve anginal pain either by improving the myocardial oxygen supply or by reducing the myocardial oxygen demand. In addition to relieving anginal pain, an ideal antianginal drug would also increase exercise performance, reduce electrocardiographic evidence of myocardial ischemia, prevent myocardial infarction, and prolong life. The following discussion will critically evaluate the efficacy of the nitrites as antianginal drugs.

I. Mechanism of Action of Sublingual Nitrates

A. Effect on Coronary Blood Flow

The mechanism of action of the short-acting sublingual nitrates in the relief of anginal pain is not clearly established (ARONOW, 1972b). Although sublingual nitroglycerin and other short-acting sublingual nitrates relax vascular smooth muscle and dilate the coronary arteries in normal people, these drugs do not increase coronary blood flow in patients with coronary artery disease either at rest (BERNSTEIN et al., 1966; GORLIN et al., 1959; PARKER et al., 1971; ROWE et al., 1961) or during exercise (PARKER et al., 1971). This is not surprising as it is difficult to conceive of a drug causing vasodilatation in diseased sclerotic coronary vessels in preference to more distensible vessels (ROWE, 1964). In fact, one wonders whether an anginal attack might be aggravated in some patients by blood being diverted from ischemic areas in the myocardium where hypoxia caused maximal vasodilatation to nonischemic areas in which the coronary vessels are capable of vasodilatation. Moreover, by inducing a drop in the systemic blood pressure, sublingual nitroglycerin and other short-acting sublingual nitrates may reduce the perfusion pressure of the diseased sclerotic vessels, actually decreasing the oxygen supply to the ischemic myocardium.

HORWITZ and his associates (1971) concluded that sublingual nitroglycerin is an effective antianginal agent because it causes redistribution of coronary blood flow so that a greater portion of the total coronary blood flow is delivered to ischemic regions, in addition to its ability to reduce myocardial oxygen demand. However, WANG and his co-workers (1971) demonstrated that nitroglycerin, while increasing total coronary blood flow, may adversely affect flow through a stenosed coronary artery. Morover, GANZ and MARCUS (1972) found that the intracoronary injection of nitroglycerin into 25 patients with pacing-induced angina pectoris did not relieve the anginal pain or decrease its intensity in any patient, whether the nitroglycerin was injected into the right or left coronary artery, into the obstructed coronary artery, or into the artery supplying collaterals to the obstructed coronary artery. Pacing-induced angina pectoris was not relieved in any patients although the intracoronary injection of nitroglycerin resulted in an increase in coronary sinus blood flow in 14 of their 25 patients. Their observations suggest that the increase in coronary blood flow did not occur in the ischemic areas but occurred in the nonischemic areas, where the arterioles were not maximally dilated. Nitroglycerin was administered intravenously to six of their 25 patients and relieved the angina in all patients. This relief of angina pectoris was associated with a fall in arterial pressure and in coronary sinus blood flow.

B. Effect on Myocardial Oxygen Demand

Sublingual short-acting nitrates such as nitroglycerin may be effective antianginal agents by decreasing the myocardial oxygen demand. By reducing venous tone, sublingual nitroglycerin causes pooling of blood in the peripheral veins (MASON and BRAUNWALD, 1961) and a reduction in ventricular volume, stroke volume, and cardiac output (WILLIAMS et al., 1965). This reduction in ventricular volume, by LaPlace's law, decreases the intramyocardial tension, reducing the myocardial oxygen demand. By causing arteriolar dilatation, sublingual nitroglycerin also lowers the arterial pressure (MASON and BRAUNWALD, 1961). By reducing systolic intraventricular pressure and the resistance to ventricular ejection, the myocardial oxygen demand is further decreased. A reduction in the arterial pressure, stroke volume, and cardiac output causes a decrease in left ventricular external work, reducing the myocardial oxygen demand.

Sublingual nitroglycerin increases myocardial oxygen demand by causing an increase in heart rate and in myocardial contractility (PARKER et al., 1971). However, the net result of the different hemodynamic effects of sublingual nitroglycerin is to decrease the myocardial oxygen demand. This decrease in myocardial oxygen demand is primarily caused by peripheral vasodilatation, causing a reduction in left ventricular volume.

II. Sublingual Nitroglycerin as an Antianginal Drug

A. Therapy of Anginal Attacks

Sublingual nitroglycerin is considered by most physicians to be effective in the treatment of angina pectoris (ARONOW, 1972c). However, MASTER et al. (1939) reported that sublingual nitroglycerin was not better than placebo in the treatment of angina pectoris in 89 anginal patients. FISCH and DEGRAFF (1963) observed in a double-blind study that nitroglycerin administered sublingually to nine anginal patients at the onset of exercise-induced angina pectoris was not significantly better than placebo in shortening the duration of the anginal attack. SANDLER et al. (1963) also demonstrated in a double-blind study that nitroglycerin administered sublingually to 15 anginal patients in doses of 0.25 mg, 0.50 mg, and 1.0 mg immediately after the onset of exercise-induced angina pectoris did not significantly change the duration of the anginal attacks or the duration of ischemic S-T segment depression in the electrocardiogram in comparison with placebo.

RISEMAN and BROWN (1937) found that the duration of exercise-induced angina pectoris without medication was less than 1 min in 18 of their 37 anginal patients (49%), between 1 and 2 min in 16 of their 37 anginal patients (43%), and between 2 and 3.5 min in three of their 37 anginal patients (8%). Almost all patients believed that their anginal attacks lasted longer. Sublingual nitroglycerin shortened the anginal episodes in 22% of the 18 patients whose anginal attacks without medication lasted less than 1 min, in 62% of the 16 patients whose anginal attacks without medication lasted between 1 and 2 min, and in all three of the patients whose anginal attacks without medication lasted between 2 and 3.5 min. These investigators (RISEMAN and BROWN, 1937) also showed that 0.3 mg of sublingual nitroglycerin was as effective as 0.6 mg of sublingual nitrolgycerin in relieving angina pectoris and was less likely to cause headache. A dose of 0.12 mg of sublingual nitroglycerin, however, was less effective than a 0.3 mg dose in relieving angina pectoris.

Using a standardized interview, HORWITZ et al. (1972) found that 37 of their 49 patients (76%) with angina pectoris due to angiographically documented significant coronary artery disease and four of their 21 patients (19%) with chest pain not due to significant coronary artery disease as documented by coronary angiography usually or always experienced relief of their chest pain within 3 min after administration of sublingual nitroglycerin. Four of their 49 patients (8%) with angina pectoris due to documented coronary artery disease and eight of their 21 patients (38%) with chest pain not due to coronary artery disease reported that sublingual nitroglycerin did not relieve their chest pain.

Our experience is that sublingual nitroglycerin is not necessary for treating mild anginal episodes which respond well to cessation of exertion with motionless standing (ARONOW, 1972c; ARONOW, 1973a; ARONOW, 1973b). However, sublingual nitroglycerin is effective in treating more severe anginal episodes. We recommend using an initial dose of 0.3 mg which often suffices to relieve the anginal episode and is less likely to induce headache or other unpleasant side effects. Care should be taken to avoid marked postural hypotension. Patients should be instructed not to take more than two to three sublingual nitroglycerin tablets over a period of 15 min for a prolonged anginal attack as the patient may be experiencing an acute myocardial infarction. In addition, the systemic hypotension and decreased coronary blood flow induced by sublingual nitroglycerin might also convert an episode of prolonged angina pectoris into an acute myocardial infarction.

A fresh supply of sublingual nitroglycerin tablets must be used (BURCH and DEPASQUALE, 1966). Sublingual nitroglycerin tablets should be kept in a tightly-stoppered, dark glass container without much cotton filler in the bottle to avoid rapid deterioration of this drug. Sublingual nitroglycerin tablets should produce a slight stinging or burning sensation when placed under the tongue and should be replaced if this does not occur.

B. Prophylactic Use

In our experience, nitroglycerin is most effective as an antianginal drug when administered sublingually 2 to 3 min prior to performing activities such as sexual intercourse or encountering stressful situations in which an anginal attack may be anticipated (ARONOW, 1972c; ARONOW, 1973a; ARONOW, 1973b). SANDLER, ILAHI, and LAWSON (1963) showed in a double-blind study that sublingual nitroglycerin administered to 12 anginal patients in doses of 0.25 mg, 0.50 mg, and 1.0 mg 3 min prior to exercise significantly increased the amount of exercise performed before angina developed in comparison with placebo. The 0.25 mg and 0.50 mg doses, but not the 1.0 mg dose, also significantly reduced the duration of the anginal attacks.

MACALPIN, ALVARO, and KATTUS (1970) demonstrated that nitroglycerin administered sublingually to 16 anginal patients in doses ranging from 0.3 mg to 0.6 mg 2 to 4 min prior to treadmill exercise increased the amount of exercise performed before the development of angina an average of 125% over the control value and increased the amount of exercise performed before the onset of ischemic S-T segment depression an average of 121% over the control value. Fourteen of their 16 patients (88%) increased their exercise tolerance prior to the onset of angina pectoris more than 50% over the control value. GOLDSTEIN and his co-workers (1971) demonstrated that sublingual nitroglycerin administered to eight anginal patients 3 min before upright bicycle ergometer exercise in doses sufficient to produce a 10 mm Hg fall in mean blood pressure and/or a 10 beat per minute rise in heart rate while at rest in the sitting position caused a significant increase in exercise capacity and a significant delay in the onset of ischemic S-T segment depression in comparison with placebo. DETRY and BRUCE (1971) found that 0.4 mg of nitroglycerin administered sublingually to 32 anginal patients at the onset of treadmill exercise significantly increased the maximal heart rate, significantly increased the product of systolic blood pressure times heart rate, and significantly reduced ischemic S-T segment depression during and after exercise in comparison with the control values. Following sublingual nitroglycerin, 12 of their 32 patients (35%) were also symtomatically limited by dyspnea and fatigue rather than by chest pain.

PARKER and his associates (1971) demonstrated that 0.5 mg of chewable nitroglycerin administered to seven anginal patients approximately 10 min prior to supine leg exercise caused only two of these seven patients to experience angina pectoris, and their angina was less severe than that experienced during the control period. However, FISCH and DEGRAFF (1963) observed in a double-blind study that nitroglycerin administered sublingually to nine anginal patients 10 min before upright bicycle exercise did not significantly improve exercise tolerance in comparison with placebo.

C. Comparison with Other Sublingual Nitrates

We (ARONOW, 1970a) found in a double-blind crossover study that 5 mg of isosorbide dinitrate administered sublingually four times daily for 4 weeks to 19 anginal patients was not better than sublingual placebo in significantly reducing the number of anginal episodes requiring nitroglycerin. Sublingual isosorbide dinitrate administered 1 hr prior to upright bicycle ergometer exercise did not significantly improve the exercise time until the onset of angina pectoris or the resting or exercise electrocardiogram in any of our 17 patients tested in comparison with placebo. Using doses of sublingual nitroglycerin and sublingual isosorbide dinitrate matched to produce equal physiologic effects at rest in patients with angina pectoris, GOLDSTEIN and his co-workers (1971) demonstrated that sublingual isosorbide dinitrate was not significantly better than sublingual nitroglycerin in improving exercise performance until angina or in delaying the onset of ischemic S-T segment depression. The magnitude and duration of the beneficial effect on exercise capacity caused by sublingual isosorbide dinitrate and sublingual nitroglycerin were indistinguishable in their study. Benefit was observed in only a minority of their 23 anginal patients tested 1 hr and in none tested 2 hrs after either sublingual isosorbide dinitrate or sublingual nitroglycerin. Therefore, since sublingual isosorbide dinitrate is ineffective as a long-acting nitrite (ARONOW, 1970a; GOLDSTEIN et al., 1971), not more effective than sublingual nitroglycerin as a short-acting nitrite (GOLDSTEIN et al., 1971), and is more expensive than sublingual nitroglycerin, there is no justification for prescribing isosorbide dinitrate.

KLAUS and associates (1973) observed in a double-blind study that the mean duration of exercise in 10 anginal patients 45 min after administration of 10 mg of sublingual erythrityl tetranitrate, 5 mg of sublingual isosorbide dinitrate, and 10 mg of pentaerythritol tetranitrate (89.1, 87.5, and 87.5 seconds respectively) was significantly improved in comparison with 60.5 seconds 45 min after placebo. However, 100 min after administration of 10 mg of sublingual erythrityl tetranitrate, 5 mg of sublingual isosorbide dinitrate, and 10 mg of pentaerythritol tetranitrate, the mean duration of exercise performance in their 10 anginal patients was not significantly different from placebo. The mean duration of exercise performance 4 min after administration of 0.4 mg of sublingual nitroglycerin to their 10 anginal patients was 89.3 sec and significantly increased in comparison with placebo. However, 50 min after administration of sublingual nitroglycerin, the mean duration of exercise performance was not significantly changed in comparison with placebo.

On the basis of the above data and our clinical experience, we feel that the sublingual nitrites are not long-acting in duration and are not preferable to the less expensive sublingual nitroglycerin. Sublingual nitroglycerin used prophylactically before stressful activities which might be expected to precipitate anginal attacks is the cornerstone of the drug therapy of angina pectoris.

D. Adverse Effects

Headache is common with sublingual nitrates. Twelve of our 19 anginal patients (63%) complained of headache due to isosorbide dinitrate administered sublingually 5 mg four times daily (ARONOW AND CHESLUK, 1970a). These headaches were severe in six of our 19 anginal patients (32%) and caused two of our 19 patients (11%) to discontinue taking this drug. Transient episodes of dizziness, weakness, and syncope may be caused by cerebral ischemia associated with postural hypotension. Sublingual nitrates may cause cutaneous dilatation with flushing, drug rash, palpatations, excessive tachycardia, and increased intraocular pressure.

III. Long-Acting Nitrates

A. Ineffectiveness

The efficacy of the long-acting nitrates in the treatment of angina pectoris has not been adequately established (ARONOW, 1972d; FREIS et al., 1970). This is not surprising as long-acting nitrites neither increase the oxygen supply to the myocardium nor reduce the myocardial oxygen demand and, therefore, are ineffective as antianginal agents.

The design of an antianginal drug study influences the results (ARONOW, 1972a). The design of the exercise study used to evaluate an antianginal drug may prejudice the results. Some of my objections to one such study evaluating sublingual isosorbide dinitrate and propranolol (RUSSEK, 1968) have been discussed in detail elsewhere (ARONOW, 1972a).

STIPE and FINK (1973) searched the literature for the period 1952 to 1972 on the efficacy of the organic nitrates and found 59 clinical studies on prophylactic therapy of angina pectoris with erythrityl tetranitrate, glyceryl trinitrate, isosorbide dinitrate, and pentaerythritol tetranitrate. Their paper contains the references for these 59 clinical studies. Long-term prophylaxis of anginal attacks was considered in 36 of these clinical studies, with 23 reporting effective and 13 reporting ineffective therapy. Table 1 from STIPE and FINK's paper (1973) shows that there was a significantly greater proportion of studies reporting effective therapy with the organic nitrates among the investigations that did not include the generally accepted elements of experimental design.

EVANS and HOYLE (1933) showed that only three of 21 anginal patients (14%) had an improvement in the number of anginal attacks on 120 mg of oral mannitol hexanitrate three times daily whereas eight of these 21 anginal patients (38%) had an improvement in the number of anginal episodes on placebo. These investigators also observed that none of 20 anginal patients had an improvement in anginal episodes on 30 mg of oral erythrol tetranitrate three times daily whereas eight of these 20 anginal patients (40%) had an improvement in anginal attacks on placebo. WILLIS and DUFF (1957) also reported that oral erythrol tetranitrate and mannitol hexanitrate were of limited usefulness. COLE and associates (1963) demonstrated that a 15 mg rapidly disintegrating buccal tablet of erythrol tetranitrate (Cardilate) prescribed four to eight times daily for 3 to 6 week periods to nine anginal patients caused no improvement in anginal attacks in six of their nine patients. None of these nine anginal patients asked that this drug be continued after its scheduled use.

FISCH and DEGRAFF (1963) demonstrated that pentaerythritol tetranitrate, isosorbide dinitrate, and itramin tosylate evaluated by blind procedures in uniform, as well as in maximally tolerated, doses were not statistically better than placebo in reducing the frequency of anginal attacks. FRIEND and co-workers (1954) found in a double-blind study that triethanolamine trinitrate administered orally 2 mg four times daily was not better than placebo in reducing the number of anginal episodes in seven anginal patients.

KALMANSON and associates (1955) demonstrated in a double-blind study that oral pentaerythritol tetranitrate administered 10 mg three times daily and 20 mg three times daily to 23 anginal patients had no beneficial effect on the number of anginal attacks or the number of nitroglycerin tablets consumed in comparison with

Table 1. Relationship between elements of experimental design and conclusion of efficacy in clinical investigations of antianginal therapy with the organic nitrates

Design elements	Number of articles		
	Effective		Ineffective
All study articles			
Blinding	21		16
No blinding	22		0
		$P<0.01$	
Controls	35		16
No controls	8		0
		$P=0.065$	
Statistics	14		12
No statistics	29		4
		$P<0.01$	
Long-term prophylaxis			
Blinding	13		13
No blinding	10		0
		$P<0.01$	
Placebo	15		13
No placebo	8		0
		$P<0.02$	
Statistics	7		9
No statistics	16		4
		$P<0.03$	
Random	9		13
Nonrandom	9		0
		$P<0.01$	
Crossover	12		13
No crossover	6		0
		$P<0.03$	
Immediate prophylaxis			
Blinding	11		6
No blinding	13		0
		$P<0.02$	
Placebo	13		6
No placebo	11		0
		$P<0.02$	
Statistics	6		6
No statistics	18		0
		$P<0.05$	
Random	7		6
Nonrandom	16		0
		$P<0.01$	
Crossover	17		6
Non crossover	6		0
		$P=0.213$	

P = probability that the proportion of effective to ineffective articles is the same between the classifications.

Reproduced with permission from the authors and *The Journal of Clinical Pharmacology*.

placebo. COLE and associates (1957) found in a double-blind study that oral peritrate administered in doses ranging from 40 to 80 mg daily was not significantly better than placebo in reducing anginal attacks in 14 anginal patients. DEWAR and associates (1959) reported in a double-blind study that pentaerythritol tetranitrate administered orally 30 mg three times daily or 60 mg three times daily did not significantly affect the number of anginal episodes or the number of nitroglycerin tablets consumed by 19 anginal patients in comparison with placebo.

ORAM and SOWTON (1961) demonstrated in a double-blind study that neither pentaerythritol tetranitrate administered orally 30 mg three times daily nor propatyl nitrate administered orally 30 mg three times daily significantly reduced the number of anginal attacks in comparison with placebo in 30 anginal patients. DAGENAIS and associates (1969) observed that pentaerythritol tetranitrate administered orally in 20 mg or 40 mg doses 90 min prior to exercise did not significantly improve the mean exercise duration or improve ischemic S-T segment abnormalities in 15 anginal patients.

In a double-blind study, we (ARONOW and KAPLAN, 1969) observed no significant difference in exercise performance until angina whether isosorbide dinitrate or placebo was administered orally to 24 anginal patients 2 hrs prior to exercise. GOLDSTEIN and co-workers (1971) analyzed the data reported by BATTOCK and associates (1969; 1971) and found that isosorbide dinitrate administered orally in doses of 10 mg four times daily to nine anginal patients and 15 mg four times daily to one anginal patient was not significantly better than placebo in improving exercise performance until angina in these 10 anginal patients.

GOLDBARG and associates (1969) demonstrated in a double-blind study that isosorbide dinitrate administered orally 10 mg four times daily to 21 anginal patients was not more effective than placebo in reducing the number of anginal episodes or the number of nitroglycerin tablets consumed. Isosorbide dinitrate was also ineffective in improving exercise performance or ischemic S-T segment depression following exercise in their 21 anginal patients. LIVESLEY and co-workers (1973) found in a double-blind study that isosorbide dinitrate administered orally 20 mg three times daily to 32 anginal patients was not more effective than placebo in affecting the number of anginal episodes experienced, the number of nitroglycerin tablets consumed, or their exercise tolerance test. Fourteen of their 32 anginal patients (44%) experienced such severe headaches from isosorbide dinitrate that even when the dose was reduced to 10 mg three times daily they had to discontinue isosorbide dinitrate therapy.

We agree with MODELL (1962) that, unlike sublingual nitroglycerin, oral nitroglycerin is of little clinical value and that none of the nitroglycerin preparations designed for delayed absorption in the gastrointestinal tract have any merit. Also, no well controlled studies of which I am aware show that nitroglycerin administered either orally in an ordinary tablet or in sustained-release form is effective as an antianginal agent.

Our attitude toward long-acting nitrites may be best summarized by quoting MODELL (1962) as follows:

The nitrites currently in use which have little merit include aminotrate, erythrityl tetranitrate, inositol hexanitrate, isosorbide dinitrate, mannitol hexanitrate, and pentaerythrityl tetranitrate. The lack of faith of the pharmaceutical industry in its long-acting nitrites is nicely demonstrated by the rash of these agents that are now being put up in special "delayed-action" forms. What is even more delayed is the proof that they have any merit whatever.

NEEDLEMAN and associates (1973, 1972) have also demonstrated that orally administered organic nitrates go directly to the liver via the portal vein and are rapidly and completely degraded by a liver enzyme before reaching the systemic circulation. Their experimental data furnish us with the rational basis why the long-acting nitrates are ineffective as antianginal agents.

B. Tolerance

NEEDLEMAN (1970) demonstrated that high doses of nitroglycerin administered three times daily to rats produced tolerance to the blood pressure response of nitroglycerin. However, MODELL (1962) stated that the development of tolerance to nitroglycerin from even unusually frequent clinical use was not common.

Several investigators (MODELL, 1962; NICKERSON, 1965; SCHELLING and LASAGNA, 1967; ZELIS and MASON, 1969) have raised the possibility that chronic administration of long-acting nitrates may lead to crossover tolerance to nitroglycerin so that nitroglycerin will become ineffective in the treatment of angina pectoris. SCHELLING and LASAGNA (1967) observed in volunteer subjects that the changes in blood pressure and in heart rate after administration of 0.3 mg of sublingual nitroglycerin were significantly decreased while the subjects were receiving pentaerythritol tetranitrate 40 to 60 mg daily for 4 weeks. ZELIS and MASON (1969) demonstrated that administration of oral isosorbide dinitrate 120 mg daily for 6 weeks reduced the venodilator response to sublingual nitroglycerin and stated that this action may be responsible for vascular tolerance and diminished effectiveness of sublingual nitroglycerin during chronic administration of long-acting nitrites.

However, we (ARONOW, 1971; ARONOW and CHESLUK, 1970b) found no significant difference in the duration of anginal pain following administration of 0.6 mg of sublingual nitroglycerin at the onset of anginal pain in 17 patients whether the anginal patients were on no medication, sublingual placebo, or on sublingual isosorbide dinitrate 5 mg four times daily for 4 weeks. We also found no significant difference in the blood pressure, heart rate, product of systolic blood pressure times heart rate, and the electrocardiographic response after complete relief of angina following sublingual nitroglycerin whether the patients were on no medication, sublingual placebo, or sublingual isosorbide dinitrate. These data indicate that sublingual isosorbide dinitrate prescribed as a long-acting nitrite in ordinary therapeutic doses of 5 mg sublingually four times daily did not cause any clinical impairment of the effectiveness of sublingual nitroglycerin for relieving angina pectoris. GOLDSTEIN and associates (1971) also found that the chronic administration of sublingual isosorbide dinitrate 5 to 10 mg four times daily did not alter either baseline exercise performance until angina or the responsiveness to sublingual isosorbide dinitrate when administered acutely.

Finally, LANGE and associates (1972) observed 200 munitions workers exposed for 12 to 48 months to nitroglycerin. Symptomatic nonatherosclerotic ischemic heart disease developed in nine of these 200 people after withrawal from nitroglycerin exposure. These data would lead us to avoid the chronic administration of ineffective long-acting nitrates and to avoid stopping nitrates abruptly after regular, frequent, heavy, long-term usage.

References

ARONOW, W. S.: Drug evaluation—Chronic trials, in ROSS, R. S. and HOFFMAN, F., editors: Myocardial Ischemia, International Congress Series No. 225, Amsterdam, 1971, Excerpta Medica, pp. 73—82.

ARONOW, W. S.: The medical treatment of angina pectoris II. Design of an antianginal drug study. Amer. Heart J. **84**, 132—134 (1972a).

ARONOW, W. S.: Medical treatment of angina pectoris. III. Pharmacology of sublingual nitrites as antianginal drugs. Amer. Heart J. **84**, 273—275 (1972b).

ARONOW, W. S.: The medical treatment of angina pectoris. IV. Nitroglycerin as an antianginal drug. Amer. Heart J. **8**, 415—418 (1972c).

ARONOW, W. S.: The medical treatment of angina pectoris. V. Long-acting nitrites as antianginal drugs. Amer. Heart J. **84**, 567—569 (1972d).

ARONOW, W. S.: The medical treatment of angina pectoris. IX. The medical management of angina pectoris. Amer. Heart J. **85**, 275—278 (1973a).

ARONOW, W. S.: Management of stable angina. New Engl. J. Med. **289**, 516—520 (1973b).

ARONOW, W. S., CHESLUK, H. M.: Sublingual isosorbide dinitrate therapy versus sublingual placebo in angina pectoris. Circulation **41**, 869—874 (1970a).

ARONOW, W. S., CHESLUK, H. M.: Evaluation of nitroglycerin in angina in patients on isosorbide dinitrate. Circulation **42**, 61—63 (1970b).

ARONOW, W. S., KAPLAN, M. A.: Evaluation of propranolol and of isosorbide dinitrate in angina pectoris. Curr. Ther. Res. **11**, 80—86 (1969).

BATTOCK, D. J., ALVAREZ, H., CHIDSEY, C. A.: Effect of propranolol and isosorbide dinitrate on exercise performance and adrenergic activity in patients with angina pectoris. Circulation **39**, 157—169 (1969).

BATTOCK, D. J., CHIDSEY, C. A.: Isosorbide dinitrate in angina. Circulation **44**, 1147 (1971) (Letter to the Editor).

BERNSTEIN, L., FRIESINGER, G. C., LICHTLEN, P. R., ROSS, R. S.: The effect of nitroglycerin on the systemic and coronary circulation in man and dogs. Myocardial blood flow measured with xenon. Circulation **33**, 107—116 (1966).

BURCH, G. E., DEPASQUALE, N. P.: Fresh nitroglycerin (glyceryl trinitrate). Amer. Heart J. **72**, 842 (1966).

COLE, S. L., KAYE, H., GRIFFITH, G. C.: Assay of anti-anginal agents I. A curve analysis with multiple control periods. Circulation **15**, 405—413 (1957).

COLE, S. L., KAYE, H., GRIFFITH, G. C.: Assay of antianginal agents. A long-acting nitrate, psychic energizers and a tranquilizer. Amer. J. Cardiol. **11**, 639—645 (1963).

DAGENAIS, G. R., MASON, R. E., FRIESINGER, G. C., WENDER, C., ROSS, R. S.: Exercise tolerance in patients with angina pectoris: Daily variation and effect of pentaerythritol tetranitrate. John Hopkins med. J. **125**, 301—311 (1969).

DETRY, J. M., BRUCE, R. A.: Effects of nitroglycerin on "maximal" oxygen intake and exercise electrocardiogram in coronary heart disease. Circulation **43**, 155—163 (1971).

DEWAR, H. A., HORLER, A. R., NEWELL, D. J.: A clinical trial of penta-erythritol tetranitrate, a khellin derivative (recordil), and iproniazid in angina of effort. Brit. Heart J. **21**, 315—322 (1959).

EVANS, W., HOYLE, C.: The comparative value of drugs used in the continuous treatment of angina pectoris. Quart. J. med. **2**, 311—338 (1933).

FISCH, S., DEGRAFF. A. C.: Coronary vasodilators. Dis Chest **44**, 533—537 (1963).

FREIS, E. D., GAFFNEY, T. E., KIRKENDALL, W., MARCUS, F. I., NICKERSON, M., PEARCE, M. L.: Report of the panels on cardiovascular drugs from the drug efficacy study. Circulation **41**, 149—151 (1970).

FRIEND, D. G., O'HARE, J. P., LEVINE, H. D.: Action of triethanolamine trinitrate in angina pectoris. Amer. Heart J. **48**, 775—779 (1954).
GANZ, W., MARCUS, H. S.: Failure of intracoronary nitroglycerin to alleviate pacing-induced angina. Circulation **46**, 880—889 (1972).
GOLDBARG, A. N., MORAN, J. F., BUTTERFIELD, T. K., NEMICKAS, R., BERMUDEZ, G. A.: Therapy of angina pectoris with propranolol and long-acting nitrates. Circulation **40**, 847—853 (1969).
GOLDSTEIN, R. E., REDWOOD, D. R., EPSTEIN, S. E.: Isosorbide dinitrate in angina. Circulation **44**, 1148—1149 (1971) (Letter to the Editor).
GOLDSTEIN, R. E., ROSING, D. R., REDWOOD, D. R., BEISER, G. D., EPSTEIN, S. E.: Clinical and circulatory effects of isosorbide dinitrate: comparison with nitroglycerin. Circulation **43**, 629—640 (1971).
GORLIN, R., BRACHFELD, N., MACLEOD, C., BOPP, P.: Effect of nitroglycerin on the coronary circulation in patients with coronary artery disease or increased left ventricular work. Circulation **19**, 705—718 (1959).
HORWITZ, L. D., GORLIN, R., TAYLOR, W. J., KEMP, H. G.: Effects of nitroglycerin on regional myocardial blood flow in coronary artery disease. J. clin. Invest. **50**, 1578—1584 (1971).
HORWITZ, L. D., HERMAN, M. V., GORLIN, R.: Clinical response to nitroglycerin as a diagnostic test for coronary artery disease. Amer. J. Cardiol. **29**, 149—153 (1972).
KALMANSON, G. M., DRENICK, E. J., BINDER, M. J., ROSOVE, L.: Pentaerythritol tetranitrate in the treatment of angina pectoris. Arch. intern. med. **95**, 819—822 (1955).
KLAUS, A., ZARET, B., PITT, B., ROSS, R. S.: Comparative evaluation of sublingual long acting nitrates in angina pectoris. Amer. J. Cardiol. **31**, 142 (1973) (Abstract).
LANGE, R. L., REID, M. S., TRESCH, D. D., KEELAN, M. H., BERNHARD, V. M., COOLIDGE, G.: Nonatheromatous ischemic heart disease following withdrawal from chronic industrial nitroglycerin exposure. Circulation **46**, 666—678 (1972).
LIVESLEY, B., CATLEY, P. F., CAMPBELL, R. C., ORAM, S.: Double-blind evaluation of verapamil, propranolol, and isosorbide dinitrate against a placebo in the treatment of angina pectoris. Brit. med. J. 1973 I, 375—378.
MACALPIN, R. N., ALVARO, A. B., KATTUS, A. A.: Effect of propranolol and nitroglycerin on exercise tolerance in angina pectoris, in KATTUS, A. A., ROSS, G., HALL, V., editors: UCLA forum in medical sciences No. 13. Cardiovascular beta adrenergic responses, pp. 191—203. Berkeley-Los Angeles-London: University of California Press 1970.
MASON, D. T., BRAUNWALD, E.: The effects of nitroglycerin and amyl nitrite on arteriolar and venous tone in the human forearm. Circulation **32**, 755—766 (1961).
MASTER, A. M., JAFFE, H. L., DACK, S.: The drug treatment of angina pectoris due to coronary artery disease. Amer. J. med. Sci **197**, 774—782 (1939).
MODELL, W.: Clinical pharmacology of antianginal drugs. Clin. pharm. Ther. **3**, 97—108 (1962).
NEEDLEMAN, P.: Tolerance to the vascular effects of glyceryl trinitrate. J. Pharmacol. exp. Ther. **171**, 98—102 (1970).
NEEDLEMAN, P.: Oral nitrates: Efficacious? Ann. intern. med. **78**, 458 (1973).
NEEDLEMAN, P., LANG, S., JOHNSON, E. M.: Organic nitrates: relationship between biotransformation and rational angina pectoris therapy. J. Pharmacol. exp. Ther. **181**, 489—497 (1972).
NICKERSON, M.: Vasodilator drugs. In GOODMAN, L. S. and GILMAN, A. (Eds.): The Pharmacological Basis of Therapeutics, p. 748. New York: Macmillan Co. 1965.
ORAM, S., SOWTON, E.: Failure of propatylnitrate and pentaerythritol tetranitrate to prevent attacks of angina pectoris. Brit. med. J. **1961 II**, 1745—1746.
PARKER, J. O., WEST, R. P., DIGIORGI, S.: The effect of nitroglycerin on coronary blood flow and the hemodynamic response to exercise in coronary artery disease. Amer. J. Cardiol. **27**, 59—65 (1971).
RISEMAN, J. E. F., BROWN, M. G.: The duration of attacks of angina pectoris on exertion and the effect of nitroglycerin and amyl nitrite. New Engl. J. med. **217**, 470—473 (1937).
ROWE, G. G.: Coronary vasodilator therapy for angina pectoris. Amer. Heart J. **68**, 691—696 (1964).
ROWE, G. G., CHELIUS, C. J., AFONSO, S., GURTNER, H. P., CRUMPTON, C. W.: Systemic and coronary hemodynamic effects of erythrol tetranitrate. J. clin. Invest. **40**, 1217—1222 (1961).
RUSSEK, H. I.: Propranolol and isosorbide dinitrate synergism in angina pectoris. Amer. J. Cardiol. **21**, 44—54 (1968).

SANDLER, G., ILAHI, M. A., LAWSON, C. W.: Glyceryl trinitrate in angina pectoris. Lancet **1963 I**, 1130—1136.
SCHELLING, J. L., LASAGNA, L.: A study of cross-tolerance to circulatory effects of organic nitrates. Clin. pharm. Ther. **8**, 256—260 (1967).
STIPE, A. A., FINK, G. B.: Prophylactic therapy of angina pectoris with organic nitrates: Relationship of drug efficacy and clinical experimental design. J. clin. Pharmacol. **13**, 244—250 (1973).
WANG, J., MATHUR, V. S., MESSER, J. V.: Nitroglycerine induced flow maldistribution in coronary stenosis. Circulation **44** (Suppl II). 59 (1971) (Abstract).
WILLIAMS, J. F., JR., GLICK, G., BRAUNWALD, E.: Studies on cardiac dimensions in intact unanesthetized man. V. Effects of nitroglycerin. Circulation **32**, 767—771 (1965).
WILLIS, P. W. III, DUFF, I. F.: Coronary vasodilating drugs. Med. clin. N. Amer. **41**, 449—469, 1957.
ZELIS, R., MASON, D. T.: Demonstration of nitrite tolerance: Attenuation of the vasodilator response to nitroglycerin by the chronic administration of isosorbide dinitrate. Circulation **40** (Suppl. III), 221 (1969) (Abstract).

Author Index

Page numbers in *italics* refer to the bibliography

Subject Index

Handbuch der experimentellen Pharmakologie/ Handbook of Experimental Pharmacology

Heffter—Heubner, New Series

Vol. IV: **General Pharmacology**
ISBN 3-540-04845-6 DM 86,—; US $35.10

Vol. X: **Die Pharmakologie anorganischer Anionen**
ISBN 3-540-01465-9 DM 255,—; US $104.10

Vol. XI: **Lobelin und Lobeliaalkaloide**
ISBN 3-540-01910-3 DM 20,—; US $8.20

Vol. XII: **Morphin und morphinähnlich wirkende Verbindungen**
ISBN 3-540-02158-2 DM 95,—; US $38.80

Vol. XIII: **The Alkali Metal Ions in Biology.** Temp. out of print

Vol. XIV:

Part 1 **The Adrenocortical Hormones I**
ISBN 3-540-02830-7 DM 290,—; US $118.40

Part 2 **The Adrenocortical Hormones II**
ISBN 3-540-03146-4 DM 90,—; US $36.80

Part 3 **The Adrenocortical Hormones III**
ISBN 3-540-04147-8 DM 170,—; US $69.40

Vol. XV: **Cholinesterases and Anticholinesterase Agents**
ISBN 3-540-02988-5 DM 360,—; US $146.90

Vol. XVI: **Erzeugung von Krankheitszuständen durch das Experiment**

Part 1 **Blut/Blood.** In preparation

Part 2 **Atemwege**
ISBN 3-540-04517-1 DM 150,—; US $61.20

Part 3 **Heart and Circulation.** In preparation

Part 4 **Niere, Nierenbecken, Blase**
ISBN 3-540-03305-X DM 180,—; US $73.50

Part 5 **Liver.** In preparation

Part 6 **Schilddrüse.** In preparation

Part 7 **Zentralnervensystem**
ISBN 3-540-02831-5 DM 150,—; US $61.20

Part 8 **Stütz- und Hartgewebe**
ISBN 3-540-04518-X DM 120,—; US $49.00

Part 9 **Infektionen I**
ISBN 3-540-03147-2 DM 180,—; US $73.50

Part 10 **Infektionen II**
ISBN 3-540-03531-1 DM 200,—; US $81.60

Part 11 A **Infektionen III**
ISBN 3-540-03840-X DM 180,—; US $73.50

Part 11 B **Infektionen IV**
ISBN 3-540-06290-4 DM 195,—; US $ 79.60

Part 12 **Tumoren I**
ISBN 3-540-03532-X DM 180,—; US $73.50

Part 13 **Tumoren II**
ISBN 3-540-03533-8 DM 110,—; US $44.90

Part 14 **Tumoren III.** In preparation

Part 15 **Kohlenhydratstoffwechsel, Fieber/Carbohydrate Metabolism, Fever**
ISBN 3-540-03534-6 DM 180,—; US $73.50

Vol. XVII:

Part 1 **Ions, alcalino-terreux I. Systèmes isolés**
ISBN 3-540-02989-3 DM 190,—; US $77.60

Part 2 **Ions, alcacino-terreux II. Organismes entiers**
ISBN 3-540-03148-0 DM 240,—; US $98.00

Vol. XVIII:

Part 1 **Histamine**
ISBN 3-540-03535-4 DM 230,—; US $93.90

Part 2 **Anti-Histaminics.** In preparation

Vol. XIX: **5-Hydroxytryptamine and Related Indolealkylamines**
ISBN 3-540-03536-2 DM 230,—; US $93.90

Vol. XX:

Part 1 **Pharmacology of Fluorides I**
ISBN 3-540-03537-0 DM 175,—; US $71.40

Part 2 **Pharmacology of Fluorides II**
ISBN 3-540-04846-4 DM 165,—; US $67.40

Vol. XXI: **Beryllium**
ISBN 3-540-03538-9 DM 48,—; US $19.60

Vol. XXII:

Part 1 **Die Gestagene I**
ISBN 3-540-04148-6 DM 370,—; US $151.00

Part 2 **Die Gestagene II**
ISBN 3-540-04519-8 DM 370,—; US $151.00

Vol. XXIII: **Neurohypophysical Hormones and Similar Polypeptides**
ISBN 3-540-04149-4 DM 230,—; US $93.90

Vol. XXIV: **Diuretica**
ISBN 3-540-04520-1 DM 290,—; US $118.40

Vol. XXV: **Bradykinin, Kallidin and Kallikrein**
ISBN 3-540-04847-2 DM 275,—; US $112.20

Vol. XXVI: **Vergleichende Pharmakologie von Überträgersubstanzen in tiersystematischer Darstellung**
ISBN 3-540-05132-5 DM 180,—; US $73.50

Vol. XXVII: **Anticoagulantien**
ISBN 3-540-05133-3 DM 225,—; US $91.80

Vol. XXVIII:

Part 1 **Concepts in Biochemical Pharmacology I**
ISBN 3-540-05134-1 DM 190,—; US $77.60

Part 2 **Concepts in Biochemical Pharmacology II**
ISBN 3-540-05389-1 DM 275,—; US $112.20

Part 3 **Concepts in Biochemical Pharmacology III.** Pharmacokinetics
ISBN 3-540-07001-X DM 248,—; US $ 101.20

Vol. XXIX: **Oral wirksame Antidiabetika**
ISBN 3-540-05554-1 DM 340,—; US $138.80

Vol. XXX: **Modern Inhalation Anesthetics**
ISBN 3-540-05135-X DM 220,—; US $89.80

Vol. XXXI: **Antianginal Drugs**
ISBN 3-540-05365-4 DM 190,—; US $77.60

Vol. XXXII:

Part 1 **Insulin I**
ISBN 3-540-05470-7 DM 275,—; US $112.20

Part 2 **Insulin II.** In preparation
ISBN 3-540-07006-0

Vol. XXXIII: **Catecholamines**
ISBN 3-540-05517-7 DM 396,—; US $161.60

Vol. XXXIV: **Secretin, Cholecystokinin-Pancreozymin and Gastrin**
ISBN 3-540-05952-0 DM 165,—; US $67.40

Vol. XXXV:

Part 1 **Androgene I**
ISBN 3-540-05706-4 DM 320,—; US $130.60

Part 2 **Androgens II and Antiandrogens / Androgene II und Antiandrogene**
ISBN 3-540-06883-X DM 398,—; US $162.40

Vol. XXXVI: **Uranium-Plutonium-Transplutonic Elements**
ISBN 3-540-06168-1 DM 374,—; US $152.60

Vol. XXXVII: **Angiotensin**
ISBN 3-540-06276-9 DM 224,—; US $91.40

Vol. XXXVIII:

Part 1 A **Antineoplastic and Immunosuppressive Agents I**
ISBN 3-540-06402-8 DM 258,—; US $105.30

Part 2 **Antineoplastic and Immunosuppressive Agents II**
ISBN 3-540-06633-0 DM 348,—; US $142.00

Preisänderungen vorbehalten / Prices are subject to change without notice